RECENT ADVANCES
IN SEXUALLY TRANSMITTED DISEASES

R. S. MORTON
MBE FRCP (Ed)

Consultant Venereologist, United
Sheffield Hospitals and Sheffield
Regional Hospital Board, Lecturer
in Venereal Diseases, University of
Sheffield

J. R. W. HARRIS
MRCP DTM&H

Consultant Venereologist,
King's College Hospital, London

RECENT ADVANCES IN SEXUALLY TRANSMITTED DISEASES

EDITED BY

R. S. MORTON AND J. R. W. HARRIS

NUMBER ONE

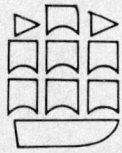

CHURCHILL LIVINGSTONE
Edinburgh London and New York
1975

CHURCHILL LIVINGSTONE
Medical Division of Longman Group Limited
Represented in the United States of America by
Longman Inc., New York and by associated
companies, branches and representatives throughout
the world.

© Longman Group Limited 1975

First published 1975
ISBN 0 443 01156 7
Library of Congress Catalog Card Number 74 77695

Printed in Great Britain

Preface

In writing this book we have been conscious of the high standards set by R. R. Willcox in his 'Progress in Venereology' (1953) and A. J. King in his 'Recent Advances in Venereology' (1964). We have aimed to match these standards and to reflect the widening spectrum of recognisable sexually transmissible diseases.

The annual output of literature concerning venereal and other sexually transmissible diseases has increased at least four-fold since the first of these reviews and currently amounts to nearly 1 000 publications per annum. For this reason we have been glad to seek the help of colleagues who have a special interest, wide experience and research involvement in a particular aspect.

For the same reason we have all had to be selective in choosing which papers to include, which to leave out, which to mention only and which to deal with more fully. Each decision has called for judgement and no doubt, like ourselves, each contributor has good reasons for setting down what he considers to have been the key references of recent years.

Each of us has aimed to thread the data together in narrative form— no easy task where a high proportion of references to text is perforce to be contained within a limited number of words. To lighten the reader's burden we have augmented our endeavours with a leavening of pictures, each of which we hope will tell a story. Also, here and there at the end of some chapters, we have added a coda or tailpiece which we hope will stimulate further thought, investigation or research and so may occasionally help to make for effective policy decisions.

R. S. MORTON
J. R. W. HARRIS

Sheffield, 1974

Acknowledgements

We are indebted to our seven colleagues for their prompt response and for their contributions. We are happy to acknowledge our debt to Mr. A. S. Foster, medical artist, the United Sheffield Hospitals, for his help with some of the illustrations. We acknowledge the help we have received from the sources listed in Appendix I.

Our thanks are due to our staffs for their understanding and to our wives for their forbearance and help.

We are grateful to Dr. T. D. Spencer for reading the proofs.

Contributors

Dr. R. D. CATTERALL, F.R.C.P.(ED.)
Director, Department of Sexually Transmitted Diseases, The Middlesex Hospital, London.

Dr. E. M. C. DUNLOP, M.D., F.R.C.P.
Senior Physician, The London Hospital, and Consultant Venereologist, Moorfield Eye Hospital, London.

Dr. J. R. W. HARRIS, M.B., CH.B., M.R.C.P., D.T.M.&H.
Consultant Venereologist, King's College Hospital, London.

Dr. A. E. JEPHCOTT, M.A., M.B., DIP.BACT., M.R.C.PATH.
Consultant Microbiologist, Public Health Laboratory Service, Northern General Hospital, Sheffield.

Prof. M. G. McENTEGART, M.D., F.R.C.PATH.
Department of Medical Microbiology, University of Sheffield.

Dr. R. S. MORTON, M.B.E., F.R.C.P.(ED.)
Consultant Venereologist, Royal Infirmary, Sheffield.

Mr. F. St. D. ROWNTREE, M.SC., F.R.S.H., M.R.I.P.H., M.I.P.R., M.I.H.E.
Health Education Officer, City of Sheffield.

Dr. A. E. WILKINSON, F.R.C.PATH.
Director, Venereal Disease Reference Laboratory, The London Hospital, London.

Dr. R. R. WILLCOX, M.D., M.R.C.P.
Consultant Venerologist, St. Mary's Hospital, London, and Edward VII Hospital, Windsor.

Contents

Part 1
GONORRHOEA

1	Epidemiological Aspects	R. S. Morton	7
2	Social Aspects	R. S. Morton	15
3	Clinical Aspects	R. S. Morton	32
4	Recent Advances in Routine Laboratory Procedures	A. E. Jephcott	44
5	Fundamental Research Developments	M. G. McEntegart	54
6	Therapy	R. S. Morton	69

Part 2
SYPHILIS

7	Epidemiological and Social Aspects	J. R. W. Harris	91
8	Clinical Aspects	J. R. W. Harris	97
9	Non-venereal Treponematoses	J. R. W. Harris	124
10	Sereological Tests for Syphilis	A. E. Wilkinson	127
11	Experimental Syphilis	J. R. W. Harris	148
12	Immunity in Syphilis	A. E. Wilkinson	155
13	Therapy	J. R. W. Harris	162
14	The Chronic Biological False Positive Reaction	R. D. Catterall	174

Part 3
CHANCROID, LYMPHOGRANULOMA VENEREUM AND GRANULOMA INGUINALE (DONOVANIOSIS)

15	Chancroid	R. R. Willcox	185
16	Lymphogranuloma Venereum	R. R. Willcox	188
17	Granuloma Inguinale (Donovaniosis)	R. R. Willcox	194

CONTENTS

Part 4
TRICHOMONIASIS

18	Epidemiological and Social Aspects	R. S. Morton	203
19	Clinical Aspects	R. S. Morton	210
20	Laboratory Aspects	R. S. Morton	214
21	Therapy	R. S. Morton	221

Part 5
CANDIDIASIS

22	Introduction, Epidemiology and Social Aspects	J. R. W. Harris	231
23	Predisposing Factors	J. R. W. Harris	235
24	Clinical Aspects	J. R. W. Harris	240
25	Laboratory Aspects	J. R. W. Harris	243
26	Therapy	J. R. W. Harris	246

Part 6
NON-SPECIFIC GENITAL INFECTION

27	Epidemiological and Social Aspects	R. S. Morton	253
28	Clinical Aspects	R. S. Morton	257
29	Laboratory Aspects	E. M. C. Dunlop	267
30	Therapy	R. S. Morton	296

Part 7
REITER'S SYNDROME

31	Epidemiology	J. R. W. Harris	303
32	Laboratory Aspects	J. R. W. Harris	304
33	Clinical Aspects	J. R. W. Harris	308
34	Therapy	J. R. W. Harris	314

Part 8
OTHER SEXUALLY TRANSMISSIBLE DISEASES

35	Herpes Genitalis	R. S. Morton	325
36	Molluscum Contagiosum	R. S. Morton	336
37	Genital Warts	R. S. Morton	338
38	Phthiris Pubis Infestation	R. S. Morton	342
39	Scabies	R. S. Morton	344
40	Virus Hepatitis B	J. R. W. Harris	350
41	Corynebacterium Vaginale Infection	J. R. W. Harris	354
42	Cytomegalovirus Infection	J. R. W. Harris	361
43	Sexually Transmitted Protozoa and Helminths	J. R. W. Harris	365

Part 9
CONTROL

44 Size and Nature of the
      Problem   *R. S. Morton*   371
45 Clinical Services   *R. S. Morton*   380
46 Health Education   *F. St. D. Rowntree*   388
47 Contact Tracing   *R. S. Morton*   402

APPENDIX   409

INDEX   411

Part 1
Gonorrhoea

Preamble

In 1963 the World Health Organisation stated that the rising incidence of gonorrhoea was affecting 53 (47·7 per cent) of 111 countries and areas making reports. The trend has continued throughout the ensuing decade and throughout the world (Table I and Fig. 1). Inevitably, more attention has been paid to clinical signs of the disease, particularly the complications of salpingitis and septicaemia. Epidemiological and social aspects have likewise received more attention and the concept of gonorrhoea as a behavioural disease emphasised. The role of a great variety of treatments as curative agents, as promotional of resistance and as tools of epidemiological control has also been stressed.

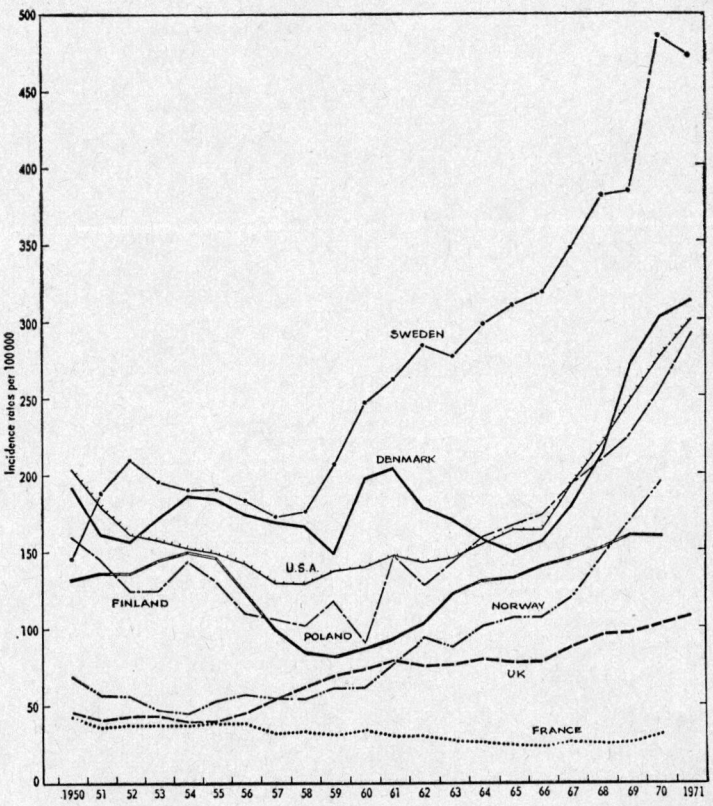

FIG. 1. Reported gonorrhoea 1950–71 incidence rates per 100 000 population. (Supplied by K. Kiraly (1973), Chief V.D.T. W.H.O., Geneva.)

3

Table I. Notified cases of gonorrhoea: number and incidence rate per 100 000 for each year 1950–67

	Country										
	Denmark		England and Wales		Finland		France		Italy		Norway	
Year	No.	Rate	No.	Rate	No.	Rate	No.	Rate	No.	Rate	No.	Rate
1950	8 485	192·8	20 304	39·1	6 629	160·0	17 888	42·9	28 976	58·6	2 415	69·0
1951	7 093	161·2	18 064	40·8	5 806	145·0	14 664	35·2	21 204	44·4	1 947	56·4
1952	7 017	156·0	19 095	43·0	5 022	125·0	15 698	37·3	21 695	44·1	1 933	56·0
1953	7 551	171·6	19 263	43·3	5 187	125·0	16 151	37·5	21 323	45·0	1 647	47·0
1954	8 215	186·7	17 536	39·4	5 685	144·0	15 959	36·5	20 429	42·5	1 560	44·3
1955	8 129	184·7	17 845	39·6	5 568	131·0	17 150	39·0	17 788	37·0	1 866	53·0
1956	7 665	174·2	20 383	45·3	4 728	110·0	16 682	38·0	14 517	30·1	2 002	56·8
1957	7 447	169·2	24 381	54·1	4 616	106·0	15 267	32·0	13 071	27·0	1 916	54·4
1958	7 314	166·2	27 887	62·0	4 474	102·0	14 611	32·9	11 582	23·6	1 910	54·2
1959	8 194	148·5	31 344	69·2	5 190	118·0	13 848	30·8	11 493	23·4	2 137	60·6
1960	9 055	197·7	33 770	73·0	4 150	90·6	15 164	33·4	8 751	17·3	2 173	61·7
1961	9 244	204·7	37 107	79·0	6 551	147·3	13 509	29·6	7 966	16·0	2 714	77·0
1962	8 502	178·3	35 438	75·5	5 702	128·2	13 563	29·5	6 921	13·9	3 320	94·2
1963	7 752	170·0	36 049	76·0	6 458	143·5	12 444	26·7	7 349	14·7	3 160	88·0
1964	7 219	157·6	37 665	79·5	7 306	159·5	12 910	26·3	7 619	15·9	3 665	102·0
1965	6 839	149·3	36 691	77·4	7 648	167·0	11 740	23·9	6 895	13·5	3 850	107·2
1966	7 162	156·3	37 483	78·5	7 987	173·6	11 607	23·2	7 270	14·2	3 862	107·2
1967	8 219	179·0	41 829	87·6	8 881	193·0	12 972	25·9	7 469	14·6	4 440	120·0

	Country										
	Poland		Sweden		United States of America		Ceylon		Japan		Cameroon	
Year	No.	Rate	No.	Rate	No.	Rate	No.	Rate	No.	Rate	No.	Rate
1950	31 549	131·5	10 212	145·6	303 992	204·0	554	11·9	178 273	214·3		
1951	32 982	132·0	13 294	188·0	270 459	179·5	532	11·4	177 774	210·2		
1952	35 013	134·7	14 963	210·0	254 633	161·3	870	18·6	158 670	184·8		
1953	38 512	133·4	14 052	195·9	343 857	157·4	585	12·5	140 458	161·7		
1954	40 052	150·0	13 717	190·2	239 661	152·0	1 149	24·6	141 416	160·0		
1955	39 039	145·6	13 852	190·7	239 787	149·2	1 120	21·7	134 571	150·3		
1956	34 403	127·9	13 810	183·8	233 333	142·4	927	17·9	116 842	129·7		
1957	27 979	101·7	12 730	172·8	216 476	129·8	796	15·4	86 195	94·7		
1958	24 209	84·1	13 038	175·8	220 191	129·3	1 088	16·5	24 367	26·7		
1959	23 408	81·4	15 421	206·9	237 318	137·6	1 049	15·9	9 970	11·4		
1960	24 974	86·4	18 473	246·8	246 697	139·6	1 045	15·8	8 736	10·0		
1961	27 829	93·8	19 712	262·1	246 665	147·8	—	—	6 364	7·0	24 793	467·8
1962	30 871	103·4	21 590	284·8	260 468	142·9	—	—	5 125	5·5	35 575	671·2
1963	36 787	123·0	21 137	277·1	270 076	145·7	2 678	25·2	4 166	4·3	33 707	716·8
1964	40 264	129·5	22 936	298·1	290 603	154·5	2 466	22·5	4 041	4·1	41 237	764·6
1965	41 389	132·8	24 100	310·1	310 155	163·8	2 516	23·0	4 663	4·7	27 122	493·1
1966	44 153	140·7	25 002	318·8	334 949	173·6	2 695	24·5	6 931	7·0	36 309	660·0
1967	45 575	145·1	26 024	347·0	375 606	193·0	3 099	28·1			44 706	812·8

Produced from: Guthe and Idsøe (1968). The Nature and Extent of Veneral Disease—World Trends, INT/VDT/68, 234.

Laboratory workers too have been increasingly active not only in seeking improved and more rapid methods of diagnosis but in exploring the hitherto neglected areas of fundamental research such as the chemical constitution of the N. gonorrhoeae, its cultural characteristics, strain identification and antigenic potential for the development of a reliable diagnostic blood test. The mechanism of development of antibiotic resistance still eludes us but monitoring has helped map the distribution of resistant strains and acts as an early warning device. Not least, efforts have been made to establish an animal model of

infection which would give increased scope for study of antibody/
antigen activity. To date success has only been possible with the
chimpanzee.

On the whole, however, medical endeavour to date is being surpassed
by social and environmental factors and the outlook regarding gonorrhoea control can only be described as bleak.

1 Epidemiological Aspects

R. S. Morton

Introduction

In the early 1960s the annual number of gonococcal infections in the
world was estimated at 60 million. Today's estimate is 200 million. In
the Western world particularly, this has been associated with relative
peace and prosperity. This is in marked contrast to the traditional
association of peak incidence with war and poverty—social conditions
which have recently applied in Bangladesh (see Table II).

The worldwide trend towards homogenicity in the structure and
functions of societies and in the attitudes and behaviour of their peoples
continues to cross barriers of colour, creed and culture. Prostitution
accounts for the great majority of infections in males in Eastern and
South American countries. By contrast, the growing freedom of
Western women, to express themselves sexually, reduces the percentage
of men in the countries concerned who attribute their infection to
prostitutes.

Dissemination of infection

The age-old, widespread and serious problems of reporting gonorrhoea
have bedevilled full epidemiological understanding in many countries
for many years. The recent past has been no exception. This and some
selected epidemiological factors are dealt with.

In two articles Willcox (1965a, b) states his belief that it is not enough
nowadays to confine epidemiological thought to the idea of the promiscuous female as a source of infection in several men. He propounds
the philosophy of these infected men as a source of 'feed-back' to
maintain the incidence of the disease in the female pool. Acceptance of
this philosophy Willcox sees as fundamental to control. He believes
that discouragement of male promiscuity, increased use of prophylaxis
by males and perfection of their early treatment have real capability as
tools of control of the incidence of gonorrhoea. These considerations

7

are further pressed by Willcox (1966a, b). He produces figures to show how even a few treatment failure cases in males can produce startling rises in the infectious pool, especially in countries and conditions with high levels of promiscuity. The second paper mentioned makes allowance for homosexual males in these calculations.

Lomholt (1965) and Lomholt and Berg (1965) outline in detail the epidemiology of gonorrhoea in Greenland and use it as a basis for a comprehensive control programme. A year later Lomholt and Berg (1966) give a résumé of their work. They investigated 309 inhabitants of Greenland all aged 14 years and over. They found that 40 per cent of male and female Eskimos had had gonorrhoea on more than three occasions; 28 per cent of the unmarried population had been infected during the previous 6 months and of 52 women aged 16–29 years, only five had not previously had gonorrhoea.

Within a single country incidence may vary from place to place. Urban areas are well recognised as having higher rates than rural ones. Seafarers, known to have an infection rate 15–20 times higher than landlubbers, play an import/export role in the epidemiology of gonorrhoea. According to Schofield (1965) this should be constantly monitored. He has shown how seafarers of several nationalities imported gonorrhoea to one port in north-east England. One hundred and forty-five exposures abroad produced 94 men requiring treatment in his department.

Problems of reporting

Writing in the South American press, Brown (1966) points out the shortcomings of case reporting. This is a problem of all countries, particularly in those where the great majority of the infected are treated in the private sector. Brown emphasises the need for reporting as a means of identifying epidemiological characteristics of the disease such as geographic distribution. He calls also for the use of standard definitions and good data registration. This last point is echoed by Juhlin and Krook (1965). Of 5 666 samples examined for gonorrhoea 978 yielded positive results either by smear or culture. They showed that 29 per cent gave positive culture results and negative smears, while 4·5 per cent gave positive smear results but negative cultures. In males, 15 per cent of those with negative or doubtful smears had positive cultures. In females, the corresponding figure was 54 per cent. The authors make the pertinent point that when reporting totals, the criteria of diagnosis should be clearly stated. They see this as vital to a rational discussion of the epidemiology of the disease.

This comparatively sophisticated approach is not mentioned in most reports so that comparisons between countries are meaningless and comparative demographers are confined to trends only.

Table II. Recorded cases of gonorrhoea in Bangladesh (reproduced from WHO/SEARO/72, 267)

	Dacca Med. Coll. Hosp.	Mitford Hosp. Dacca	Skin and Social Hygiene Centre, Chittagong	Chittagong Med. Coll. Hosp.	V.D. Clinic Sadat Hosp., Khulna	Total
1962	1 126	1 059	228	—	—	—
1963	895	1 713	570	—	—	—
1964	911	2 401	454	—	512	—
1965	946	1 435	92	—	750	—
1966	1 068	3 409	52	603	662	5 794
1967	991	2 813	96	654	845	5 399
1968	987	1 292	47	532	1 270	5 128
1969	724	785	82	506	1 164	3 261
1970	1 208	776	52	1 251	1 385	3 464
1971	941	598	67	1 656	217‡	2 528
1972	—	2 221*	140†	3 048†	1 250§	6 659

* Period 1 January 1972–18 October 1972
† Period 1 January 1972–25 October 1972
‡ Period 1 January 1972–25 March 1972
§ Period 25 March 1972–31 October 1972

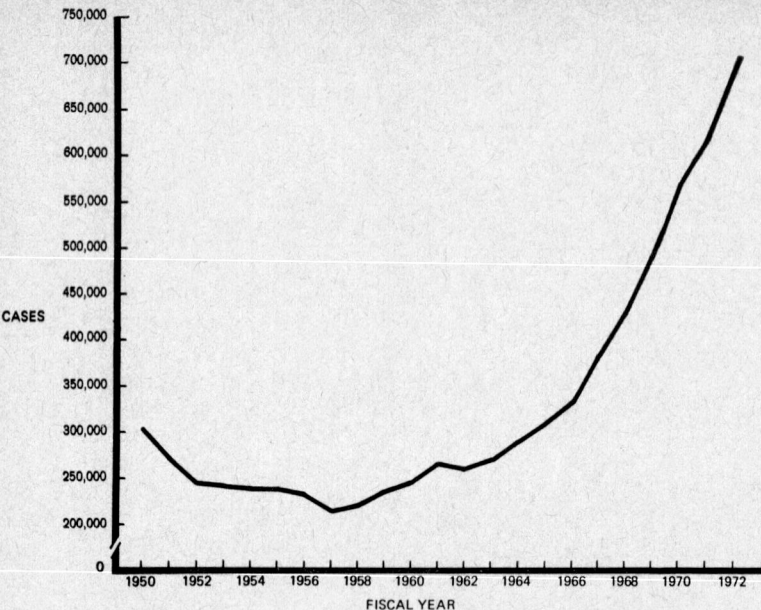

FISCAL YEAR

FIG. 2. Gonorrhoea—reported cases, U.S.A., fiscal years, 1950–72. (As depicted in 'Today's V.D. Control Problem" (1973), published by the American Social Hygiene Association.)

Papers considering the problems of reporting incidence include those by Shanhultz (1967), from Virginia, who showed that private physicians in that area reported only 17·2 per cent of the gonorrhoea treated. Adams (1967) reviewed the situation in Sydney, Australia, and Siboulet and Egger (1966) the situation in France. On a nationwide basis, Fleming et al (1970) questioned all private physicians in the U.S.A. regarding treatment of gonorrhoea. The reply response was 65·3 per cent (134 633 doctors). Of these, 39 392 treated 185 548 infections. Only 16·9 per cent of these had been officially reported. This was listed as a marginal improvement over 1962. Reviewing the American fiscal year 1971 'Today's V.D. Control Program' (1972) states that, although gonorrhoea is now the country's most frequently reported communicable disease, when the estimated unreported cases are added, then the morbidity rate rises 4·5 fold and reaches 800 infections per 100 000 population per annum (see Figs. 2 and 3).

International variables

'Today's V.D. Control Program' (1973) shows that the annual increase in gonorrhoea returned to its more usual proportions with an

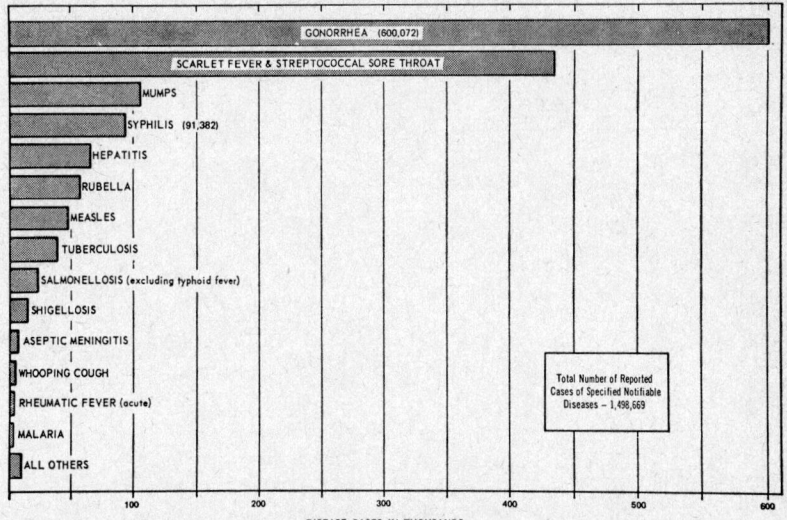

FIG. 3. Communicable diseases—number of reported cases U.S.A., calendar year 1970. (Reproduced from 'Today's V.D. Control Problem' (1973) published by the American Social Hygiene Association.)

increase of 15·1 per cent in 1972 over 1971. It is of interest to find some measure of parallelism in England where in 1972 there was a reversal of the upward incidence trend. The indications are that 1973 will again see a renewal of the upward trend. That these variations are to some extent dictated by economics seems likely. Both countries have employed a phased attack on inflation, the U.S.A. before the U.K. In each country, Phase I with its associated fall in investments, reduction of ready cash and rising unemployment has been accompanied by deceleration or reversal in the growing incidence of gonorrhoea; whereas endeavours making for economic stability, as in the introduction of Phase II, have in each country been accompanied by a return to the trend which started with post-war economic recovery around the early/mid-1950s.

A report from the U.S.S.R. by Litvinova and Cherepovitch (1966) deals with the role of women in dictating demographic data. They found that, in 1958, women with gonorrhoea formed 9·8 per cent of the total. In 1964, the figure was 27·9. Gedicke (1967) found a similar trend in Western Germany. Morton (1970a) showed the growing preponderance of females in public clinic populations in England. He found this applied to all categories of patients, that is, those with gonorrhoea, those with other conditions and those found free of infection. He viewed the trend towards a male : female ratio of 1 : 1 as evidence of greater freedom of sexual expression, an important epidemiological change and one altering the face of medical practice. Dunlop et al (1971) published a paper with similar observations. The technical and scientific innovations of the intra-uterine contraceptive device and the contraceptive pill have paralleled and augmented the changing attitudes and behaviour patterns mentioned. Freedom from fear of pregnancy allied to much public indifference to gonorrhoea appears, according to Juhlin (1968), to have increased sexual activity and the rate of partner change in pill takers, when compared with their non-pill taking sisters. Juhlin sees these changes as enhancing the chances of acquiring infection.

Willcox (1967) discusses growing antibiotic resistance as a reason for the worsening epidemiological situation. This aspect is also dealt with by Danbolt (1967), the *Lancet* (1968) and by Warren (1968). Warren shows the association between treatment failure and relatively resistant strains of gonococci. He found that a significantly higher incidence of partially resistant strains were isolated from patients infected overseas. This work was carried out in the port of Southampton in England. How such resistance has built up to alarming proportions in the Western Pacific and in South-east Asia is given by Willcox (1969) in the 'Report of the Second Symposium on V.D. Control in the Western Pacific'. His graphic form of the development is reproduced.

Morton (1970b) shows that in Singapore only one case of gonorrhoea in every four or five is treated in a public clinic. He found that nearly 97 per cent of infected men attributed their infection to a prostitute. Some indication of the size of the resulting reservoir of occult gonorrhoea in married women is apparent in the finding that one baby in every 500 develops gonococcal ophthalmia. Holmes et al (1970) used the visit of a U.S. aircraft carrier to a naval base in the Philippines to conduct an epidemiological study. Of the ship's crew, 2 191 men admitted sexual intercourse with 'hostesses' while ashore. The mean number of consorts per man was 1·2. Of this total 77 per cent used no prophylaxis, and 88 were infected with gonorrhoea. By a series of calculations Holmes and his colleagues declare that the risk of infection is 22 per cent. This work, while not beyond criticism, is a useful attempt to establish the kind of epidemiological index which should be commonplace.

The seasonality of gonorrhoea in the U.S.A. was studied by Cornelius (1971). He used quarterly incidence returns from both private and public sources for the years 1950–69. These revealed that the third quarters consistently showed the highest morbidity rates. There was a consistent rise from the first to third quarters each year. Seasonal variation was identical for both sexes and all latitudes, even for those where climatic conditions varied little from one part of the year to another. It correlated with reverse seasonality of births, both legitimate and illegitimate. Not all the factors operating are fully understood.

Three general reports are worthy of note. Guthe and Idsøe (1968) insist on the lack of reliance which can be placed on data from some countries. They have, however, more confidence in the trend shown by figures from individual countries, each using its own method of reporting. Thus between 1957–67 they are able to show morbidity trends as follows:

Sweden	172·8 to 347·0/100 000
England and Wales	54·1 to 87·6/100 000
U.S.A.	129·8 to 193·0/100 000
Ceylon	15·4 to 28·1/100 000
Japan	94·7 to 7·0/100 000

This last is attributed to a drift to care in the private sector (which has come with prosperity) and a subsequent decline in reporting.

The 'W.H.O. Report on the Second Seminar on V.D. Control in the Western Pacific' was published in 1969. It is packed with epidemiological data concerning the 15 participating countries. How this, with clinical, laboratory and pharmacological data, can be correlated and the whole deployed to fulfil the aims of V.D. control is clearly set out. This document is probably the most comprehensive and practically useful one published in the late 1960s. The facts and principles given have worldwide application.

The *British Journal of Venereal Diseases* published a 'Report of an International Meeting on Gonorrhoea' (1971). Epidemiological data gives some idea of the dynamics at work in Sweden, Belgium, Italy, Austria, Senegal and the Lebanon to produce increasing infection rates.

The varying relevance of all factors in different countries can also be appreciated by reference to Catterall (1970), Lindman (1970), Micheal (1971), Siboulet (1969), Morton (1971) and 'W.H.O. Assignment Report on V.D. in Bangladesh' (1973).

Coda

Future epidemiological studies should concern themselves primarily with organisational ways and means of improving reporting. It is clear that data gathering should be an active rather than a passive exercise. The quality of data also calls for improvement. The geography of gonorrhoea requires attention. Is there evidence, for example, of centrifugal spread within a country's boundaries, from metropolis, to big cities, to towns and so to rural areas? Can we be more accurate in the make-up of national import/export balance sheets? If poverty and prosperity are both associated with increased prevalence of gonorrhoea what is the optimum economic state of affairs for maximum control?

There is scope not only for informative indices, but for evaluative and predictive indices also. These are essential to an understanding of the nature of the epidemiology of gonorrhoea in any area and to the planning and operation of an effective V.D. control programme.

REFERENCES

ADAMS, A. (1967). *Med. J. Aust.*, **1**, 145.
BROWN, W. J. (1966). *Bol. Sanit., Pan-am.*, **60**, 93.
CATTERALL, R. D. (1970). *Brit. J. Hosp. Med.*, **3**, 55.
CORNELIUS, C.S. III (1971). *H.S.M.M.A. Hlth. Rep.*, **86**, 157.
DANBOLT, M. (1967). *Triangle*, **8**, 2.
DUNLOP, E. M. C., LAMB, A. M. and KING, D. M. (1971). *Brit. J. vener. Dis.*, **47**, 192.
FLEMING, W. L., BROWN, W. J., DONOHUE, J. F. and BRANIGAN, D. W. (1970). *J. Amer. Med. Ass.*, **211**, 1827.
GEDICKE, K. (1967). *Gesundheit. dienst.*, **29**, 28.
GUTHE, T. and IDSØE, O. (1968). W.H.O. Document INT/VDT/**68**, 234.
HOLMES, K. K., JOHNSON, P. W. and TROSTLE, H. J. (1970). *Amer. J. Epiderm.*, **91**, 170.
JUHLIN, L. and KROOK, G. (1965). *Acta derm.-venereol., Stockh.*, **45**, 142.
JUHLIN, L. (1968). *Acta derm.-venereol., Stockh.*, **48**, 75 and 82.
LANCET (1968). Annotation, **1**, 675.
LINDMAN, C. (1970). *J. Maine med. Ass.*, **61**, 162.
LITVINOVA, N. N. and CHEREPOVICTH, E. V. (1966). *West. derm. vener.*, **40**, 70.
LOMHOLT, G. (1965). *Ugeskr. Haeg.*, **127**, 485.
LOMHOLT, G. and BERG, O. (1965). *Ugeskr. Haeg.*, **127**, 457.
LOMHOLT, G. and BERG, O. (1966). *Brit. J. vener. Dis.*, **42**, 1.
MICHEAL, M. (1971). *Harefauh.*, **80**, 229.
MORTON, R. S. (1970a). *Brit. J. vener. Dis.*, **46**, 103.
MORTON, R. S. (1970b). Singapore Assigment 0021, WHO/WPRO/**70**, 328.
MORTON, R. S. (1971). *Brit. J. vener. Dis.*, **47**, 48.
REPORT OF INTERNATIONAL MEETING ON GONORRHOEA (1971). *Brit. J. vener. Dis.*, **47**, 377.
SCHOFIELD, C. B. S. (1965). *Brit. J. vener. Dis.*, **41**, 51.
SHANHULTZ, M. I. (1967). *Virginia med. Monthly*, **94**, 188.
SIBOULET, A. and EGGER, L. (1966). *Buol. Inst. Nat. Santi.*, **21**, 737.
SIBOULET, A. (1969). *J. Urol. Nephrol.*, 75 Suppl., **12**, 557.
'TODAY'S V. D. CONTROL PROGRAM' (1972). *Amer. Soc. Hyg. Ass.*
'TODAY'S V.D. CONTROL PROGRAM' (1973). *Amer. Soc. Hyg. Ass.*
WARREN, R. M. (1968). *Brit. J. vener. Dis.*, **44**, 80.
W.H.O. (1969). Report on Second Symposium on V.D. Control in Western Pacific Region. Document WHO/WPRO/VDT/**69**, 0144.
W.H.O. (1973). Assignment Report, Bangladesh. WHO/SEARO/**73**, 83 (R. S. Morton).
WILLCOX, R. R. (1965a). *Brit. J. vener. Dis.*, **41**, 287.
WILLCOX, R. R. (1965b). *Acta derm-venereol., Stockh.*, **45**, 302.
WILLCOX, R. R. (1966a). *Acta. derm.-venereol., Stockh.*, **46**, 95.
WILLCOX, R. R. (1966b). *Acta derm.-venereol., Stockh.*, **46**, 250.
WILLCOX, R. R. (1967). *Brit. J. clin. Pract.*, **21**, 165.
WILLCOX, R. R. (1969). W.H.O. Document WPRO/VDT/**69**, 0144

2 Social Aspects

R. S. Morton

Post-World War II population growth has been spectacular and many people born in the decade 1945–55 are now in their most sexually active years. The rising incidence of gonorrhoea, however, far exceeds that which can be accounted for by young people forming a high proportion of national populations. Sexual activity appears to begin earlier than formerly in many countries; improved nutrition and social conditions as well as earlier financial independence all play a part. Greater economic prosperity in many parts of the world has encouraged immigration on a huge scale. Sea trade and tourist traffic has likewise increased at a rapid rate. The twin processes of industralisation and urbanisation have encouraged many millions of young people to move away from their home environment in search of work and education. Countries and continents have been affected. Densely populated urban areas offer the prostitute and the homosexual anonymity and the opportunity for easy contact of partners.

The restraints and constraints on behaviour, imposed by family, religion, custom, neighbours and public opinion have declined. Prosperity has brought leisure to many and has given time and impetus to demands for even greater freedom of expression both generally and sexually. Increased alcohol consumption in some areas of the world has further facilitated sexual activity and the partner change process. The contraceptive pill has made the exercise of sexual freedom a practical reality for some women. Such trends are welcomed by many as a healthy change from the two-standard morality of much of the last century and the beginning of this one. Others fear that liberal views will be interpreted as licence and that irresponsible rates of partner change will precipitate medico-social problems, such as sexually transmitted disease and pre-marital conception, in such numbers that dealing with them will eventually prove too costly in individual, social and financial terms (Morton, 1971).

General view

Shapiro and Lentz (1965) reviewed the ancient history of gonorrhoea and in the light of this considered the present epidemic. Their only firm conclusions were that there was a need for doctors to have a high index of suspicion about the disease and that this should be supported by adequate laboratory facilities. Bent (1965) of Canada listed what he considered to be the social background and problem areas in gonorrhoea. He listed them as follows: apparent increase in moral laxity, inadequate reporting, inadequate legislation, homosexuals and teenagers, asymptomatic females, antibiotic resistance, inadequate follow-up, inadequate health education and the influence of alcohol and narcotics. Fleming (1966) also reviewed the operation of environmental factors in the spread of gonorrhoea. He discussed the dynamics and changing emphasis of some factors.

Papers from Africa pointed to the influence of social changes on that continent. Maffreeba et al (1965) writing from Dakar in West Africa blame recent increases in infection rates on economic evolution, changing customs and the complex migration/urbanisation movement of endogenous peoples. Kibukamusoke (1965) from the study of 1 000 consecutive patients seen in a -7week period in East Africa found 665 with gonorrhoea. He gave special regard to the breakdown of tribal customs and migration as factors facilitating the dissemination of the infection. Sieff (1966) showed that in South Africa the teenagers formed 3·8 per cent of gonorrhoea cases in 1953. In 1965 the figure was 7·9 per cent. Schaller (1968) quoting writings from Ethiopia demonstrated how in that country acquired infection is widely regarded as a sign of sexual maturity. Prostitutes were commonly used and 50 per cent of them were infected.

Guthe and Idsøe (1968) discussing world trends emphasise the complex of balances—ecological, human and environmental—facilitating and restraining gonorrhoea rates (see Fig. 4). The authors give a list of those factors which they consider are currently tipping the balance in favour of recrudescence:

(a) Unprecedented demographic and economic change, technological development, industrialisation, urbanisation and population movement, both civil and military.
(b) Socio-psychological changes as exemplified in emergence of permissive behaviour patterns in both males and females and new attitudes towards both prostitution and homosexuality.
(c) Easy treatment leading to less concern by patients, potential patients and no less amongst medical administrators.

Catterall (1968) in a survey states 'The emergence of the behavioural diseases as the most important group of conditions threatening con-

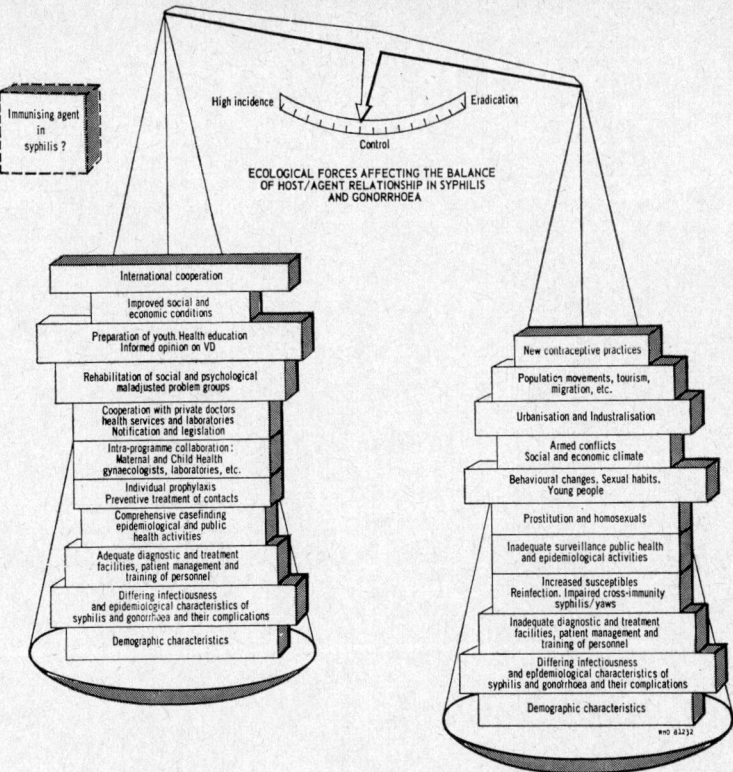

FIG. 4. Ecological forces in V.D. (Reproduced from Idsøe, O. and Guthe, T. (1968). "Some epidemiological aspects of venereal diseases." Document INT/WHO/DVT/68/235.)

temporary mankind during the best years of life is an unexpected and disappointing development in the medical and social history of our time'.

The following year Willcox (1969) refers to 1968 as a gloomy year. He senses that in many countries there is increasing realisation that the influences of social and behaviouristic patterns are beginning to out-weigh those of health workers. Guthe (1971) concludes from a global evaluation that, in spite of national and international measures, upward trends have prevailed the world over for at least a decade. The multiple, interdependent and interlocking forces encouraging the propagation of gonorrhoea are assessed by Guthe and Willcox (1971). They see these forces as promoting attitudinal and behavioural changes, and the whole process as commensurate with the growing prevalence of gonorrhoea for some time to come.

YOUNG PEOPLE

Catterall (1965) pointed to the earlier physical maturity of young people, and the large part played by sex in periodicals, advertisements, radio and television. He believes that paternally based sex education would have a better influence. Although fear of pregnancy remains, fear of sexually transmitted disease no longer deters the young from casual relationships. Hitchens and James (1965), on the contrary, are less disturbed. While admitting reason for disquiet they find no evidence that teenagers are more promiscuous or acquire more infections than earlier generations. They consider that writers would be better employed drawing attention to regional differences as has already been done in the case of illegitimacy. Morton (1966a) drew attention to the increasing role of the young female as a feature of the rising infection rate and Lourie (1966) expressed the view that scientific progress had occurred without sufficient education of the individual. Distortions he saw as leading to gang activities, promiscuity and violence. In the U.S.A., Blaine (1967) and Dalrympale (1967) both discussed sex and the adolescent and this at a time when Frichot and Evertet (1967) were pointing out that the annual number of gonococcal infections exceeded 1·5 million.

Two papers from Uppsala, Sweden, are noteworthy. They are companion pieces by Juhlin (1968a) and 1968b). The first is mainly concerned with sexual behaviour at different ages, and is based on a study of 205 female gonorrhoea contacts of whom 175 were found infected. Points emerging from the series were:

1. 25 per cent were students.
2. 34 per cent came from broken homes.
3. 39 per cent were being observed by juvenile authorities.
4. Alcohol was a common problem amongst non-students, particularly males aged 20–25 years and females of 25 years and over.
5. The income of the non-students was higher than average for Sweden.
6. Fear of infection played little or no part in the life of the group.
7. 18 per cent possessed little information about venereal disease.

The companion paper showed:

1. That patients with gonorrhoea had generally started on a full sex life at an earlier age and that non-students make an earlier start than students.
2. Sexual intercourse occurred on average 1·5 times per week.
3. 25 per cent of infected males recorded 11 to 70 sex partners in the month prior to interview.

4. 44 per cent of the total males in the series used a condom but only 15 per cent of those with 11 or more partners did so.
5. 33·5 per cent of the students and 13 per cent of the non-students were taking contraceptive pills.

Juhlin concluded from these comprehensive studies that the increase in gonorrhoea in students was probably due to them coming from a broader distribution of social classes than formerly, the availability of contraceptive pills and the growth of sexual freedom.

Similar work has been carried out in Denmark by Ekstom (1966, 1970). He found in the earlier paper that young people with gonorrhoea generally had a poor home background, left school early and subsequently had a poor job record. They were usually unskilled and showed evidence of emotional disturbance; 12 per cent had already been under the care of a psychiatrist. Measured by pre-marital pregnancies and reported infections the female teenagers in the group emerged as promiscuous. Ekstrom concluded that these young people were products of their time and that gonorrhoea was a social disease. His second paper is a detailed psychosocial study of 202 girls and 100 boys aged 14–19 years all attending a venereal disease clinic. A significantly high per-

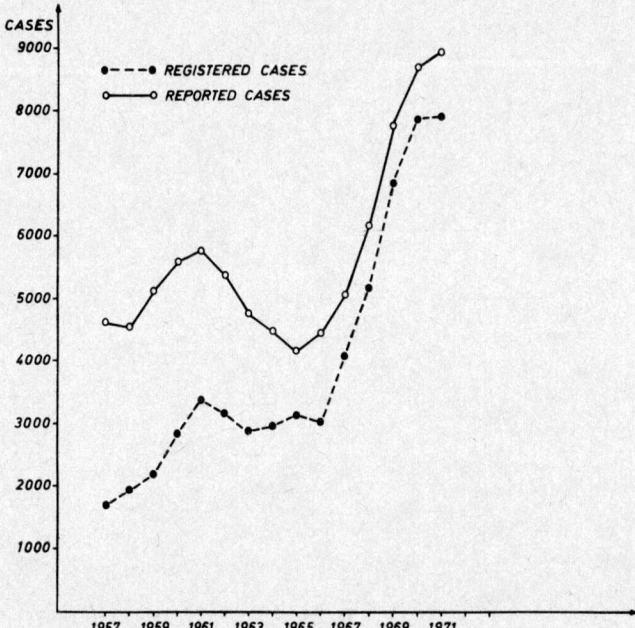

FIG. 5. Male gonorrhoea in Denmark. Annual number of cases reported to the National Health Service compared with those registered at the Neisseria Department, Statens Seruminstitut. (Reproduced from Inga Lind (1972). Document WHO/VDT/72/383.)

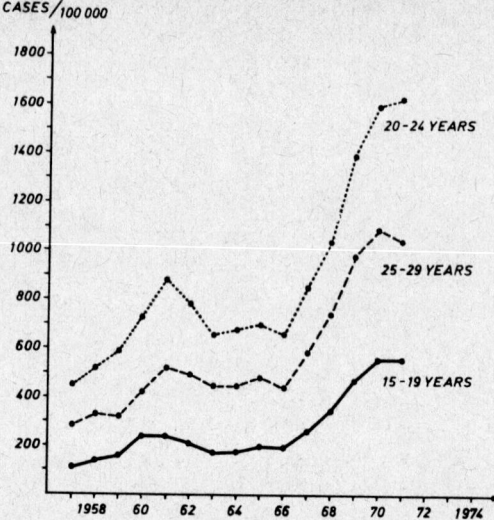

FIG. 6. Male gonorrhoea in Denmark. Comparison of number of cases per 100 000 inhabitants in the three predominant 5-year age-groups 1957–1971. (Reproduced from Inga Lind (1972). Document WHO/VDT/72/383.)

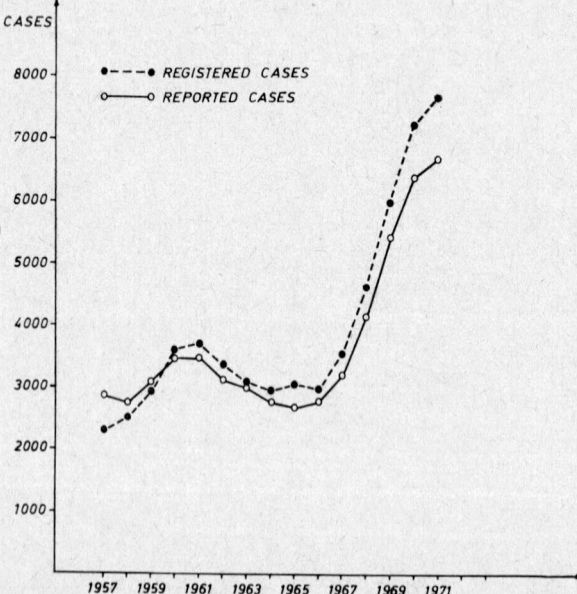

FIG. 7. Female gonorrhoea in Denmark. Annual number of cases reported to the National Health Service compared with those registered at the Neisseria Department, Statens Seruminstitut. (Reproduced from Inga Lind (1972). Document WHO/VDT/72/383.)

centage had poor contact with home and parents, had had frequent changes of both school and job, made frequent sex partner changes and had high frequency concerning pregnancy, abortion, criminal offences, alcohol abuse, etc. Ekstom sees the lesson to be learned from these findings very clearly. It is essential to prevent inheritance of the same social environment by the next generation (see Figs. 5, 6, 7 and 8).

Karolyi (1969) of Hungary noted that the recrudescence of gonorrhoea was mainly due to population mobility, growing international traffic, changes in sexual behaviour and modification of moral concepts. The latter he saw as manifesting itself in an increasing measure of promiscuous behaviour amongst the young and homosexuals. He showed the spread of infection to be not so much between one young person and another as between one teenage group and another (see Figs. 9 and 10).

From the U.S.A. Kampmeier (1971) noted that the gonorrhoea morbidity rate for these under 24 years was 372 per 100 000 and for

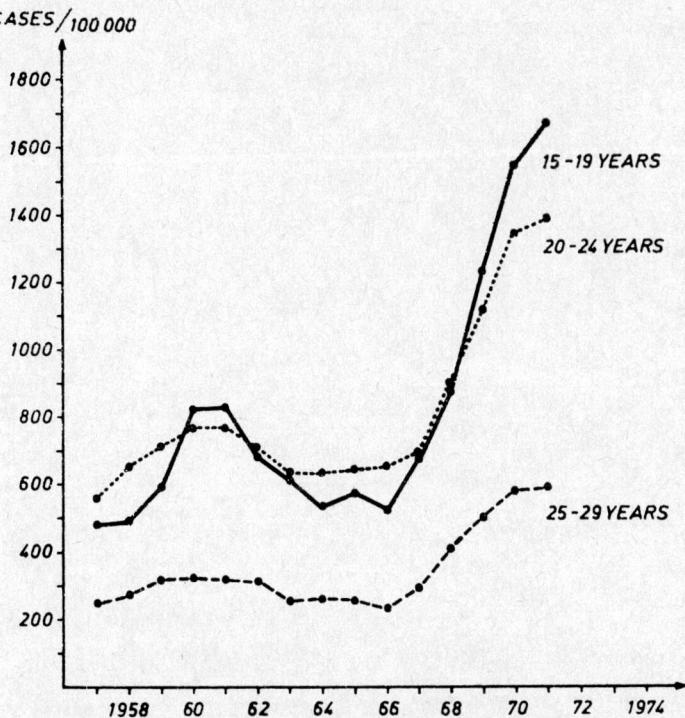

Fig. 8. Gonorrhoea in Denmark. Comparison of number of cases per 100 000 female inhabitants in the three predominent five-year age groups. (Reproduced from Inga Lind (1972). Document WHO/VDT/72/383.)

2

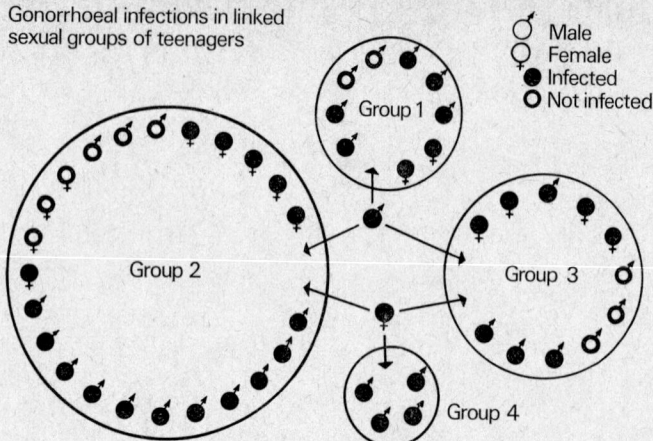

FIG. 9. Gonorrhoea in Hungary. (Reproduced from I. Karolyi (1969). Document INT/WHO/VDT/69/253.)

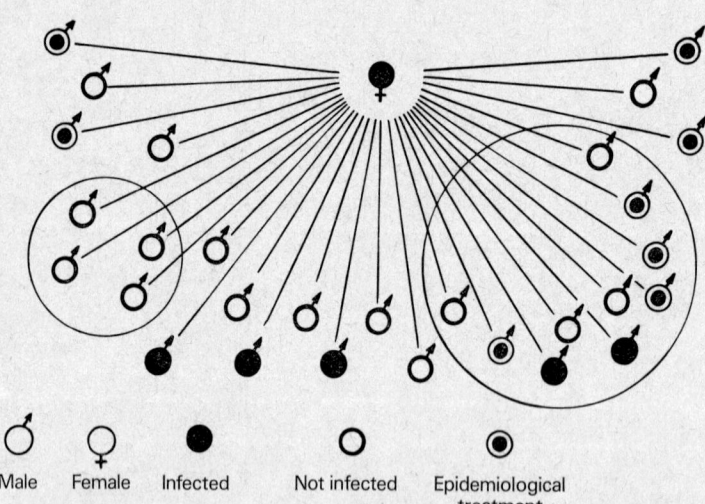

FIG. 10. Gonorrhoea in Hungary. (Reproduced from I. Karolyi (1969). Document INT/WHO/VDT/69/253.)

those over 24 years was 179 per 100 000. Delune (1971) reported 'sexual vagabondage' in Belgium. By this he meant that young girls ever more commonly made themselves available as casual sex partners and were now ahead of prostitutes as the principal disseminators of gonorrhoea.

An editorial in the *British Medical Journal* (1973) discussed the legal aspects of dealing with venereal diseases in those under 16 years of age. It is noted that in the U.S.A. the law has been altered in many states to permit doctors to act *in loco parentis*. In the U.K. the Family Law Reform Act of 1969 is judged to be adequate protection for all concerned.

FEMALES

Guthe (1966) suggested that a new factor which would soon be added to those already at work was the increasing use of the intra-uterine contraceptive device and the contraceptive pill. He believed these innovations could lead to more active sexual behaviour patterns and to multiple sex contacts.

The British Co-operative Clinical Group (1968) reviewed 95 per cent of all reported gonorrhoea in England and Wales and showed how the male : female ratio was steadily moving towards unity. In 1966 it was 2·0 : 1. Even in London where disparity was always greatest it had moved from a ratio of 4·1 : 1 in 1965 to 3·4 : 1 in 1966. The trend was confirmed by Willcox (1970). He pointed out with reference to the 1968 figures for gonorrhoea that those for males represented 88·3 per cent of the post-war peak year whilst those for females represented 106·6 per cent. 'Thus', says Willcox, 'the considerable gains which followed the introduction of antibiotics have now been virtually dissipated.'

In a well-documented study Juhlin (1968a, b) investigated the use of the contraceptive pill amongst 522 female patients attending the venereal diseases clinic in Uppsala, Sweden, between September 1967 and February 1968. Married women numbered 272. Of the 250 single women 71 were students and 179 non-students. Of the whole group 141 (53 per cent) were pill takers; 50 students (70 per cent of 71) and 91 non-students (50·8 per cent of 179). Questioning of all the single women revealed that the number of their sex partners and the frequency of their intercourse had increased after pill taking began. The incidence of gonorrhoea in the pill-taking group was marginally higher. Juhlin concluded that pill taking probably increased the risk of infection and encouraged the spread of gonorrhoea. Hewitt (1970) in England found that 11·9 per cent of his V.D. clinic patients took contraceptive pills. This was twice that for the general population and compared with 15·1 per cent for patients with gonorrhoea. The author cautiously concludes that the availability of the pill may be a factor prompting promiscuity in recent years. Cohen (1970) in Wales found in 1965 that the proportion of his pill-taking patients with gonorrhoea was 25 per cent. In 1968 this figure was 40 per cent. This compares with 14 and 20 per cent for their non-pill taking sisters. Over the study years the incidence of gonorrhoea increased in the total clinic population by 6 per cent.

Such observations have prompted special screening studies of young women. Zackler et al (1970) submitted 32 470 cervical specimens for Gram-staining and culture on Thayer–Martin medium over a 12-month period. Women attending 22 private, public and non-profit making clinics in the Chicago area were involved. Positive findings were made in 1 782 or 5·5 per cent. Another 'blind' mass survey by Allen (1970) in Arkansas brought appreciation of changing behavioural standards and population mobility. Of 841 women attending a family planning clinic 101 (12 per cent) were found to have gonorrhoea. All were asymptomatic carriers. Women seeking abortion were viewed as an 'at risk' group by Geizer and Kopecky (1972). They cultured gonococci from 33 (8 per cent) of 414 women seeking legal termination. Gallagher (1970) in England found 8·8 per cent of 716 girls on remand to have gonorrhoea.

Thompson and Rutherford (1972) reviewed the records of females attending the V.D. clinic at Aberdeen in Scotland during the years 1960–69. The clinic population increased 2·5 times and this paralleled the illegitimacy rate. There were changes in the type of female attending. They were largely unmarried teenagers and in the later years non-manual workers began to form an important group. In 1969 some 22 per cent of the patients were 'on the pill'. Over the study years there had always been a small group having a close association with foreign sailors. These women tended to have a history of multiple hospital admissions, a record of attempted suicides, alcoholism and vicious behaviour. This latter point was emphasised by Pemberton et al (1972) in a study carried out in Belfast, Northern Ireland.

Schofield (1969) from a review of the mothers of 48 infants who developed gonococcal ophthalmia neonatorum pointed to the importance of social data. He sees that there are social as well as medical indications for making a search for the gonococcus in the pregnant, *eg* an unmarried pregnant patient especially if she has previously been pregnant, any girl with a history of promiscuous behaviour or any form of sexually transmitted disease, lack of co-operation in ante-natal or other care and a teenager marrying in the last months of pregnancy.

SEAFARERS

Wheldon (1964) analysed the results obtained from the administration of a detailed questionnaire to the crew of a British naval cruiser stationed in the Far East. Amongst some of the points to emerge were these:

1. Men in the British Royal Navy generally see chastity as no longer a matter of merit.
2. There is virtual absence of social stigma about venereal disease.
3. Alcohol abuse is still a major factor leading to infection.

Guthe and Idsøe (1964) showed that the higher prevalence rate of infection in seafarers was of the order 15–20 times that of landlubbers. Schofield (1965a, b) drew attention to the fact that in one clinic on the north-east English coast 53·6 per cent of the patients were mariners and that 44·5 per cent of the gonorrhoea was imported.

Idsøe and Guthe (1967) noted that the world merchant shipping tonnage had increased from 76 690 thousand tons in 1945 to 150 347 in 1963. They do not relate this to the number of seafarers and the number of stop-over days in ports, but the inference is clear. When dealing with air traffic they note that in 26 countries, arrivals increased from 55·25 millions in 1958 to 128 millions in 1966.

Idsøe et al (1972) reported a joint study by W.H.O. and the International Radio-Medical Centre at Rome. This centre dealt by radio with 227 cases of V.D., 80 per cent of them gonorrhoea. All cases were diagnosed in one calendar year during 1968–69. The infections were found in a total of 3 818 crew aboard Italian ships. The incidence of infection was twice as high in freighters as in tankers and the rate in officers, half that in the men. The age range 20 to 29 years predominated This paper defines more precisely than ever before the nature and extent of a well-known 'at risk' group.

PROSTITUTES

The Committee of Public Health in New York (1965) commented on the high percentage of prostitutes amongst prisoners and narcotic addicts. In view of the occult nature of much V.D. in women generally, they considered that making tests for V.D. should be approved practice for women prisoners. De Amorin (1966) examined 202 arrested prostitutes in Brazil and found 55·9 per cent with gonorrhoea. Wren (1967) in Australia found 44 per cent of prostitutes infected. This was 10 times greater than the infection rate in 276 other prisoners.

Johnson et al (1969) examined 702 'hostesses' in the Philippines. Using cervical cultures they found an infection rate of 8·5 per cent. This was raised to 19·7 per cent by weekly testing. The positivity rate in 163 named contacts of gonorrhoea was 22 per cent, a figure which also doubled by repeated weekly testing. Luger (1971) reported that gonorrhoea in Austria is 10 to 15 times more frequent in unregistered prostitutes than in the registered. The morbidity rate in this last group is said to be not significantly higher than that of the population of Vienna. In the years 1960 to 1968 the average age of patients fell by 2·5 years. Kokoshka et al (1972) also writing from Vienna found 152 (76 per cent) of 200 prostitutes to have gonorrhoea. Twenty-one per cent had salpingitis. Repeated infections were frequent.

Verhagen and Gemmett (1972) showed the social forces at work in determining a growing frequency of gonorrhoea in Kenya. Featuring high on the list were the morbidity of promiscuous males and their association with prostitutes.

HOMOSEXUALS

Michael Schofield (1964) pleaded on the basis of a review of the social aspects of homosexuality and venereal infection, for a freer and franker exchange of contact data between homosexuals and venereologists. This could be the basis for a more enlightened legal and social attitude towards the problem.

Fluker (1966) noted that 15·5 per cent of all gonorrhoea in males at the West London Hospital occurred in homosexuals. Pedder (1970) found the typical male homosexual in the V.D. clinic to be a single, U.K.-born man between 20 and 40 years. His motivation for help with his homosexuality was low. Only 0·3 per cent of the group wished to be referred for psychiatric help. A British Co-operative Clinical Group study looked at the incidence of gonorrhoea in homosexuals. In clinics in Scotland, England and Wales, excluding London, homosexuals contributed between 3·1 and 5·6 per cent. In London the figure was 19·9 per cent. In five clinics in London's West End the incidence was 27·6 per cent and this compared with 7·7 per cent for the other 15 London clinics. The ratio of active : passive homosexuals was 1·2 : 1.

IMMIGRANTS

Willcox (1966) noted that the gonorrhoea rate in West Indians in London was 10 times that of U.K.-born males of the same age. The British Co-operative Clinical Group study (1967), referring to the year 1966 noted, as in the previous three years, a fall in the contribution of immigrants to the rising gonorrhoea rate. Oller and Wood (1970), from Bradford, England, reviewed the case notes of 5 000 males with gonorrhea seen in the decade 1959–68. In the first 7 years 80 per cent were immigrants. A decline in their numbers and proportion followed the arrival of wives and families.

STUDENTS

Morton (1966b) reviewed students as V.D. clinic patients year by year over a 5-year period. He showed that the growth of patients far outstripped the expansion in student population and that immigrant students were markedly affected. In the earlier years there was little requiring comment. In the fourth year of the study numbers doubled but infections per 1 000 students was stationary. In the fifth year of the study the number of patients again doubled and so did the infection rate. An attempt is made to explain these changes. Arya and Bennett (1967) writing from Makerere Medical School, Uganda, stated that they found 23 per cent of all attendances at the student health department to be on account of venereal disease. About one quarter of those at risk were infected annually. Of all faculties, medicine produced the fewest cases. Freshmen tended to have repeated attacks. Faye (1971) from Senegal showed that the progressive increase of gonorrhoea in that country was largely among the lower socio-economic groups. Migration and urbanisation especially, affected the attitudes and sex habits of students.

'REPEATERS'

This aspect has received scant attention. Glass (1967) brought evidence to support his view that upwards of 50 per cent of patients with gonorrhoea have more than one episode. He believes that education can reduce the 'repeater' caseload. Karolyi (1969) also considered the 'repeater'. He points to the need for thorough understanding of hetero-sexuals if the percentage of 'repeaters' is to be reduced.

MISCELLANEOUS

Singh et al (1966) saw the typical V.D. patient in India as a young bachelor of poor education, the product of an upbringing in a large family. Hartman and Nicolay (1966) commented on the deviant behaviour of the expectant father, a social phenomenon long recognised by venereologists, occasionally by wives but rarely by the expectant mother. Seale (1966) considered the wives of infected husbands. He found that their individual reactions and feelings of depression, guilt or shame were largely dependent on their knowledge of the facts. Mbanefo (1968) also discussed the emotional problems associated with gonococcal infection. Statham (1968) pointed out that 12 (3 per cent) of 336 con-secutive males with urethral gonorrhoea had had their urethral discharge for 2 to 10 weeks before attending for diagnosis and treatment. This was a worse state of affairs than that pertaining 5 and 10 years previously.

Rawlins (1969) in a study at St. Mary's Hospital, London, found that 50 per cent of 186 patients attending the V.D. department had taken drugs at some time. Cannabis, amphetamines, and sleeping pills were those used. All social strata were concerned. The sex distribution was 45 per cent of males interviewed and 63 per cent of females. Smith and Rose (1968) found a higher incidence of V.D. in drug addicts than in controls in San Francisco.

How the increasing prevalence of gonorrhoea has been accompanied
and paralleled by other manifestations of social pathology in England
and Wales is shown in Table III.

Table III. Incidence of certain social phenomena in England and
Wales (reproduced from Morton, R. S. (1973). *Brit. J. vener. Dis.*, **49**,
155)

Year	1963	1968	1969	1970
Indictable offences	978 076	1 289 090	1 488 638	1 555 995
Non-indictable offences	1 154 073	1 387 724	1 372 584	1 426 059
Juveniles found guilty	128 394	117 537	119 928	123 166
Violence against the person	12 832	18 338	20 855	23 443
Breaking and entering	47 249	51 897	—[a]	—[a]
Sexual offences	6 120	6 343	6 497	6 656
Consumption of spirits[c]	17·3	18·6	17·5	20·1
Drunkenness	79 598	75 225	77 007	78 748
Prostituion offences	1 982	2 452	2 318	2 347
Suicides	5 715	4 584	4 326	3 939
Attempted suicides	Estimated to be six to eight times suicide rate[b]			
Legitimate births	796 206	731 966	711 589	720 000
Illegitimate births	59 104	69 806	67 041	64 744
Legal abortions[e]		22 000[f]	54 000	83 000[g]
Divorces filed	36 385	54 036	60 134	70 575
Divorces decrees absolute	31 405	45 036	50 063	57 421
Vehicles with current licence (thousands)[d]	11 446	14 446	14 753	14 950
Total casualties in road accidents	356 179	349 208	353 194	363 348
Deaths in road accidents	9 622	6 810	7 383	7 501
Deaths from lung cancer	24 434	28 836	29 768	30 281
Cases of gonorrhoea	36 049	44 962	50 037[h]	53 617[h]

[a] Deleted with changes in legal terminology, [b] See Stengel (1964). [c] Million proof
gallons. [d] Great Britain. [e] Round figures only. [f] Eight months only. [g] 1971—126,000.
[h] England only. (Compiled mostly from the 'Annual Abstract of Statistics' (1971).
H.M.S.O., London.)

INDIVIDUAL PREDISPOSITION

This section started with the social pressures making for high and
rising infection rates. What about the predisposition of the individual?
Wells (1969, 1970), a clinical psychologist in Glasgow, defined the
personality characteristics of the venereally infected. The basis of his
work was 326 successive patients exposed to the Eysenck inventory of
psychoticism, extroversion and neuroticism. Wells found that infected
males tend to be significantly more extroverted than controls. Infected
females tend to be substantially more introverted and neurotic than
controls. Female scores deviate to such a degree as to resemble those

of in-patient psychotics on the psychoticism measure and to resemble those of clinical neurotics on the neuroticism dimension. Wells and Schofield (1972) applied the Eysenck personality inventory to 109 male homosexuals successively presenting at a V.D. clinic. As a group, homosexuals scored lower for extroversion than heterosexuals. Passive homosexuals were significantly more neurotic than the general male population. Thus like V.D. clinic patients generally, homosexuals have a tendency to emotional instability.

Coda

Regular review of the part played by social changes in altering how 'at risk' groups feature in any national situation requires to be continued. The migration of unattached males is now widely recognised as inseparably associated with a rise in V.D. morbidity. Governments who encourage this type of migration should prepare for the consequences. It is to be hoped that nowadays a more enlightened social policy, which encourages families to migrate rather than individuals, will prevail.

In spite of many countries being signatories to the 1959 U.N. Convention on Prostitution—which prohibits registration of women for this purpose—the practice still continues. It is to be hoped that in the countries concerned man's social awareness will soon prompt him to join those nations which are prepared to treat women as people.

It becomes increasingly clear that the social structure and function of any country determines its V.D. rate. So much is this so that a demographically minded epidemiologist should, with detailed study, be able to determine fairly accurately the gonorrhoea morbidity rate of any nation, without ever visiting the country concerned.

REFERENCES

ALLEN, E. S. (1970). *Brit. J. vener. Dis.*, **46**, 336.
ARYA, O. P. and BENNETT, F. J. (1967). *Brit. J. vener. Dis.*, **43**, 275.
BENT, W. I. (1965). *Canad. J. Publ. Hlth*, **56**, 137.
BLAINE, G. B. (1967). *N.Y. J. Med.*, **67**, 1967.
BRITISH CO-OPERATIVE CLINICAL GROUP (1967). *Brit. J. vener. Dis.*, **43**, 25.
BRITISH CO-OPERATIVE CLINICAL GROUP (1968). *Brit. J. vener. Dis.*, **44**, 55.
BRITISH CO-OPERATIVE CLINICAL GROUP (1973). *Brit. J. vener. Dis.*, **49**, 329.
BRITISH MEDICAL JOURNAL (1973). Editorial, **1**, 129.
CATTERALL, R. D. (1968). *Practitioner*, **195**, 620.
CATTERALL, R. D. (1965). *Nurs. Times*, **64**, 1041.
COMMITTEE ON PUBLIC HEALTH (1965). *Bull, N.Y. Acad. Med.*, **41**, 1104.
COHEN, L. (1970). *Brit. J. vener. Dis.*, **46**, 108.
DALRYMPALE, W. (1967). *J. Amer. Coll. Hlth Ass.*, **15**, 279.
DE AMORIN, P. J. (1966). *Hospital, Rio de Janeiro*, **70**, 1739.
DELUNE, H. (1971). *Brit. J. vener. Dis.*, **17**, 377.
EKSTROM, K. (1966). *Brit. J. vener. Dis.*, **42**, 162.
EKSTROM, K. (1970). *Brit. J. vener. Dis.*, **46**, 93.

FAYE, A. J. (1971). *Brit. J. vener. Dis.*, **47**, 378.
FLEMING, W. L. (1966). *Arch. Envir. Hlth*, **12**, 101.
FLUKER, J. L. (1966). *Brit. J. vener. Dis.*, **42**, 48.
FRICHOT, B. C. and EVERETT, M. A. (1967). *J. Oklahoma med. Ass.*, **60**, 597.
GALLAGHER, E. (1970). *Brit. J. vener. Dis.*, **46**, 129.
GEIZER, E. and KOPECKY, K. (1972). W.H.O. Document VDT/72, 379.
GLASS, L. H. (1967). *Brit. J. vener. Dis.*, **43**, 128.
GUTHE, T. and IDSØE, O. (1964). *Tidssk. Norske. Laegeforen.*, **84**, 1262.
GUTHE, T. (1966). *Bol. Soviet. Pan-am.*, **60**, 235.
GUTHE, T. and WILLCOX, R. R. (1971). *Roy. Soc. Hlth J*, **91**, 122.
GUTHE, T. (1971). *Bol. Soviet. Pan-am.*, **70**, 6.
GUTHE, T. and IDSØE, O. (1968). W.H.O. Document VDT/68, 234.
HARTMAN, A. A. and NICOLAY, R. C. (1966). *J. Abnorm. Soc. Psychol.*, **72**, 232.
HEWITT, A. B. (1970). *Brit. J. vener. Dis.*, **46**, 106.
HITCHENS, R. A. M. and JAMES, E. B. (1965). *Publ. Hlth*, **79**, 258.
IDSØE, O. and GUTHE, T. (1967). *Brit. J. vener. Dis.*, **42**, 31.
IDSØE, O. et al (1972). W.H.O. Document VDT/72, 378.
JOHNSON, D. W., HOLMES, K. K., KVALE, P. A., HALVERSON, R. W. and HIRSCH, W. P. (1969). *Amer. J. Epiderm.*, **90**, 438.
JUHLIN, L. (1968a). *Acta derm-venereol., Stockh.* **48**, 75.
JUHLIN, L. (1968b). *Acta derm.-venereol., Stockh.*, **48**, 82.
KAMPMEIER, R. H. (1971). *Amer. intern. Med.*, **75**, 793.
KAROLYI, I. (1969). W.H.O. Document VDT/69, 253.
KIBUKAMUSOKE, J. W. (1965). *Roy. Soc. Trop. Med. Hyg.*, **59**, 642.
KOKOSHKA, E. M., SOLTZ-SOLTZ, J. and THURNER, J. (1972). *Z. Haut. Geschl.-Kr.*, **47**, 243.
LOURIE, R. S. (1966). *Arch. Envir. Hlth*, **12**, 684.
LUGER, A. F. (1971). *Brit. J. vener. Dis.*, **47**, 378.
MAFFREEBA, H., MATTERN, P., BAYLET, R., GUEYE, C. and WONE, I. (1965). *Bull. Soc. Med. Afr. Hibiri Lang. Fr.*, **10**, 603.
MBANEFO, S. E. (1968). *J. Roy. Coll. Gen. Pract.*, **15**, 272.
MORTON, R. S. (1966a). *Med. Gynaec. Social.*, **1**, 2.
MORTON, R. S. (1966b). *Brit. J. vener. Dis.*, **42**, 280.
MORTON, R. S. (1971). 'Sexual Freedom and Venereal Disease'. Peter Owen, London.
MORTON, R. S. (1973). 'Venereal Diseases', 2nd ed. Penguin Books Ltd., London.
OLLER, L. Z. and WOOD, T. (1970). *Brit. J. vener. Dis.*, **46**, 96.
PEDDER, J. R. (1970). *Brit. J. vener. Dis.*, **46**, 54.
PEMBERTON, J. McCANN, J. S., MAHONEY, J. D. H., MacKENZIE, G., DOUGAN, H. and HAY, I. (1972). *Brit. J. vener. Dis.*, **48**, 391.
RAWLINS, D. C. (1969). *Brit. J. vener. Dis.*, **45**, 238.
SCHALLER, K. F. (1968). Quoting 'Problems of Medicine and Gynaecology in Ethiopia', by Heiber and Bold, Academic Press, London.
SCHOFIELD, M. (1964). *Brit. J. vener. Dis.*, **40**, 129.
SCHOFIELD, C. B. S. (1965a). *Brit. J. vener. Dis.*, **41**, 51.
SCHOFIELD, C. B. S. (1965b). *Acta derm.-venereol., Stockh.*, **44**, 445.
SCHOFIELD, C. B. S. (1969). W.H.O. Document VDT/69, 362.
SEALE, J. R. (1966). *Brit. J. vener. Dis.*, **42**, 31.
SHAPIRO, L. H. and LENTZ, J. W. (1965). *J. Einstein med. Cent.*, **13**, 3.
SIEFF, B. (1966). *Med. Proc.*, **12**, 224.
SINGH, K., MOHAMED, E. and SUKHIJA, C. L. (1966). *J. Indian med. Ass.*, **46**, 270.
SMITH, D. E. and ROSE, A. J. (1968). *Clin. Pediat.*, **7**, 313.
STATHAM, R. (1968). *J. Inst. Hlth Educ.*, **6**, 29.
STENGAL, E. (1964). 'Suicide and Attempted Suicide.' Pelican Books Ltd., London.
THOMPSON, B. and RUTHERFORD, H. W. (1972). *Brit. J. vener. Dis.*, **48**, 209.
VERHAGEN, A. R. and GEMMETT, W. (1972). *Brit. J. vener. Dis.*, **48**, 277.

WELLS, B. W. D. (1969). *Brit. J. Soc. Clin. Psychol.*, **8**, 246.
WELLS, B. W. D. (1970). *Brit. J. vener. Dis.*, **46**, 498.
WELLS, B. W. D. and SCHOFIELD, C. B. S. (1972). *Brit. J. vener. Dis.*, **48**, 75.
WHELDON, G. R. (1964). *J. Roy. Mar. Serv.*, **50**, 109.
WILLCOX, R. R. (1966). *Brit. J. vener. Dis.*, **42**, 225.
WILLCOX, R. R. (1969). *Abstr. Hyg.*, **44**, 945.
WILLCOX, R. R. (1970). *Abstr. Hyg.*, **45**, 993.
WREN, B. G. (1967). *Med. J. Aust.*, **1**, 847.
ZACKLER, J., BROLNITSKY, O. and ORBACH, H. (1970). *Publ. Hlth. Rep.*, *Wash.*, **84**, 681

3   Clinical Aspects

R. S. Morton

Introduction

The most outstanding feature of the clinical field in recent years has
been the increased incidence of complicated infection. It has been both
relative and real. Relative, because gonorrhoea is again so very common;
and real, because an increasing proportion of the infected are women,
so many of whom go undetected in their early asymptomatic phase.

Asymptomatic males.

The phenomenon of the male 'carrier' was recently emphasised by
Roberts speaking at the Second International V.D. Symposium (*Lancet*,
1972). He states that asymptomatic males have become more frequent
and now constitute between 5 and 10 per cent of all patients with
gonorrhoea.

Two other facets have also been receiving increasing attention;
proctitis in women and pharyngeal/tonsillar gonorrhoea.

Gonococcal proctitis in females

A series of publications in recent years has revealed the importance
of bacteriological examination of rectal material from female contacts
of men with gonorrhoea. Sparling et al (1965) were amongst the first,
during the present epidemic, to draw attention to the frequency of
rectal infection. They found gonococci in the rectum of 44 per cent of 44
women with gonorrhoea elsewhere. Olsen (1971) claimed that inclusion
of such specimens increased the yield of diagnosed contacts by 2–6 per
cent. Oödegaard (1971) showed that in a series of 221 females with
gonorrhoea, 118 (53 per cent) had positive rectal specimens. In six (2·7
per cent) rectal specimens only were positive. Schroeter and Reynolds
(1972) claimed that 65 per cent of 779 women with gonorrhoea had
rectal involvement and that failure to cure this complication—usually
the result of auto-inoculation—provides a reservoir of latent disease.
Their failure rate was 10·6 per cent. Nearly one-third of their therapeutic

failures would have been missed if only cervical specimens had been tested. Owen and Hill (1972) caution that rectal infection may have neither signs nor symptoms.

Battacharyya and Jephcott (1974) took specimens for Gram-staining and culture from the anal canal and from the rectal wall of 107 named female contacts of men with gonorrhoea. Seventy-one of them were found infected. Anal canal samplings revealed nothing not detected by urethral, endocervical or rectal specimens. Rectal cultures detected three times more infections than Gram-stained rectal smears. Four patients (5·6 per cent) were found positive in rectal specimens only. Of the 32 (43 per cent) with ano-rectal infection none had symptoms and only seven had signs of proctitis. The authors conclude that the time has come to view rectal examination and rectal samplings as an essential part of the investigation of all named female contacts.

Pharyngeal/tonsillar infection

Fiumara et al (1967) reported one confirmed and two probable cases of gonococcal pharyngitis. The writers suggested that the possibility of this type of primary site should always be entertained if contacts show no evidence of genito-urinary or rectal gonorrhoea. All three patients in this series were homosexuals and one had gonococcal urethritis. Iqbal (1971) reported a case of gonococcal tonsillitis in a heterosexual male. Smears but not cultures showed the organism. The consort had positive cervical cultures. Pharyngitis due to gonorrhoea and complicated by arthritis was described by Metzger (1970).

Bro-Jorgensen and Jensen (1971) carried out cultures for gonococci using tonsillar exudates from patients with genito-urinary gonorrhoea. Positive results were found in six (6 per cent) of 95 men and six (9 per cent) of 66 women. Ten of the 12 patients were without throat symptoms or signs. Oro-genital contact was admitted with the last sex partner by 80 per cent of males and 61 per cent of females. A control group of 186 men and 77 women all gave negative culture results with tonsillar exudates. Hallgren (1971) in a similar study found that 50 patients, 30 men and 20 women, out of 200 had had oro-genital contact with their last sex contact. One man and one woman in the series were found to have gonococcal tonsillitis. He had mild sore throat; she had neither symptoms nor signs. Rodin et al (1972) described three cases of gonococcal pharyngitis. All were homosexuals and one was asymptomatic. The authors recommend throat samplings from all infected homosexuals. Owen and Hill (1972) remark on the frequency of absence of signs and symptoms. Pharyngeal cultures were positive in 11 patients: only three had symptoms.

Weisner et al (1973) have confirmed much that has been written about this subject in a larger series. They isolated *N. gonorrhoeae* on selective

medium from the pharanx of 150 patients, 125 of them during a prospective study over a 9-month period. Of 2 224 patients who had
pharyngeal specimens cultured:

17·2 per cent had *N. meningitidis*
5·6 per cent had *N. gonorrhoeae*
1·9 per cent had *N. lactamicis*

Gonococcal pharyngitis was found in:

20·9 per cent of homosexual men
10·3 per cent of women
3·2 per cent of heterosexual men.

Positive pharyngeal cultures and presence of sore throat both correlated positively with the practice of fellatio.

In five patients gonococcal pharyngitis was the only apparent source
of disseminated infection.

COMPLICATED INFECTION
Salpingitis

Rees (1964) drew attention to the rising incidence of gonococcal
salpingitis. In Liverpool, it was 6·5 per cent of cases in 1960 and 11·6
per cent in 1962. That gonococcal salpingitis predisposes women to
ectopic pregnancy finds confirmation in Elizabeth Rees's paper. The
number of deaths from ectopic pregnancy in England and Wales during
the same years was 12 and 22. Similar reports from other parts of the
world followed. In South Africa, Riberio (1965) found 64 (11·6 per cent)
of 553 women with gonorrhoea to have salpingitis. Hedberg and Anberk
(1965) looked at this complication in Sweden with particular attention
to its aftermath. They performed air insufflation of 200 patients treated
for gonococcal salpingitis during the years 1956–62. They found both
Fallopian tubes patent in 105; one tube sealed in 57 and both tubes
sealed in 38 (19 per cent). The last figure is lower than many venereologists would have expected. It is perhaps of note in this respect that 70
of the women had prednisolone as well as penicillin therapy.

Dietrich et al (1965) found gonococci in the adenexal exudate in 11
cases of chronic salpingo-oophoritis. Lip and Burgoyne (1966) cultured
gonococci from material in the Pouch of Douglas in cases of acute
salpingitis. In some patients this method was positive when endocervical
cultures were negative. Statham and Morton (1968), while noting that
in general pelvic infection in women wearing an intra-uterine contraceptive device (I.U.C.D.) was rare, described three cases. All were
gonococcal. The detailed histories suggest that in cases of endocervical
gonorrhoea the I.U.C.D. becomes a dangerous foreign body, increasing
the severity of infection, speeding its spread and interfering with the

expected response to specific treatment. The authors recommend practice of the surgical principle that any foreign body found in uncomplicated or complicated gonorrhoea should be removed before antibacterial treatment commences.

Rees and Annels (1969) found salpingitis in 61 (10·6 per cent) of 606 consecutive cases of gonorrhoea. The pathology and symptomatology is described in detail and well illustrated. It is pointed out that hydrosalpinx is generally the result of recurrent, subacute attacks. The authors believe that the increasing incidence of salpingitis is partly due to increasing antibiotic resistance engendered by giving antibacterials for other infections in dosages which do not cure asymptomatic gonorrhoea. Particular mention is made of sulphonomides which are so commonly used in preference to antibiotics for urinary tract infections.

At the Second International V.D. Symposium, Weisner (*Lancet*, 1972) reported that in some hospitals in the U.S.A. 20 per cent of gynaecological inpatients had gonococcal salpingitis and between 16 and 20 per cent of them were sterilised by it.

Acosta et al (1971) give details of four pregnant patients with co-existent pelvic infection. Two miscarried. The need to consider gonorrhoea as a possibility in cases of acute abdomen in pregnancy is emphasised. Holmes (*Lancet*, 1972) reported that gonococci had been isolated from amniotic fluid and that amnionitis was believed to be responsible for intra-uterine infection, small babies and deaths.

Lassus and Kousa (1973) writing from Finland, described an 18 year old girl with gonococcal salpingitis, hepatitis and concomitant skin lesions.

Septicaemia

Gonococcal septicaemia has been variously described as gonococcaemia, gonococcal septicaemia and disseminated gonococcal infection. All authors are concerned to get away from the narrow, deceiving and unhelpful concept of 'gonococcal arthritis'.

Descriptions of single cases appeared in the early 1960s, for example, that of Bjornberg and Gisslen (1965). Niles and Lowe (1966) described one of the first large series. It consisted of 50 females with arthritis of whom 14 were pregnant. Taylor et al (1966) saw 103 cases of gonococcal arthritis over a period of 10 years. No less then 30 (28 per cent) were pregnant. The authors judged that pregnancy, like menstruation, was often a predisposing or precipitating factor in the onset of generalised spread of gonorrhoea. They judged from a review of 66 000 pregnancies that gonococcal arthritis occurred in 0·04 per cent.

Danielsson and Michaelson (1966) in Sweden, described another manifestation of gonococcal septicaemia. They called it the 'gonococcal dermatitis syndrome'. It manifested itself with intermittent fever, arthralgia and a haemorrhagic, vesiculo-papular rash. Skin lesions often have to be looked for as they are usually few in number and give little cause for complaint. Diagnosis in the three cases described was primarily by bacteriological examination of genito-urinary material. In two cases gonococci were found in the skin lesions. In five cases described by Vietzki (1966) two had E.C.G. changes consistent with pericarditis.

Portain and Cohen (1968) reported 26 cases of culture-proven gonococcal arthritis. They studied their patients in terms of age, sex, and the interval between infection and onset of arthritis, mode of presentation, pattern of joint involvement and synovial fluid analysis. The chief features of the series were:

1. In 21 cases the arthritis was suppurative, multiple joints were affected and response to penicillin was rapid.
2. In five cases the arthritis was non-suppurative, polyarticular and non-responsive to treatment. In two of these, Reiter's disease was a possibility.
3. The majority of patients were female and this is believed to be due to the asymptomatic nature of much uncomplicated gonorrhoea in women.

Contrary to the general view Keiser et al (1968) believed that gonococcal arthritis was less common and less crippling since the antibiotic era. They described 30 cases seen by them in the 4 years to 1967. Almost all were female and skin lesions were the clue to diagnosis in 15. Early cases had chills, fever and several joints affected. Later the arthritis tended to be mono-articular. Apart from culture-positive skin lesions, positive cultures were obtained from joints in nine cases, blood in six cases and genito-urinary tract in eight cases. Sharp et al (1968) discussed the differential diagnosis in 94 patients in whom gonococcal arthritis and Reiter's disease were the strongest possibilities. Although of a general nature, this paper offers many observations by a widely experienced group of rheumatologists. Altwan (1969) reported 31 cases of disseminated gonorrhoea and noted that the onset of complications correlated positively with the onset of menstruation. Useful observations are offered on the culture diagnosis from blood, joint fluid and genito-urinary material.

Cowan (1969) reported on a female patient with gonococcal arthritis, dermatitis and ulceration of the tongue. Cultures from all sites were positive. In reviewing the literature the author calls for revision of the classical concept that disseminated gonorrhoea is a disease of females. He believes this could be shown to be spurious if gonorrhoea was sought by culture in all young men presenting with polyarthritis. Metzger (1970) reported the first case of a male where culture proven gonococcal pharyngitis was associated with gonococcal septicaemia.

Svandom et al (1970) reported 15 females and one male with the triad of recurring fever, mild arthritis and skin lesions. All had gonorrhoea. The authors draw attention to the need to consider gonorrhoea in all cases of pyrexia of unknown origin in young people. Wolff et al (1970) add a further four cases and call the syndrome 'benign gonococcaemia'. They point out that it can only be differentiated from Reiter's disease and meningococcal or staphlococcal septicaemia by bacteriological methods. In their cases blood culture was positive in three, joint fluid culture in one and genito-urinary tract cultures in three.

A further report from Danielsson (1971) in Sweden stated that routine skin examination of all patients with gonorrhoea showed that 1·9 per cent had skin lesions, 3 per cent of females and 0·7 per cent of males. In 23 patients with gonococcal dermatitis the presenting symptom was arthritis, arthralgia or bouts of fever. Skin lesions gave the clue to the diagnosis. The types of scar left by the lesions are illustrated. Barr and Danielsson (1971) described gonococcal skin lesions in detail. They are usually few in number and violaceous maculo-papular, versiculo-papular or haemorrhagic. Kushner (1970) stated that in septicaemic cases more than 70 per cent had several joints affected; tenosynovitis and skin lesions were encountered in 50 per cent and chills and fevers were common. As in most other series some 90 per cent of those affected were females.

By 1971 such reports are a commonplace, e.g. *British Medical Journal* editorial (1971), *Californian Medical Journal*, editorial (1971), Jacobsen and Tidsjröm (1971), Wheeler et al (1970) and Bjornberg (1970). Perhaps the most remarkable series was published by Holmes et al (1971) under the heading 'Disseminated gonococcal infection'. The cases included two with meningitis, two with endocarditis and a fatal case of pericarditis. Women comprised 79 per cent of the cases and dissemination occurred in many of them during pregnancy or menstruation. The authors describe a 'bacteraemic stage' characterised by poly-arthalgias, skin lesions and positive blood culture, followed by a 'septic stage' with positive joint fluid culture and joint destruction. Under the heading 'Gonococcal arthritis—a common rarity', Harris et al (1973) from Northern Ireland describe five cases. The authors point out the relative absence of reports in the literature of the U.K. as compared with North America and Europe and call for a greater index of suspicion and improved communication between venereologists and specialists in other fields.

Ophthalmia neonatorum

Gransström et al (1965) reported the return of neo-natal gonococcal conjunctivitis to the clinical scene after a relative absence of 16 years. They saw eight cases between 1960 and 1964, ie 0·06 per cent of all newborn babies. The infections occurred despite the use of Crede's method. All the mothers had gonorrhoea. Kober (1967) reported from Kiel that 17 cases had occurred there in recent years in spite of the regular use of 10 per cent silver nitrate solution used as for Crede's method. The author calls for stricter observance of preventive methods as gonorrhoea becomes increasingly common. He believes that all cases of inflamed eyes in infants are a clear indication for pre-treatment bacteriological investigation.

Schofield and Shanks (1971) from a review of 48 cases of gonococcal ophthalmia neonatorum note that 36 had their first symptom at 4 days of age. One of the lessons to be learned from this study is that a 'sticky eye' which calls for antibiotic treatment automatically calls for thorough bacteriological testing. Morton (1971) in a review of the V.D. problem in Singapore found that in a 5-year period, up to and including 1969, one baby in every 500 born in the republic developed gonococcal ophthalmia. This was an average of 100 cases per annum. Mother and baby were both immediately admitted to hospital for bacteriological examination and treatment.

In parts of the world where gonorrhoea morbidity rates are high Waters and Roulston (1969) believe there is need to screen ante-natal patients. They found gonorrhoea in 207 (6·1 per cent) of 3 375 in a $3\frac{1}{2}$-year period.

Other complications

Rees (1967) found gonococci in Bartholin ducts of 52 women or 28·4 per cent of 182 named contacts. In two women no other site gave positive cultures.

Bartholin 'abscess' and its treatment received attention from Mayer (1970) and Goldberg (1970).

Elebute (1966) found 69 men with post-gonococcal urethral stricture. One in three of them had a blood pressure reading in excess of 140/90 mmHg. A matching control sample of 100 showed only 15 per cent similarly affected. Of those with stricture 90 per cent had a history of genito-urinary infection other than gonorrhoea. It was judged that this had led to pyelonephritis, kidney damage and so to hypertension.

Beilby et al (1968) isolated the genital herpes virus from eight (3·8 per cent) of 209 consecutive patients attending a London V.D. clinic. Fifty-five patients had endo-cervical gonorrhoea and seven of the eight cases of herpes occurred in these. The authors suggest that genital herpes may be reactivated by gonorrhoea. The association is certainly statistically significant.

Gonorrhoeal infection of a congenital duct of the median raphé of the penis was described by Dlabalova et al (1969) and acute penile ulceration associated with regional adenitis and culture of gonococci was reported by Haim and Merzbach (1970).

Amongst others, Kimball and Knee (1970) reported a case of gonococcal perihepatitis (Fitzheigh–Curtis syndrome). The patient had been ineffectively treated for gonorrhoea 3 weeks prior to presenting with symtoms of cholecystitis. The liver was enlarged with a sausage-shaped swelling at its lower edge. Cultures of biopsy material revealed gonococci. This is claimed to be the first report of a case of the syndrome in a male. Francis and Osoba (1972) describe a further case in a man.

Voigt et al (1970) reported the successful replacement of an aortic valve on the seventh day of treatment for gonococcal endocarditis. Their surgical approach was justified as a means of avoiding left ventricular failure.

Taubin and Landsberg (1971) reported the twenty-ninth case of gonococcal meningitis. The patient also had arthralgia and skin lesions. The infection was at least of 6 months' duration. Sayed et al (1972) described three cases of gonococcal meningitis. Culture, biochemical and fluorescent methods of diagnosis were used. One patient had arthritis and pericarditis. Satisfactory genital specimens were not obtained.

Burgess (1971) detailed a case of gonococcal tynosynovitis without urethritis. Kushner (1970) stated that this complication was common in those with disseminated disease.

Fiumara (1972) in the U.S.A. described the transmission of gonorrhoea during artificial insemination with donor semen. Another case was reported from Holland by Bakker (1972).

GONORRHOEA IN CHILDREN

Sersiron (1965) judged that only 5 per cent of cases of vulvo-vaginitis were due to the gonococcus.

Fink (1965) described five female children aged 2–13 years with gonococcal arthritis. All came from an area with a high gonorrhoea prevalence rate amongst adults. The disease was poly-articular, migrating early, but later becoming mono-articular. As in the adult, the organism was most readily found in the genito-urinary system but two of the four joints tested gave positive culture results. There was indirect evidence of familial contact in the three youngest girls.

Sersiron and Roiron (1967) reported on the examination of 872 children with leucorrhoea. Twenty-one (2·4 per cent) had gonorrhoea. It was always acute with purulent discharge and commonest in the 2–5 year olds. The authors warn against inadequate diagnosis. They found another 1·5 per cent with Neisseriae other than biochemically proven gonococci. Nazarian (1967) saw nine children under 15 years of age with gonorrhoea: two aged 2–4 years, had vulvo-vaginitis: one aged 1 month had ophthalmia, while her brother had urethritis; five, aged 9–14 years, had venereally acquired disease. The writer concludes that the dividing line between socially contacted and sexually contacted infection is around 9 or 10 years of age. Mausner and Gezon (1967) described a phantom epidemic of gonorrhoea. It occurred in a school of 174 girls. Fifty were alleged, on the evidence of Gram-stained smears alone, to have gonococcal vulvo-vaginitis. The absence of confirmatory culture methods as well as poor communication led to spread of rumours and closure of the school.

Shore and Winkelstein (1971) drew attention to the high incidence of gonorrhoea in children in parts of the world where morbidity rates in adults are high and rising. Their report comes from Alaska where the morbidity of gonorrhoea is 2 182 per 100 000 population per annum. Fourteen children, aged 1–12 years, were seen with gonorrhoea in a single year. Of six boys, three had conjunctivitis and three urethritis. Of eight girls with vulvo-vaginitis one also had conjunctivitis. Seven of the children had been sleeping with infected parents. Three of the girls had been raped. The authors consider that gonorrhoea in children should be viewed as a by-product of poor environmental conditions.

Burry and Thorn (1971) studied 15 boys and 38 girls with gonorrhoea. They were seen in the years 1963–70. Five boys and 31 girls were aged less than 10 years. A history of sexual exposure was obtained from three girls and suspected in three others. None of the boys gave a history of sexual exposure.

Burry (1971) reported four cases of peritonitis complicating gonococcal vulvo-vaginitis. He claimed that this represented 10 per cent of all such cases seen between 1963 and 1970. Doyle (1972) reported two children, aged 2 and 3 years, with gonococcal conjunctivitis. He believed both were infected by wet towels used communally by their infected parents. Gregory et al (1972) described a culture proven case of gonococcal arthritis in an infant, and Swierczewski et al (1970) a fulminating case of gonococcal meningitis with Waterhouse–Friedrichsen syndrome in a 3 month old baby. Gonococci were cultured from the external ear of a baby whose mother's lochia also gave positive culture results.

DIAGNOSTIC PROBLEMS

Pariser et al (1964) discussed the asymptomatic male carrier of gonorrhoea. Anderson (1966) examined the blood of 34 patients attending a V.D. clinic. He found evidence of previous therapy with penicillin or sulpha drugs in three women and nine men. One man admitted taking tablets left over from a previous visit to the department and one man and two women admitted taking tablets prescribed for their spouse.

Molin and Danielsson (1970) examined accessory gland material from males treated for gonorrhoea. In 40 per cent of them immunofluorescence revealed gonococci for up to 2–3 weeks after treatment. This observation led them to examine seven asymptomatic named male contacts prospectively. All had had urethritis 1–2 years earlier. Six men gave positive immunofluorescent findings, although in all but one routine tests made by smear and culture from a variety of sites were negative. The sole positive findings were smear and culture specimens from the prostate in one man. The authors suggest that the antibacterial properties of prostatic secretions reduce the virulence of gonococci and that the organisms become infective again when their environment changes.

Increasing awareness of just how common gonorrhoea has become in the U.S.A. is reflected in a paper by Cave et al (1969). They investigated 875 patients from an urban community and found positive culture results in 72 (8·2 per cent). A further eight had positive smear results only. Endometrial curettage by Novak's method and search for gonococci did not increase the yield of positive findings.

Bhattacharyya et al (1973) have shown how one named contact in three would fail to be diagnosed if only high vaginal smears and culture tests are done—a recommendation commonly found in British textbooks of gynaecology.

Coda

Several clinical problems seem worthy of study, for example, how often is 'cystitis' really gonorrhoea? What about treated or partially treated gonorrhoea? Can immunofluorescence diagnose it with sufficient accuracy to allow of confident contact tracing? What of the varying names—pharyngitis and tonsillitis—for throat gonorrhoea; from where should specimens be taken?

REFERENCES

ACOSTA, A. A. et al (1971). *Obstet. Gynaecol., N.Y.*, **37**, 282.
ALTWAN, R. D. (1969). *J. Florida med. Ass.*, **56**, 318.
ANDERSON, K. (1966). *Brit. J. vener. Dis.*, **42**, 44.
BAKKER, P. (1972). Personal communication.
BARR, J. and DANIELSSON, D. (1971). *Brit. med. J.*, **1**, 482.
BEILBY, C. H. *et al.* (1968). *Lancet*, **1**, 1065.
BHATTACHARYYA, M. N., JEPHCOTT, A. E. & MORTON, R. S. (1973). *Brit. med. J.*, **2**, 748.
BHATTACHARYYA, M. N. and JEPHCOTT, A. E. (1974). *Brit. J. Vener. Dis.* (50, 109. press).
BJORNBERG, A. (1970). *Acta derm.-venereol, Stockh.*, **50**, 313.
BJORNBERG, A. and GISSLEN, H. (1965). *Brit. J. vener. Dis.*, **42**, 100.
BRITISH MEDICAL JOURNAL (1971). Editorial. **1**, 472.
BRO-JORGENSEN, A. and JENSEN, T. (1971). *Brit. J. vener. Dis.*, **47**, 100.
BURGESS, J. A. (1971). *Brit. J. vener. Dis.*, **47**, 40.
BURRY, V. F. (1971). *Amer. J. Dis. Child.*, **121**, 536.
BURRY, V F. and THORN, P. M. (1971). *Missouri med. J.*, **68**, 691.

CALIFORNIA MEDICAL JOURNAL (1971). Editorial, **114**, 18.
CAVE, V. G., BLOOMFIELD, R. D., HURDLE, E. S., GORDON, E. W. and HAMMOCK, D. Jr. (1969). *J. Amer. med. Ass.*, **210**, 309.
COWAN, L. (1969). *Brit. J. vener. Dis.*, **45**, 228.
DANIELSSON, D. and MICHAELSON, G. (1966). *Acta derm.-venereol., Stockh.*, **46**, 257.
DANIELSSON, D. (1971). *Brit. med. J.*, **1**, 482.
DLABALOVA, H., KRAUS, Z. and DIABL, K. (1969). *Acta derm.-venereol., Stockh.*, **40**, 202.
DIETRICH, H., LODENKÄMPER, H. and NICKEL, H. (1965). *Geburtsh, Frauen-heilk.*, **25**, 822.
DOYLE, J. O. (1972). *Brit. med. J.*, **1**, 88.
ELEBUTE, A. E. (1966). *Trans. Roy. Soc. Trop.-med. Hyg.*, **60**, 676.
FINK, C. W. (1965). *J. Amer. med. Ass.*, **194**, 237.
FIUMARA, N. J., WISE, H. M. Jr. and MANY, M. (1967). *New Engl. J. Med.*, **276**, 1248.
FIUMARA, N. J. (1972). *Brit. J. vener. Dis.*, **48**, 308.
FRANCIS, T. L. and OSOBA, A. O. (1972). *Brit. J. vener. Dis.*, **48**, 187.
GOLDBERG, J. E. (1970). *Obstet. Gynec., N.Y.*, **35**, 109.
GRANSSTRÖM, K. O. et al (1965). *Opusuc. med.*, **10**, 8.
GREGORY, J. E., CHISOM, J. L. and MEADOWS, A. T. (1972). *Brit. J. vener. Dis.*, **48**, 306.
HAIM, S. and MERZBACH, D. (1970). *Brit. J. vener. Dis.*, **46**, 336.
HALLGREN, L. (1971). *Svenska. Läk-Tiden.*, **68**, 569.
HARRIS, J. R. W., McCANN, J. S. and MAHONEY, J. D. H. (1973). *Brit. J. vener. Dis.*, **49**, 42.
HEDBERG, E. and ANBERK, A. (1965). *Fertil. Steril.*, **16**, 125.
HOLMES, K. K., COUNTS, G. W. and BEATY, H. N. (1971). *Ann. intern. Med.*, **74**, 979.
IQBAL, Y. (1971). *Brit. J. vener. Dis.*, **47**, 144.
JACOBSEN, M. and TIDSJRÖM, B. (1971). *Ugeskr. Laeg.*, **133**, 6.
KEISER, H., RUBEN, F. L., WOLINSKY, E. and KUSHNER, I. (1968). *New Engl. J. Med.*, **279**, 234.
KIMBALL, M. W. and KNEE, S. (1970). *New. Engl. J. Med.*, **282**, 1082.
KOBER, P. (1967). *Med. Klin.*, **62**, 424.
KUSHNER, I. (1970). *Med. Times, Manhasset.*, **98**, 111.
LANCET (1972). Editorial, **1**, 1109.
LASSUS, A. and KOUSA, M. (1973). *Brit. J. vener. Dis.*, **49**, 48.
LIP, J. and BURGOYNE, Y. (1966). *Obstet. Gynec., N.Y.*, **28**, 561.
MAUSNER, J. S. and GEZON, H. M. (1967). *Amer. J. Epiderm.*, **85**, 320.
MAYER, H. G. (1970). *Med. Klin.*, **65**, 200.
METZGER, A. L. (1970). *Ann. intern. Med.*, **73**, 267.
MOLIN, L. and DANIELSSON, D. (1970). *Brit. med. J.*, **1** 257.
MORTON, R. S. (1971). *Brit. J. vener. Dis.*, **47**, 48.
NAZARIAN, J. F. (1967). *Paediatrics*, **39**, 372.
NILES, J. H. and LOWE, F. W. (1966). *Med. Ann.*, **35**, 69.
ÖDEGAARD, K. (1971). *Tidsskr. Laegeforen.*, **91**, 1474.
OLSEN, G. A. (1971). *Brit. J. vener. Dis.*, **47**, 102.
OWEN, R. L. and HILL, L. J. (1972). *J. Amer. med. Ass.*, **220**, 1315.
PARISER, H., FARMER, A. D. and MARINO, A. F. (1964). *Sth. Med. J.*, **57**, 688.
PORTAIN, E. S. C. and COHEN, A. S. (1968). *Ann. rheum. Dis.*, **27**, 156.
REES, E. (1964). *Bull. Inst. Tech. Venereol.*, **6**, 87.
REES, E. (1967). *Brit. J. vener. Dis.*, **43**, 150.
REES, E. and ANNELS, E. H. (1969). *Brit. J. vener. Dis.*, **45**, 205.
RIBERIO, F. D. (1965). *S. Afr. J. Obstet. Gynaec.*, **3**, 16.
RODIN, P., MONTEIRO, G. E. and SCRIMGEOUR, G. (1972). *Brit. J. vener. Dis.*, **48**, 182.
SAYED, Z. A., BHADURI, U., HOWELL, E. and MYERS, H. L. (1972). *J. Amer. med. Ass.*, **219**, 1703.
SCHOFIELD, C. B. S. and SHANKS, R. A. (1971). *Brit. med. J.*, **1**, 257.

SCHROETER, A. I. and REYNOLDS, G. (1972). *J. infect. Dis.*, **125**, 499.
SERSIRON, D. (1965). *Med. Infart.*, **72**, 229.
SERSIRON, D. and ROIRON, V. (1967). *Brit. J. vener. Dis.*, **43**, 33.
SHARP, J. T., LIDSKY, M. D. and RILEY, W. A. (1968). *Arthritis Rheum.*, **11**, 569.
SHORE, W. B. and WINKELSTEIN, J. A. (1971). *J. Pediat.*, **79**, 661.
SPARLING, P. F., BILLINGS, T. E. and HACKNEY, J. F. (1965). *Antimicrob. Agents Chemother.*, **5**, 689.
STATHAM, R. and MORTON, R. S. (1968). *Brit. med. J.*, **4**, 623.
SVANDOM, M., BENGTSSON, E., STRANDELL, T. and TUNEVALL, G. (1970). *Scand. J. infect. Dis.*, **2**, 191.
SWIERCZEWSKI, J. A. et al (1970). *Ann. J. clin Path.*, **54**, 202.
TAUBIN, H. L. and LANDSBERG, L. (1971). *New Engl. med. J.*, **285**, 504.
TAYLOR, H. A., BRADFORD, S. A. and PATTERSON, S. P. (1966). *Obstet Gynec. N.Y.*, **27**, 776.
VIETZKE, W. M. (1966). *Arch. intern. Med.*, **117**, 270.
VOIGT, G. C., BENDER, H. W., BUCKELS, L. J., DE MEESTER, R. and MACDONALD, W. (1970). *Johns Hopkins med. J.*, **126**, 305.
WATERS, J. R. and ROULSTON, J. M. (1969). *Amer. J. Obstet. Gynec.*, **103**, 532.
WEISNER, P. J., TRONCA, E., BONIN, P., PEDERSEN, A. H. B. and HOLMES, K. K. (1973). *New Engl. J. Med.*, **288**, 181.
WHEELER, J. K., HEFERON, W. A. and WILLIAMS, R. C. Jr. (1970). *Ann. J. med. Sci.*, **260**, 150.
WOLFF, C. B., GOODMAN, H. V. and VAHRMAN, J. (1970). *Brit. med. J.*, **2**, 271.

4 Recent Advances in Routine Laboratory Procedures

A. E. Jephcott

Introduction

The previous edition of this review was written at the end of an era of gradual refinement and consolidation of long-established methods. Such fundamental innovations as had been published at that time were not yet sufficiently developed for routine application.

Rapid presumptive diagnoses were made by inspection of smears stained by Gram's method, and were confirmed by cultural diagnoses made from plates inoculated either directly in the clinic, or after the specimen had been held in Stuart's transport medium (Stuart, 1946). Highly nutrient media, such as McLeod's heated blood agar (McLeod et al, 1934) were popular and other enriched media such as Møller and Reyn's H.Y.L. (Møller and Reyn, 1965) represented improvements on the same theme.

Confirmatory identification, which was by means of Gram stain, oxidase reaction, and production of acid from glucose, but not from maltose or sucrose, frequently took 1 week to achieve. Overgrowth of a proportion of cultures with yeasts and bacteria must have resulted in many diagnostic failures.

Sensitivity testing was not common and a variety of methods were in vogue. The W.H.O. Expert Committee on Antibitiotics in its Second Report (1961) had commented on the desirability of a standard test.

Serological investigation of the patient was limited to the Gonococcal Complement Fixation Test (G.C.F.T.) (Price, 1930). This test was regarded as a 'mere shadow of its former self' (Price, 1949) and was of real value only in the complicated case (Ramanarayana et al, 1961). It was not capable of detecting all infections (Magnusson and Kjellander, 1965) and could give positive reactions in cases of meningococcal infection and in many chronic bronchitics and bronchiectatics (Reyn, 1969; Lange et al, 1965).

FLUORESCENT ANTIBODY TESTING

Deacon's original description of a method for demonstrating gono-cocci by a fluorescent antibody technique was made in 1959 (Deacon et al, 1959) and was mentioned in the previous edition of this review as a promising method requiring evaluation and development. Its feasibility for routine use has now been demonstrated. The test hinges on the principle that antibody to gonococci, when coupled (or con-jugated) with fluorescein isothiocyanate produces a highly specific stain for gonococci. If stained with this, gonococci can be visualised as fluorescent rings when using a suitable microscope. Spurious fluores-cence of unwanted elements in the field has proved the major difficulty in practice. This has now been reduced to acceptable levels.

Selection of appropriate filters and counterstaining with naphthalene black (Sommerville, 1968) have overcome autofluorescence. Lind (1964) found that non-specific staining of cells could be prevented by carefully controlled conjugation procedure. Others, to the same end, have ab-sorbed the conjugate with tissue powders (Coons and Kaplan, 1950) and have used a variety of counterstains including lissamine rhodamine label-led albumin (Smith et al, 1969), Evans blue (Fry and Wilkinson, 1963), and flazo orange (Hall and Hansen, 1962; Hokenson and Hansen, 1966).

Staphylococci absorb serum globulins in a non-specific manner (Lind, 1968), which leads to their becoming spuriously stained. This artefact can be avoided by pretreating the smear with normal rabbit serum (Bergman et al, 1966), or by a one-step inhibition technique using conjugate mixed with unlabelled rabbit anti-staphylococcal antiserum (Lind, 1964), or with human serum (Thin, 1970). Danielsson employs a rhodamine conjugated anti-staphylococcal serum with good effect (Danielsson, 1965a).

Antigenic cross-reactions with other Neisseriae can be removed by absorption with meningococci (Deacon et al, 1959). Lind (1967), however, observed simultaneous abolition of staining of some gonococcal strains and she considers such absorbed conjugates unsuitable for routine diagnostic procedures.

The fluorescent antibody technique can be used, as it was originally described, as a 'Direct' or 'Undelayed' test on smears made from materials taken directly from the patient (Deacon et al, 1959). This method offers the possibility of a very rapid and specific diagnosis. In practice, Thin (1970) and other workers (Fry and Wilkinson, 1964; Danielsson, 1965b) reported favourably on the method but Lind (1967) found it no more reliable than the Gram film and pointed out some of its theoretical disadvantages. Danielsson and Molin (1971) have shown that the technique can prove useful in demonstrating gonococci which have been killed by previous antibiotic therapy and it has been used to demonstrate gonococci in skin lesions (Kahn and Danielsson, 1969).

The technique is most advantageously used as an 'Indirect' or 'Delayed' test (Deacon et al, 1960). With this method, 18- or 30-hour plate-cultures are spread on to slides, stained and examined. This gives a more rapid answer than the usual biochemical identification and in many hands has proved as sensitive. Furthermore, it is less susceptible to contaminant interference and seems particularly useful in the diagnosis of rectal cultures (Danielsson, 1965b; Lind, 1967).

CULTURE MEDIA

Conventional culture has been revolutionised by the introduction of effective selective media. These suppress the non-specific flora which tend to occur at sites of infection. If allowed to grow freely—as happens on conventional media—this flora can overgrow any gonococci present and can prevent their recognition. Use of selective media has led to an improvement in isolation rates from the urethral and cervical sites, and has had a dramatic effect on isolations from heavily contaminated sites such as the rectum and pharynx (Wilkinson, 1965; Reyn and Bentzon, 1972; Roepstorff and Hammarström, 1966). Examination of the rectum has now become a much more worthwhile procedure (Bhattacharyya and Jephcott, 1974); Olsen (1971) demonstrated that even vaginal cultures can now be of value if cervical specimens cannot be taken.

There have been many attempts to devise a selective medium for gonococci. Early media using crystal violet, nile blue, thallium acetate and boric acid were not satisfactory (Wilkinson, 1965). The first successful medium was described by Thayer and Martin (1964). This contained polymixin B which had previously been advocated by Crookes and Stuart (1959) and by Reyn et al (1960), with ristocetin which had been recommended in another neisserial selective medium by Berger (1961). When the supply of ristocetin became difficult, the medium was reformulated to contain vancomycin, colistin and nystatin (Thayer and Martin, 1966). This medium proved as successful as its predecessor. Unfortunately both media inhibit a small percentage of gonococcal strains (Wilkinson, 1965; Reyn and Bentzon, 1972) which has led Reyn to recommend the use of a combination of a selective and a non-selective medium for each specimen (Reyn, 1969) and to reduce the concentration of vancomycin in her plates.

Riddell and Buck (1970) and Seth (1970) improved the performance of this medium still further by the addition of trimethoprim. This prevents overgrowth and swarming of *Proteus* species contaminants—a problem experienced particularly in rectal culture examinations, and one which has been responsible for diagnostic failures with the unmodified Thayer–Martin medium (Reyn and Bentzon, 1972).

The combined use of selective media with the delayed fluorescent antibody technique has proved particularly successful, especially in coping with samplings from highly contaminated sites. Lind (1969) in particular has reported favourably on this technique.

New non-selective media have also been reported. Thus Ellner et al (1966) described a new base, which is available commercially as Columbia Blood Agar Base. Also available is Iso Vitalex (Martin et al, 1967)—a chemically defined supplement containing vitamin B_{12}, L-glutamine, adenine, guanine, p-aminobenzoic acid, L-cystine, glucose, diphospho-pyridine nucleotide, co-carboxylase, ferric nitrate, thiamine hydro-chloride and cysteine hydrochloride. Both are in widespread use at present.

The commercial availability of reliable incubators providing atmos-pheres of predetermined carbon dioxide concentration and humidity has also facilitated cultural practice, and the description of a simpler model has been published (Scruton, 1971). Such aids make for greater con-venience and speed in diagnostic work.

Cultural methods for the isolation of L forms of gonococci have been described. Holmes and co-workers (1971) have reported an isola-tion from synovial fluid and Gnarpe et al (1972) have detected them in the genital area. Infections with L forms are not diagnosable by con-ventional culture techniques, and this ability to recognise L forms represents a very real advance.

BIOCHEMICAL TEST MEDIA

Confirmation of identity of Neisseria is usually carried out by acidification of sugar-containing media. In the past, serum-containing basal media have been favoured in Britain (Cruickshank, 1965). Difficulties, including the presence of maltase in the sera of certain species of animal, have stimulated the description and use of serum-free media with incorporated sugars (Flynn and Waitkins, 1972), and have led to a test where a paper disc, impregnated with indicator and sugar, is laid on the surface of a culture plate (Stacey and Warner, 1973). In other parts of the world different sugar-containing media find favour. Cystine trypticase agar (Vera, 1948) is relied on by many and Reyn (1965) described a medium based on placental extract, a more complex version of which was introduced by Juhlin (1963). White and Kellogg (1965) described a medium containing their defined supplement and Kellogg and Turner (1973) have developed a very rapid test system using aqueous sugar solutions.

These methods, with the exception of the last, are all relatively slow and delay the result by 1 or 2 days. Further, some strains of gonococci fail to acidify glucose when grown on particular bases (Reyn, 1965), and all tests are subject to artefacts due to contaminated cultures.

These difficulties can all be avoided by use of fluorescent antibody identification techniques, provided the sera used are specific enough to be relied upon for this purpose.

TRANSPORT MEDIA

The survival of gonococci whilst the specimen is in transit to the laboratory has also received attention. Stuart's excellent carrier medium has been modified by Amies (1967). He reduced the sodium chloride ionic concentration to one more suited to the gonococcus, and substituted a non-metabolisable phosphate buffer for the glycerophosphate system which allows overgrowth of some bacteria during transit. He also added charcoal to the medium instead of applying it to the swab.

Martin and Lester (1971) made a more fundamental change of attack with their description of Transgrow Medium. This consists of a 'chocolate' agar medium inside a bottle. It is inoculated immediately the specimen is taken from the patient, and may be sent to the laboratory for examination, either before or after incubation. This was the principle behind the outdated McLeod–Reyman medium (Reyman, 1944), on which gonococci would survive adequately, but which failed because it allowed other bacteria to overgrow them. This problem has been overcome in the Transgrow system by the use of a modified Thayer–Martin medium—more recently with trimethoprim—and, as a refinement, an atmosphere of carbon dioxide is included in the bottle.

This system has been evaluated by Toshach et al (1972) who found it gave no better isolation rates than Stuart's medium, even when the original formulation had been modified to include trimethoprim. However they commented on Transgrow's advantages of speed, ease of reading and elimination of subculture procedures. It can easily be arranged that incubation is begun immediately after inoculation, so that growth has occurred by the time of arrival at the examining laboratory. A considerable saving in time taken to establish diagnosis is thus effected. Furthermore, the highly selective nature of the medium allows identification of *N. gonorrhoeae*, based on Gram stain and oxidase reaction only, to be made much more reliably than when the same diagnostic criteria are used in conjunction with non-selective media.

ANTIBIOTIC SENSITIVITY TESTING

Antibiotic sensitivity testing methods have also been scrutinised. Reyn et al (1965) demonstrated that differences in method of testing and of medium employed, could both produce variations in the result of a sensitivity test. Further, they showed that any disparity became wider with increasing antibiotic resistance of the strain involved. They suggest that these difficulties could be overcome by use of international reference values for standard reference strains. Local results could then be 'corrected' by comparison of concurrently obtained results for the reference strains with their international reference values. This would allow for meaningful comparison of results from different laboratories and a more certain picture of the resistance pattern throughout the world would emerge. It is to be hoped that greater use will be made of this facility in the future.*

ROUTINE SEROLOGICAL TESTS FOR GONORRHOEA

A serological test for gonorrhoea which is more sensitive and more reliable than the G.C.F.T. as currently performed is still being sought. The advantages of a simple, socially acceptable test for establishing a diagnosis, instead of the slow, repeated, cumbersome and embarrassing genital site cultural procedure, are obvious. However, serological testing does have certain drawbacks which may limit its usefulness. There is an initial period during the course of the infection before antibodies appear in the blood and, unless levels fall rapidly after cure, previous infections will confuse the diagnostic picture. Furthermore, cross-reacting antibodies produced to other but related bacteria are common and tend to reduce the specificity of the test. Nevertheless even with these limitations, a test could find a place, particularly in the diagnosis of the chronic case and the asymptomatic carrier, and in population screening surveys—all situations where, for different reasons, cultural methods present problems. A certain proportion of false positive reactions (as in the Wasserman reaction) would not necessarily nullify the value of a test.

Several tests have been devised and tried. Some offer the advantages of the simplicity and speed of a slide test, some lend themselves to automation, and some, by careful selection or purification of the antigen or by identification of the class of antibody involved in the reaction, are designed to improve specificity without loss of sensitivity. All require further development and assessment before they can be taken into routine use. The situation appears promising and has prompted Willcox (1971) to conclude that a useful serological test for gonorrhoea is almost within sight and should become a reality within the next few years.

Chacko and Nair (1969) described a precipitin test using a lipopolysaccharide antigen extracted from the allantoic fluid of infected chick embryos. They claimed high specificity with good sensitivity. Detectable antibody response appeared early. Sixty per cent of culture-proven cases with urethral discharge of up to 3 days' duration were reactive, and the figure increased to 100 per cent by the time the discharge had been present for a week. This test was developed from the microprecipitin test of Reising and Kellogg (1965), which employed endotoxin

* Lyophilised reference strains (3) can be obtained from Dr. Alice Reyn, Neisseria Dept., State Serum Institute, Amager Boulevard, Copenhagen, Denmark.

antigen made from a phenol/water extract of type 1 colonies of gonococcus strain F62. Again 62 per cent of proven gonorrhoea cases reacted. Control personnel were uniformly unreactive.

Maeland (1968, 1969) investigated the serological reactions of aqueous ether extracts of gonococcal endotoxin and identified both carbohydrate and protein antigenic determinants. Using indirect haemagglutination and antiglobulin techniques Maeland and Larsen (1971) showed that sera from normal persons as well as from infected patients contained antibodies of IgM class whereas IgG antibodies were limited to the sera of infected patients.

Ward and Glynn (1972) used lipopolysaccharide haemagglutination tests with unfractionated serum. With several antigens, each extracted from a different strain of gonococcus, they were able to detect up to 84 per cent of females and 46 per cent of males in an infected group, with only 2 per cent positives among their controls. Logan et al (1970) using a composite antigen adsorbed on to tanned red cells have obtained broadly similar results.

A slide flocculation test has been described by Lee and Schmale (1970). It employs a protoplasmic antigen and offers possibilities of automation in a test similar to the Automated Reagin Test for syphilis. The system appears adequately sensitive but the 12 per cent reactivity in the normal control group requires reduction. Wallace et al (1970) report another slide test—using a sensitised bentonite particle. They employed a phenol-extracted antigen and detected antibody in about 77 per cent of cases with only 4 per cent of controls reacting.

The G.C.F.T. has been improved by use of a 'protoplasmic' antigen made in a Ribi press with subsequent fractionation on Sephadex columns. Using this technique Reising et al (1969) obtained reaction rates of 72 per cent with infected females and 20 per cent with infected males and none with normal sera. Peacock (1971) has automated this test.

Buchanan and co-workers (1972) have developed a test using gonococcal pili. This offers a chance of testing with a gonococcal virulence factor which could prove to be the most specific antigenic determinant for this organism. Preliminary trials augur well, but the radio-isotope technique currently employed must be considered a disadvantage.

The fluorescent antibody technique also lends itself to the demonstration of antibody in the serum of the patient, and allows the class of antibody to be determined. This could prove a most useful facility, for it is accepted as a general principle that most 'natural' antibodies (and it is probably these which produce the bulk of the false positive reactions) are of the IgM class, and that the bulk of serum immune antibodies fall into the IgG class. If this should prove to be the case in gonococcal infections then much of the non-specificity of the test could be eliminated. Using this method Cohen and his co-workers

(Cohen, 1967; Cohen et al 1969) detected antibodies in patients and also in normal subjects, but were able to differentiate between the two groups in terms of titre, type, and class of antibody concerned. The reliability of this technique is also influenced by the strain of gonococcus used as antigen. O'Reilly and his co-workers have identified a suitable strain and have assessed its reliability (Welch and O'Reilly, 1973; O'Reilly et al, 1973).

Another approach has been to search for *local* antibodies. This is logical as, by and large, gonorrhoea is a membrane infection, and it is likely that local antibody levels will far exceed spill-over levels in the blood. The method has the great advantage that any antibody detected is likely to be significant and be produced early in the course of the disease. It has the disadvantage that specimens are not as easily obtained as they are for blood testing.

Hirschberg (1970) examined vaginal washings by haemagglutination and indirect immunofluorescence methods and Kearns et al (1973) examined urethral exudate by an indirect fluorescent antibody technique. Both reported encouraging results and future experience with these methods may well produce a very valuable test.

General conclusions

During the last decade great strides have been made in the routine laboratory diagnosis of gonorrhoea.

Problems of contamination and culture overgrowth have been overcome by the availability of good selective media. Rapid detection of gonococci, either on smear or culture plate (with varying degrees of sensitivity) can be achieved with the fluorescent antibody technique. Some of the advantages of both systems could be gained by use of the Transgrow culture medium combined with fluorescent antibody identification.

Serological testing has also developed apace, and whilst no test has yet achieved universal acceptance, much useful data on the relevance and nature of various antigens and the class of antibody response concerned has been accumulated. Tests suitable for slide techniques and automation procedures hold promise. Investigation of local antibody production is also proving a rewarding occupation, and whilst this will not fill the need for a blood test, it could well find a very useful place in our diagnostic armamentarium.

These improvements and developments add up to an increased diagnostic ability, more accurate and speedier laboratory reporting, and to good prospects of a blood test in the near future.

REFERENCES

AMIES, C. R. (1967). *Canad. J. Publ. Hlth*, **58**, 296.
BHATTACHARYYA, M. and JEPHCOTT, A. E. (1974). *Brit. J. vener. Dis.* (50, 109.).

BERGER, U. (1961). *Zbl. Bakt. I. Abt. Orig.*, **183**, 135.

BERGMAN, S., FORSGREN, A. and SWAHN, B. (1966). *J. Bact.*, **91**, 1664.

BUCHANAN, T. M., SWANSON, J. and GOTSCHLICH, E. C. (1972). *J. Clin. Invest.*, **51**, 17a.

CHACKO, C. N. and NAIR, G. M. (1969). *Brit. J. vener. Dis.*, **45**, 33.

COHEN, I. R. (1967). *J. Bact.*, **94**, 141.

COHEN, I. R., KELLOGG, D. S. JR. and NORINS, L. C. (1969). *Brit. J. vener. Dis.*, **45**, 325.

COONS, A. H. and KAPLAN, M. H. (1950). *J. exp. Med.*, **91**, 1.

CRUICKSHANK, R. (1965). 'Medical Microbiology', 11th ed., p. 816. E. and S. Livingstone Ltd., Edinburgh and London.

CROOKES, EILEEN M. L. and STUART, R. D. (1959). *J. Path. Bact.*, **78**, 283.

DANIELSSON, D. (1965a). *Acta derm.-venereol., Stockh.* **45**, 61.

DANIELSSON, D. (1965b). *Acta derm-venereol., Stockh.*, **45**, 74.

DANIELSSON, D. and MOLIN, L. (1971). *Acta derm.-venereol., Stockh.*, **51**, 73.

DEACON, W. E., PEACOCK, W. L., FREEMAN, E. M. and HARRIS, A. (1959). *Proc. Soc. exp. Biol., N.Y.*, **101**, 322.

DEACON, W. E., PEACOCK, W. L., FREEMAN, E. M., HARRIS, A. and BUNCH, W. L. (1960). *Publ. Hlth Rep., Wash.*, **75**, 125.

ELLNER, P. D., STOESSEL, C. J., DRAKEFORD, E. and VASI, F. (1966). *Amer. J. clin. Path.*, **45**, 502.

FLYNN, J. and WAITKINS, SHEENA, A. (1972). *J. clin. Path.*, **25**, 525.

FRY, C. S. and WILKINSON, A. E. (1963). *Brit. J. vener. Dis.* **39**, 190.

FRY, C. S. and WILKINSON, A. E. (1964). *Brit. J. vener. Dis.*, **40**, 125.

GNARPE, H., WALLIN, J. and FORSGREN, A. (1972). *Brit. J. vener. Dis.*, **48**, 496.

HALL, C. T. and HANSEN, P. A. (1962). *Zbl. Bakt. I. Abt. Orig.*, **184**, 548.

HIRSCHBERG, N. (1970). *Hlth Lab. Sci.*, **7**, 84.

HOKENSON, EDNA O. and HANSEN, P. A. (1966). *Stain. Technol.*, **41**, 9.

HOLMES, K. K., GUTMAN, LAUVA, T., BELDING, M. E. and TURCK, M. (1971). *New Engl. J. Med.*, **284**, 318.

JUHLIN, I. (1963). *Acta path. microbiol. scand.*, **58**, 51.

KAHN, G. and DANIELSSON, D. (1969). *Arch Derm.*, **99**, 421.

KEARNS, D. H., O'REILLY, R. J., LEE, LINDA and WELCH, B. G. (1973). *J. infect. Dis.*, **127**, 99.

KELLOGG, D. S. JR. and TURNER, E. M. (1973). *Appl. Microbiol.*, **25**, 550.

LANGE, P. K., REYN, ALICE, BENTZON, M. W. and LIND, INGA. (1965). *Ugeskr. Laeg.*, **128**, 409.

LEE, LINDA and SCHMALE, J. D. (1970). *Infect. Immunity*, **1**, 207.

LIND, INGA (1964). *Proc. XIV Scand. Congr. Path. Microbiol.*, Oslo, p. 255.

LIND, INGA (1967). *Acta path. microbiol. scand.*, **70**, 613.

LIND, INGA (1968). *Acta path. microbiol. scand.*, **73**, 624.

LIND, INGA (1969). *Acta path. microbiol. scand.*, **76**, 279.

LOGAN, LESLIE C., COX, PATRICIA M. and NORINS, L. C. (1970). *Appl. Microbiol.* **20**, 907.

McLEOD, J. W., COATES, J. C., HAPPOLD, F. C., PRIESTLEY, D. P. and WHEATLEY, B. (1934). *J. Path. Bact.*, **39**, 221.

MAELAND, J. A. (1968). *Acta path. microbiol. scand.*, **73**, 413.

MAELAND, J. A. (1969). *Acta path. microbiol. scand.*, **76**, 475.

MAELAND, J. A. and LARSEN, B. (1971). *Brit. J. vener. Dis.*, **47**, 269.

MAGNUSSON, B. and KJELLANDER, J. (1965). *Brit. J. vener. Dis.*, **41**, 127.

MARTIN, J. E. JR. and LESTER, A. (1971). *H.S.M.H.A. Hlth Rep.*, **86**, 30.

MARTIN, J. E. JR., BILLINGS, T. E., HACKNEY, J. F. and THAYER, J. D. (1967). *Publ. Hlth Rep. Wash.*, **82**, 361.

MØLLER, V. and REYN, ALICE (1965). *Bull. Wld Hlth Org.*, **32**, 471.

OLSEN, G. A. (1971). *Brit. J. vener. Dis.*, **47**, 102.

O'REILLY, R. J., WELCH, B. G. and KELLOGG, D. S. JR. (1973). *J. infect. Dis.*, **127**, 77.

PEACOCK, W. L. (1971). *H.S.M.H.A. Hlth Rep.*, **86**, 706.
PRICE, I. N. O. (1930). *J. Path. Bact.*, **33**, 493.
PRICE, I. N. O. (1949). *Brit. J. vener. Dis.*, **25**, 67.
RAMANARAYANA, MURTI B. RAJYALKSHMI and PERIN, DEVI B. (1961). *Indian J. Microbiol., Calcutta*, July-Sept., **2**, No. 3, 107.
REISING, G. and KELLOGG, D. S. JR., (1965). *Proc. Soc. exp. Biol. Med.*, **120**, 660.
REISING, G., SCHMALE, J. D., DANIELSSON, D. G. and THAYER, J. D. (1969). *Appl. Microbiol.* **18**, 337.
REYMANN, F. (1944). *Acta derm-venereol., Stockh.*, **25**, 9.
REYN, ALICE (1965). *Bull. Wld Hlth Org.*, **32**, 461.
REYN, ALICE (1969). *Bull. Wld Hlth Org.*, **40**, 245.
REYN, ALICE and BENTZON, M. W. (1972). *Brit. J. vener. Dis.*, **48**, 363.
REYN, ALICE, KORNER, B. and BENTZON, M. W. (1960). *Brit. J. vener. Dis.*, **36**, 243.
REYN, ALICE, BENTZON, M. W., THAYER, J. D. and WILKINSON, A. E. (1965). *Bull. Wld Hlth Org.*, **32**, 477.
RIDDELL, R H. and BUCK, A. C. (1970). *J. clin. Path.*, **23**, 481.
ROEPSTORFF, S. O. and HAMMERSTRÖM, E. (1966). *Acta path. microbiol. scand.*, **67**, 563.
SCRUTON, M. W. (1971). *J. clin. Path.*, **24**, 757.
SETH, A. (1970). *Brit. J. vener. Dis.*, **46**, 201.
SMITH, C. W., MARSHALL, J. D. JR. and EVELAND, W. C. (1969). *Proc. Soc. exp. Biol. Med., N.Y.*, **102**, 179.
SOMMERVILLE, R. G. (1968). *Bull. Wld Hlth Org.*, **39**, 942.
STACEY, P. and WARNER, GILLIAN (1973). *J. clin. Path.*, **26**, 303.
STUART, R. D. (1946). *Glasg. med. J.*, **27**, 131.
THAYER, J. D. and MARTIN, J. E. JR. (1964). *Publ. Hlth Rep., Wash.*, **79**, 49.
THAYER, J. D. and MARTIN, J. E. JR. (1966). *Publ. Hlth Rep. Wash.*, **81**, 559.
THIN, R. N. T. (1970). *Brit. J. vener. Dis.*, **46**, 27.
TOSHACH, SHEILA, KADIS, EILEEN and DIADO, MARGO (1972). *Canad. J. publ. Hlth*, **63**, 261.
VERA, HARRIETTE, D. (1948). *J. Bact.*, **55**, 531.
WARD, M. E. and GLYNN, A. A. (1972). *J. clin. Path.*, **25**, 56.
WALLACE, R., DIENA, B. B., YUGI, H. and GREENBERG, L. (1970). *Canad. J. Microbiol.*, **16**, 655.
WELCH, B. G. and O'REILLY, R. J. (1973). *J. infect. Dis.*, **127**, 69.
WHITE, L. A. and KELLOGG, D. S. JR. (1965). *Hlth Lab. Sci., N.Y.*, **2**, 238.
WILKINSON, A. E. (1965). *Brit. J. vener. Dis.*, **41**, 60.
WILLCOX, R. R. (1971). *Abstr. Hyg.*, **46**, 913.
W.H.O. EXPERT COMMITTEE ON ANTIBIOTICS (1961). *Wld Hlth Org. Techn. Rep. Ser.*, **210**, 18.

5   Fundamental Research Developments

M. G. McEntegart

Introduction

For years research into fundamental problems of gonococcal infection was inadequate. Clinical staff, even when they were not busy, seldom had the facilities needed for basic research and as they became ever busier there was little time left for such work. Fortunately, in the last 10 years, experienced bacteriologists have become increasingly involved in fundamental problems and today, more well-equipped and skilled research workers than ever before are seeking answers to long neglected problems of gonococcal infections. This involvement of the laboratory specialist has been the real development of this last 10 years and its success has been in the new areas of gonococcal research which have been opened up. The results so far obtained advance our understanding of the pathogenesis of the disease.

CULTIVATION

The first problem anyone undertaking gonococcal research meets is that of obtaining an adequate growth of the organism on laboratory media in a form which accurately reflects the tissue forms. Unlike many other pathogens the gonococcus is a difficult organism to grow in bulk without degradation. Despite the various developments in culture media for routine laboratory work, it is not easy to grow gonococci in bulk. Until recently both fluid cultures and biphasic media have been disappointing. These problems have been overcome by Buchanan and his co-workers (Buchanan et al, 1973b) who have successfully grown a strain of gonococcus type 2 in bulk. They report the growth of this organism in 60 litre quantities in a Biogen fermenter using a defined meningococcal medium. At the end of log phase growth, their cultures contained about 5×10^8 organisms per ml.

The problem of preserving strains of gonococci has been largely overcome by freezing in liquid nitrogen (Brookes and Heden, 1966; Ward and Watt, 1971).

Type variation and virulence

In 1963 Kellogg and his co-workers recorded their observations on type variation in gonococcal cultures. Their description of four recognisably different colonial types gave a major stimulus to research. These colonial types (Fig. 11a, b, c, d) can be distinguished under a plate microscope using an appropriate system of illumination (Jephcott and Reyn, 1971). An additional large colony type, type, 5 was observed by these latter authors. Gonococcal colonies of types 1 to 4 can be maintained by selective transfer so that subcultures of type 1 colonies give rise to a pure growth of type 1 colonies with an occasional colony of other types arising as a result of degradation. If, however, non-selective subcultures are made, the less fastidious and faster-growing type 4 variants become dominant within a few transfers and type 1 strains for all practical purposes disappear. This change probably explains the well-known degradation of old laboratory strains. Indeed, Tulloch in his account of gonococci in 'The System of Bacteriology', published in 1929 (Tulloch, 1929) described large and small colony forms which may well be examples of Kellogg's types 1 and 4. By using very large doses of cultured type 1 organisms, Kellogg and his co-workers were able to produce clinical gonorrhoea in volunteers whereas similar doses of type 4 were without effect (Kellogg et al, 1963). By a series of similar inoculations using samples of the various colony types they established beyond doubt that the change from type 1 to type 4 was associated with a loss of virulence for the human host. Here at last was a new starting point for studies on the mechanism of the virulence of gonococci.

Ward et al (1970) compared gonococci recovered from the discharge of patients with acute gonorrhoea with strains from culture. They found that gonococci from exudates were more resistant to the destructive action of antibody than culture strains. This effect was observed with both human serum antibody and a polyvalent rabbit antibody plus complement.

Although the nature of the 'virulence factor' which determines this difference in resistance is not known, Watt et al (1972) observed that if gonococci were grown on a medium containing human prostatic extract they retained their resistance to the destructive action of antibody. This resistance factor may not be directly equated to virulence as it may occasionally be absent from type 1 strains.

Thongthai and Sawyer (1973) found that types 1 and 2 gonococci were significantly more resistant to phagocytosis by rabbit polymorphonuclear leucocytes *in vitro* than less virulent strains. They regarded this as a character of the bacterial surface and showed that the difference "in ease of phagocytosis" persisted even when heat-killed, formalin-treated, organisms were used in the test. Similar differences in phagocytosis are suggested by the observations of Flynn and Waitkins (1973):

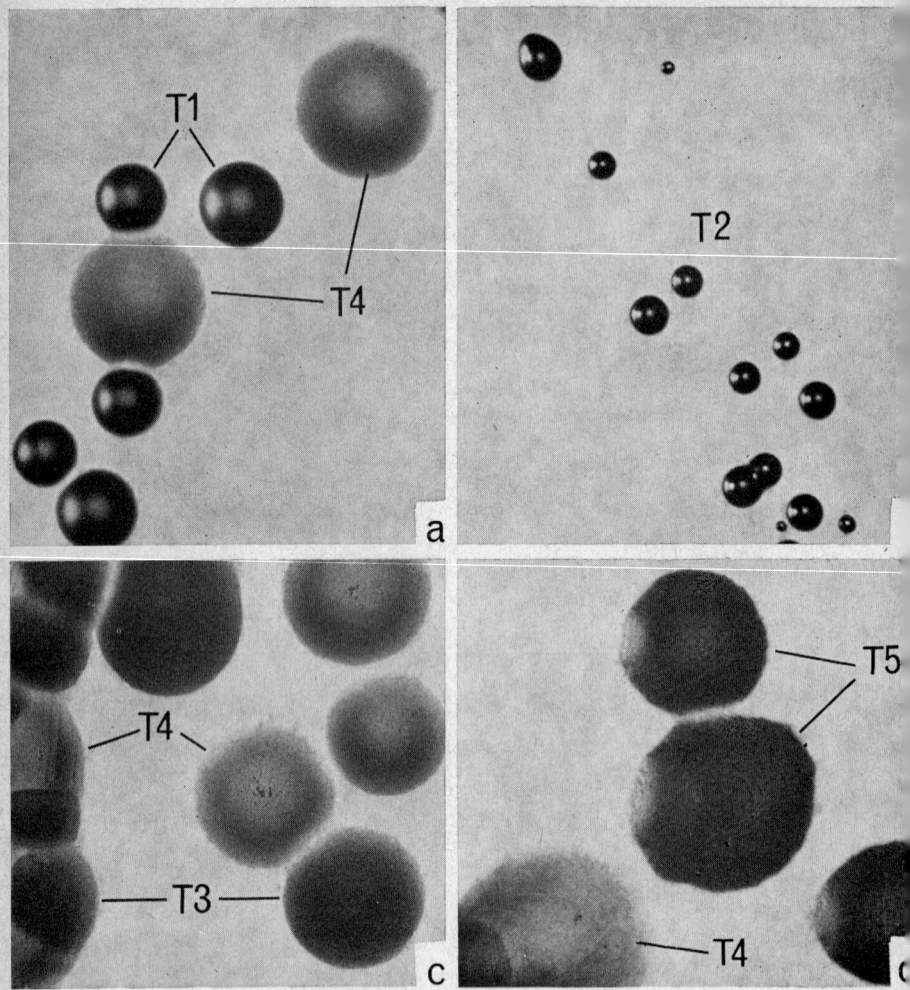

FIG. 11. Gonococcal colony types.

(a) Types 1 and 4 colonies. Strain F62.
(b) Type 2 colonies. Strain F62.
(c) Types 3 and 4 colonies. Stain F62.
(d) Types 4 and 5 colonies. Strain 43562/SS 1944.

(From a paper by A. E. Jephcott and Alice Reyn, *Acta path. microbiol. scand.* (1971). Reproduced by kind permission of the authors and the Editor of the journal).

that when gonococci are introduced into subcutaneous chambers in mice type 4 strains cannot be recovered at a time when live type 1 strains are still persisting in the chamber.

Virulence—the possible role of fimbriae

In 1971 Jephcott and Reyn made a comparative study of Kellogg's types in an attempt to determine the nature of any virulence factor that might be present. In the course of this study they examined sections of gonococcal colonies under the electron microscope and noted the

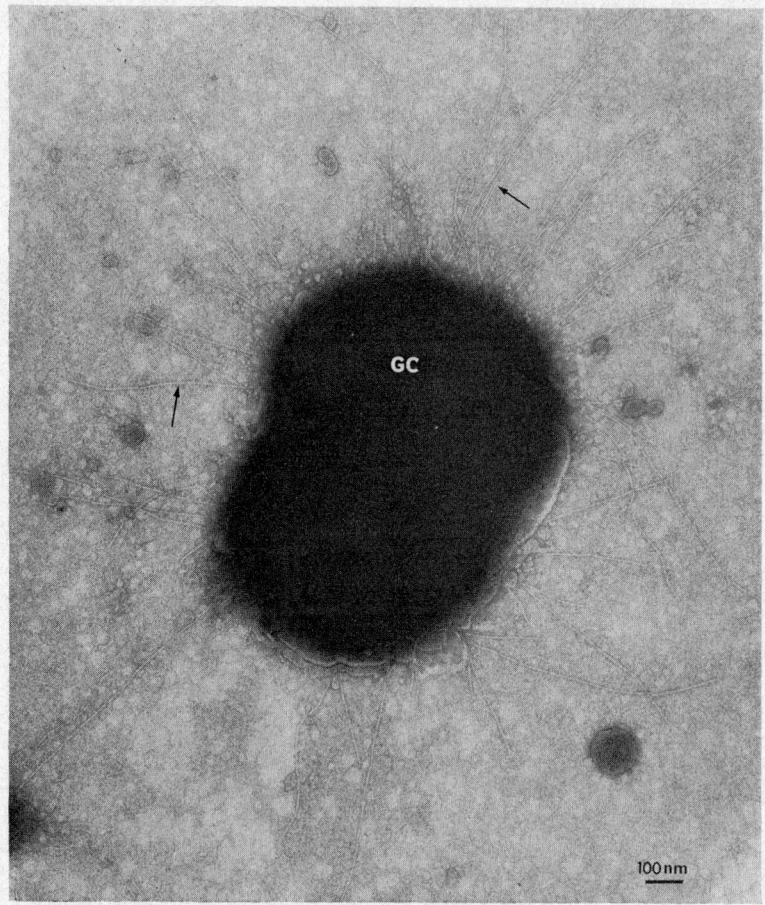

FIG. 12. Electron microscope photograph of the gonococcus showing fimbriae (pili), The specimen was negatively stained with phosphotungstic acid. (The photograph by courtesy of Alice Reyn and Birch Andersen (1973) of the Serum Institut, Copenhagen, Denmark).

presence of structures (subsequently identified as fimbriae) in virulent type 1 colonies which were very rarely seen in type 4 colonies (Jephcott et al, 1971). In the same year Swanson et al (1971) independently recorded detailed studies on these structures and suggested a possible relation between the pili (or fimbriae) and the successful attachment of the organism to the host cells. In an electron microscopic study of urethral mucosal cells from patients with gonorrhoea, zones of adherence between gonococci and epithelial cells were seen although pili were not identified (Ward and Watt, 1972). Swanson (1973), using cultures of human amnion cells, compared the attachment of pilated and non-pilated gonococci. He found the presence of pili increased the attachment of the organisms to the tissue cells. Electron microscopy photographs of thick sections suggest that the pili are the means of attachment. In thin sections no pili could be recognized but a fine space was seen between the organism and the cell membrane. This gap was not seen in thin sections of adherent non-pilated gonococci. Fimbriae may be a necessary factor in the establishment of gonococcal infection

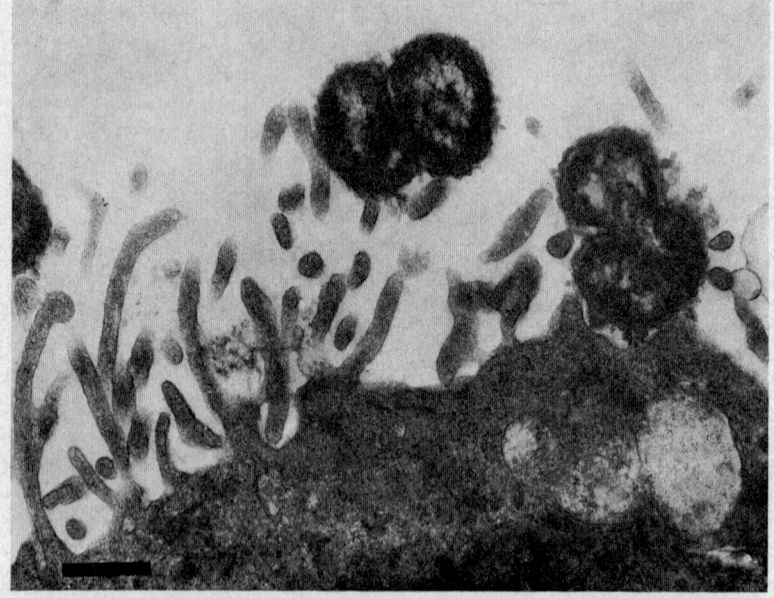

FIG. 13. Ingestion of gonococci by epithelial cells in a specimen of urethral discharge from a male patient with acute urethritis. Electron microscope photograph of a thin section showing gonococci close to the cell surface from which numerous microvilli project towards the organism. (By kind permission of P. Norris, Dept. of Pathology, Weston Park Hospital, Sheffield.) The bar represents 500 nm.

but it is unlikely that the attachment of the organisms alone is sufficient to initiate infection, as it has been demonstrated that some commensal neisseriae also have fimbriae (Weistreich and Baker, 1971). It appears that the attachment of gonococci to the surface of epithelial cells stimulates the cell to throw out pseudopodial processes (Fig. 13) and to ingest the organisms. Such ingestion differs from the phagocytosis of polymorphonuclear cells (Fig. 14a, b, c, d) in that the organisms do not seem to be subject to the action of lysozomal enzymes and so survive

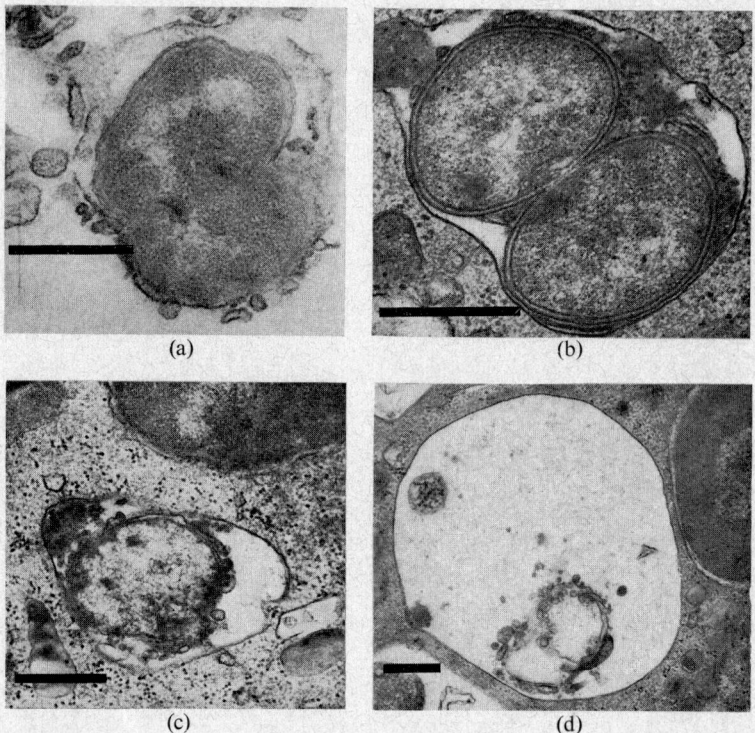

(a)   (b)

(c)   (d)

Fig. 14. Polymorphs in urethral pus. A series of photographs to show stages in the destruction of gonococci by polymorphs. The bars represent 500 nm. (Reproduced from Ward, Glynn and Watt (1972) *Brit. J. exp. Path.*, **53**, 289, by kind permission of the authors and the Editor.) (a) Extra-cellular gonococci showing intact cell wall and ribosomes evenly scattered throughout the cytoplasm. (b) A phagosome containing a diplococcus with triple layered cytoplasmic membrane and cell wall still intact. A lysosome has just discharged into the phagosome. (c) A phagosome containing a damaged gonococcus. There is a local bulge of the cell wall with detachment from the cytoplasmic membrane. Ribosomes have been lost and a reticular network is apparent in the cytoplasm. (d) A phagosome containing a gonococcus with the cell wall and cytoplasmic membrane destroyed and the cell contents lost.

within the cells at least for some hours. Within epithelial cells gonococci not only survive but appear to be protected against adverse conditions. This can be demonstrated not only *in vitro* but also when tissue culture cells containing gonococci are put into subcutaneous chambers in mice (Waitkins, 1973). Electron microscope studies of gonococci ingested by tissue cells, such as cells of the urethral mucosa obtained from an acute gonococcal discharge, suggest that the intraepithelial gonococci break down after about 12 hours. Some cells containing ingested cocci are shed in the normal process of cell loss. At present the clinical significance of intracellular gonococci is not clear. It seems unlikely that such organisms persist for long periods within cells, at least in acute infections, or we would find very many more patients 'resistant' to antibiotic treatment or showing clinical relapse. It is possible, however, that the intracellular survival of small numbers of cocci plays a part in chronic infections and may perhaps be common in chronic symptomless carriers.

Phagocytosis and the destruction of gonococci

One of the ideas which stimulated the interest of workers at the beginning of the current period of research was that gonococci might be resistant to killing by phagocytes and might even 'take refuge' within polymorphs. In this way the appearance of pus cells crammed with gonococci could have been explained as micro-colonies of surviving ingested organisms. This attractive hypothesis did not survive investigation. Several workers have shown, by a variety of methods, that ingested gonococci are rapidly destroyed within polymorphs. Watt (1970) compared the destruction of gonococci by human and guinea-pig polymorphs and found no evidence for any intrinsic difference in their ability to kill gonococci. In a study of the fate of gonococci following ingestion (Ward et al 1972), sequential electron microscope photographs show the breakdown of the gonococcal cell wall (Fig. 14). The authors concluded from these observations that gonococci degenerate within $\frac{1}{2}$–1 hour of phagocytosis. In a similar way phase contrast studies of gonococci following ingestion by polymorphs fail to show any growth of the ingested organisms. The fate of gonococci in macrophages is less clear and it is surprising that such an obvious site for survival should have been so little studied. Flynn (1972a) made some observations on the fate of gonococci in mouse peritoneal macrophages and was able to demonstrate survival of ingested gonococci for up to 7 hours.

Waitkins and Flynn (1973) found the uptake and subsequent survival of gonococci in tissue culture cells to be similar in each of the four cell lines they tested, *ie* Vero monkey kidney, LLC-MK$_2$ monkey kidney, 3T3 mouse fibroblast and human epithelial cells (HeLa). The growth curves obtained in all these cells were similar for both type 1 and type

4 strains of gonococci. There was an initial fall in the total count of the organism in the supernatant of the tissue culture cells due to active phagocytosis of organisms by the cells. The low point of the count was reached at 8 hours and thereafter the count rose again as a result of the release of organisms which had grown within the cells.

When fimbriated commensal neisseriae are added to tissue culture cells under the same conditions as the gonococci, there are obvious differences. The non-pathogenic cocci remain attached to the surface of the cell but are not phagocytosed. The difference in the location of the cocci can be demonstrated by treating the tissue culture cells with rat serum which rapidly kills organisms unless they are protected within a cell. When cells which have been incubated for 8 hours with gonococci are washed and then treated with rat serum, organisms can be recovered subsequently only when the cells are broken up. When cells plus commensal strains are tested in the same way, no such survival can be observed. Direct studies by electron microscopy show a clear difference in that there is a halo around ingested gonococci suggesting an intracellular position, whereas no such halo can be seen around commensal neisseriae attached to the surface of tissue culture cells. Ward and Watt (1973) noted the effect of cytochalasin on the ability of cells to ingest gonococci. When the mobility of the cell wall in their experimental system was inhibited by this substance there was no phagocytosis of the gonococci. This adds weight to the view that once a gonococcus has become attached to a cell by means of its fimbriae, it stimulates the production of pseudopodial processes, perhaps by some toxic action on the cell wall and so becomes ingested.

Experimental infections in man and animals

Human infection with a pure culture was first produced by Bumm in 1885. Most animal experiments were unsuccessful and even when success was claimed the experiment could seldom be repeated by other workers. Altogether the history of animal experimental infections is one of confusion and contradiction. From our present knowledge it seems probable that this was in part due to variation in the virulence of the strains of gonococci employed which ranged from organisms in fresh urethral pus to established laboratory cultures, many of which were, without doubt, avirulent. A second cause of confusion may have been the potent endotoxic effect of gonococci which accounted for the deaths of small laboratory animals (Wasserman, 1898; Flynn and McEntegart, 1973). The earlier animal experiments are reviewed by Hill (1944).

A new phase in experimental infections began in 1963 with the observations of Kellogg and his colleagues on the variation of virulence of gonococci associated with changes in colony type. The virulence of the various types was established by the urethral inoculations of volunteers in a United States prison. In this way it was demonstrated that type 1 colonies retained their virulence when selectively passed, even after 69 passages. In contrast, when subcultures were made without selection, types 3 and 4 rapidly became the predominant organisms and these cultures proved to be avirulent in volunteers. Although Kellogg demonstrated the virulence of cultured gonococci, it is important to note that the size of the infecting dose he used was very much greater than that likely in the natural transmission of the disease. It still seems likely, therefore, that there are other virulence or protective factors associated with the transmission of gonorrhoea which are absent from the organisms in pure cultures. Infection by culture was never as consistently successful as the inoculation of urethral pus from an infected patient. In 1968 Kellogg and his colleagues published the continuation of their work on colonial types and virulence in which they showed that the same type 1 strain had retained its virulence after 17 months and 440 selective passages—and even after 35 months during which it underwent 720 selective passages the strain was capable of producing infection in volunteers!

In 1971, Lucas et al produced gonococcal urethritis in three male chimpanzees infected with discharge from human male cases. They isolated *Neisseria gonorrhoeae* from the chimpanzees' urethrae and were able to transfer infection, by the inoculation of discharge, from animal to animal. It seems that these workers succeeded where others had failed because they placed their inoculum at a higher level in the urethra, that is beyond the anterior part, which in the chimpanzee consists of squamous epithelium and of course is not susceptible to infection. One of the chimpanzees in this series developed a gonococcal conjunctivitis as a result of auto-inoculation. The following year Brown et al (1972) employed similar methods of inoculation to produce infection in a male chimpanzee with pure cultures of type 1 *Neisseria gonorrhoeae*. Moreover the infection was transmitted venereally to a female chimpanzee.

It is of interest to note that the same group of workers, Brown et al (1973), subsequently recorded the natural occurrence of a urethral infection due to meningococci in a male chimpanzee which was a chronic nasopharyngeal carrier of meningococci.

Work with chimpanzees will always be limited by cost and no general laboratory investigations of experimental gonococcal infections are likely unless infection can be produced in some convenient, small, laboratory animal. So far attempts to produce such infections in small rodents have been consistently unsuccessful. Attempts to potentiate infection by immunosuppression (Flynn, 1972a, b) have met with no better success. A great deal of interest was aroused, therefore, when Arko (1972) described a method for establishing a circumscribed experimental infection in the rabbit, and recorded a small series of similar experiments in guinea-pigs, hamsters, rats and mice. In the rabbit, gonococci were introduced into an artificial, subcutaneous chamber created by the implantation of a plastic, practice golf ball below the skin. The space so created became lined with granulation tissue and partly filled with fluid. Following the introduction of gonococci, samples of fluid from the chamber could be taken on successive days and the duration of survival of the organisms assessed. Arko was able to show the survival of gonococci within these chambers for 9 months.

A similar chamber can be created in the mouse by means of a small PVC cylinder (Flynn and Waitkins, 1973) and similar, though briefer, survival of gonococci demonstrated. The survival time of the gonococci in the mouse chamber can be extended by the direct inoculation of tissue culture cells infected with gonococci (Waitkins, 1973).

Studies on serological tests for the diagnosis of gonorrhoea

An ideal serological test would give an absolute correlation with active infection so that a positive result indicated a potential source of infection irrespective of evidence of clinical disease. It could be applied as a routine in mass surveys or to any person named as a contact. In recent years many experienced laboratory workers have begun to take an interest in the search for a better, even if not ideal, test for gonococcal infection. Reyn (1965, 1969) reviews earlier work on serological investigations. Any test for serum antibody depends for its success on the antigen employed. If the antigen is pure and highly specific the chance of developing a useful test will be good. If the antigen is crude and contains antigens common to several organisms the chance of a specific reaction will be poor.

It is, therefore, not surprising that much of the work in this field has been concentrated on the problem of gonococcal antigens. The hope of workers devising a useful diagnostic test seems better since studies of experimental infections in volunteers have shown that an early antibody response does occur (Cohen et al 1969).

Three possible antigens have been prepared and characterised. Maeland (1968) studied gonococcal endotoxin as antigen and showed that an aqueous ether extract of gonococci gave a preparation of endotoxin which was characterised as a lipopolysaccharide, some 80–90 per cent of the complex being a protein derivative, whilst the carbohydrate component amounted to some 5 per cent only (Maeland, 1969a, b, c). The protein fraction of this endotoxin has been shown to contain antigenic determinants in common with the meningococcus. Samples of the carbohydrate fraction of the endotoxin also cross-reacted with commensal neisseriae. Using a different extraction process wherein the organisms were treated with phenol water (Maeland and Kristoffersen,

1971; Maeland et al, 1971) an endotoxin preparation was isolated which, in contrast to the aqueous ether extract, contained much more carbohydrate (80 per cent) and relatively much less protein (14 per cent).

The application of the endotoxin antigen to human sera was investigated by Maeland and Larsen (1971). Using sheep erythrocytes sensitised with either the carbohydrate or the protein antigen, sera from 30 patients and 30 controls were tested. Both direct agglutination and antiglobulin agglutination (to distinguish the immunoglobulin class of antibody) were employed. All patients and controls showed some IgM antibody. Following treatment with mercapto-ethanol (to disrupt the macroglobulin molecules (IgM)) the control sera no longer gave any positive results whereas one-third of the sera from patients showed IgG antibody suggesting that the specific antibody belonged to this immunoglobulin class.

In addition to the endotoxin antigens, gonococcal protoplasmic antigens have been investigated (Schmale, et al, 1969) but these have not been shown to offer any major advantage for the development of a diagnostic test.

As the significance of the fimbriae of type 1 gonococci became clear, they were an obvious choice for the preparation of a specific 'pathogenicity' antigen. There remained the very daunting technical problem of trying to amass a sufficient quantity of fimbriae to make any test possible. Buchanan et al (1973a) purified fimbriae in sufficient quantity to study their possible role as antigen. They used the fimbrial antigen to immunise rabbits. The anti-fimbrial antibody was then used by the immunofluorescent method and shown to stain fimbriated gonococci but not non-fimbriated ones. The fimbrial antibodies were specific and did not stain fimbriated meningococci. This group also developed an antigen-binding test for anti-fimbrial antibodies in human sera and preliminary results based on the study of 561 human sera are encouraging (Buchanan et al, 1973b). A control group was shown to have significantly lower levels of antibody activity than asymptomatic patients or clinical cases. The highest levels of antibody activity were shown by asymptomatic females. When the results of culture and antibody levels were compared in a group of 103 high risk females, 58 were found to have raised antibody levels and this group included 89 per cent of the culture positives. This method may therefore provide a useful test for the detection of symptomless carriers of gonococci.

Watt et al (1971) used sera from male and female cases of gonorrhoea and from a control group to compare four different tests for antibody to gonococcal antigens. Although some of their results may have been useful in confirming clinical suspicion, all of the methods they tested gave a level of false positive results which ruled them out as possible screening methods for the detection of asymptomatic patients. Similarly, Ward and Glynn (1972) used the agglutination of human red cells coated with gonococcal lipopolysaccharide to measure antibody in human sera from patients and controls. Although there was a significantly higher titre demonstrated in patients than in controls, and a low level of non-specific positives (2 per cent), there was a rather high incidence of false negatives (16 per cent) in females who were clinically positive. It seems doubtful, therefore, if the test would be helpful in asymptomatic cases.

Most workers who have studied the problem of serological methods of diagnosis have concentrated on devising a simple, specific and sensitive test for serum antibody. Given the appropriate antigen it still seems reasonable to expect radiobioassay, with its very much greater sensitivity, to provide the best possible diagnostic test. Furthermore, we should not forget that the sensitivity of the radioimmunoassay method could equally be applied to the detection of antigen in clinical specimens from suspected cases of gonorrhoea. It might be possible to devise a test which would identify specific gonococcal antigen in extracts of vaginal swabs or cervical cytology specimens even when no intact organisms were seen and no gonococci isolated on culture. Although less than ideal, such an approach might give an indication of infectivity which would be of value in the problem of control of spread.

The idea of a vaccine

Sooner or later in any discussion on the control of gonorrhoea the possible value of a prophylactic vaccine is likely to be raised. The clinical history of the disease, which shows little or no evidence of the development of effective immunity, does not encourage the hope that a vaccine would do any better. From time to time patients with repeated infections seem to show less and less in the way of acute symptoms. Indeed, it is not unknown today for a symptomless and 'signless' male patient to come to the clinic as a result of contact tracing, following the recognition of gonorrhoea in an infected consort. This in itself suggests that even the immune would remain transmitters of infection.

What little support can be mustered for the feasibility of an effective gonococcal vaccine comes from studies on vaccines in the prevention of meningococcal meningitis. It is possible that current W.H.O. investigations of vaccines in Africa will demonstrate that meningococcal vaccines are effective in preventing the disease. Before these results generate any optimism about the prospects for a gonococcal vaccine it is worth noting the probable mode of protection in meningitis. Vaccination gives rise to serum antibody which is able to destroy meningococci in the blood stream *before* they reach the target area of the meninges.

From the observations on the mode of infection by gonococci it can be seen that even if it were possible to achieve a level of serum antibody it is unlikely that it would be effective. For a vaccine to work it would be necessary for it to give rise to an effective level of IgA in the urethra. In this context it is interesting to note that in 1900 Scholtz reported that the introduction of killed gonococci into the urethra gave rise to transient purulent inflammation. This is probably a further demonstration of the endotoxic effect of gonococci.

For our knowledge of the practical application of vaccines in the control of gonorrhoea we depend upon the work of Greenberg and his colleagues (1971, 1972). In the first of these reports (Greenberg et al, 1971) 54 volunteers were given a somatic gonococcal vaccine of approximately 70 per cent autolysis. Three doses were given with 3 weeks interval between doses and the antibody response assessed by a flocculation test and a tissue culture protection test. Although there was a rise in antibody titres in most volunteers, there was still a substantial number in whom there was no response. No attempt was made to assess the development of any clinical protection.

In the second report (1972) Greenberg and his colleagues give some details of a small vaccine trial in progress in Inuvik, a small village in north-west Canada. The village was a suitable centre for the trial in having for many years a high incidence of gonorrhoea. The investigation followed a similar pattern to the first trial except that the interval between vaccine doses was reduced to 1 week and a placebo was used along with the vaccine. Within the first 3 months of study, gonorrhoea was diagnosed and confirmed in four vaccinated and three control patients. None of the cases showed any tissue culture neutralising antibodies. The investigation is continuing. Some possible reasons for the general failure of immunoprophylaxis are discussed by Kiraly (1973) in a review of various immunoallergic aspects of gonorrhoea.

Markers for epidemiological study

It is surprising, in view of the importance of case tracing and clinical epidemiology in gonorrhoea, that so little attention has been paid to strain markers. Sometimes the chance emergence of a strain of gonococci with an unusual antibiotic resistance provides a useful guide to its spread. Hutchinson (1970) suggested the trial of a simple serological typing method similar to that used for streptococci. This has, however, not been successful. Glynn and Ward (1970) investigated the complement dependent serum bactericidal action of normal human and hyperimmune rabbit sera. They tested 60 strains of *N. gonorrhoeae* and were able to divide them into four main groups on the basis of their resistance to killing. Further sub-groups could probably be defined within the four main groups but the test is too difficult to standardise and is unlikely ever to be usefully adapted as a means of sub-division of the gonococci.

Although a phage typing system would be ideal no clear evidence of bacteriophage acting on gonococci has been reported. Following the observations of Kingsbury (1966) on the bacteriocines of meningococci, Flynn and McEntegart (1972) recorded preliminary results on a similar phenomenon in gonococci. It has, however, not so far been possible to establish the nature of the phenomenon and at present the results are not sufficiently reproducible to offer a reliable typing system.

General conclusions

Without doubt one of the most exciting developments of the past few years has been the way in which research workers with special bacteriological and immunological skills have become interested in the various research problems of gonococcal infections. Credit for this is due in many countries to the various research councils and other grant-giving bodies who have made the extension of research possible.

Gonococcal research today is not only respectable, it has gained considerable momentum and there is every reason to hope that it will continue to attract able bacteriologists for many years to come. It may be true that no purely medical or clinicopathological solution will solve a problem that is symptomatic of social pathology. No one will, however, dispute that a full understanding of the tissue pathology of gonococcal infections will give us information which may be used to prevent infection; or at least limit the spread of infections in the community.

REFERENCES

ARKO, R. J. (1972). *Science, N.Y.*, **177**, 1200.

BROOKES, R. and HEDEN, C. G. (1966). *Biotech. Bioeng.*, **7**, 315.

BROWN, W. J., LUCAS, C. T. and KUHN, U. S. G. (1972). *Brit. J. vener. Dis.*, **48**, 177.

BROWN, W. J., KRAUS, S. J. and ARKO, R. J. (1973). *Brit. J. vener. Dis.*, **49**, 88.

BUCHANAN, T. M., SWANSON, J. and GOTSCHLICH, E. C. (1973a). W.H.O./V.D.T./R.E.S./G.O.N.., **73**, 72.

BUCHANAN, T. M., SWANSON, J., HOLMES, K. K., KRAUS, S. J. and GOTSCHLICH, E. C. (1973b). W.H.O./V.D.T./R.E.S./G.O.N., **73**, 79.

BUMM, E. (1885). *Dt. med. Wschr.*, **11**, 508.

COHEN, I. R., KELLOGG, D. S. and NORINS, L. C. (1969). *Brit. J. vener. Dis.*, **45**, 325.

FLYNN, J. (1972a). *Brit. J. vener. Dis.*, **48**, 293.

FLYNN, J. (1972b). M.D. Thesis, University of Sheffield.

FLYNN, J. and MCENTEGART, M. G. (1972). *J. clin. Path.*, **25**, 60.

FLYNN, J. and MCENTEGART, M. G. (1973). *J. med. Microbiol.*, **6**, 371.

FLYNN, J. and WAITKINS, S. A. (1973). *Brit. J. vener. Dis.*, **49**, 432.

GLYNN, A. A. and WARD, M. E. (1970). *Infect. Immunity*, **2**, 162.

GREENBERG, L., DIENA, B. B., KENNY, C. P. and ZNAMIROWSKI, R. (1971). *Bull. Wld IIIth Org.*, **45**, 431.

GREENBERG, L., DIENA, B. B., ASHTON, P. A., WALLACE, R., KENNY, C. P., ZNAMIROWSKI, R. and FERRAR, H. (1972). W.H.O./V.D.T/R.E.S/G.O.N. **72**, 68.

HILL, J. H. (1944). *Amer. J. Syph. Gonor. Vener. Dis.*, **28**, 334.

HUTCHINSON, I. (1970). *Br. med. J.*, **3**, 107.

JEPHCOTT, A. E. and REYN, A. (1971). *Acta path. microbiol. scand.*, **79**, 609.

JEPHCOTT, A. E., REYN, A. and BIRCH-ANDERSON, A. (1971). *Acta path. microbiol. scand.*, Section B., **79**, 437.

KELLOGG, D. S., PEACOCK, W. L., DEACON, W. E., BROWN, L. and PIRKLE, C. L. (1963). *J. Bact.*, **85**, 1274.

KELLOGG, D. S., COHEN, I. R., NORINS, L. C., SCHROETER, A. L. and REISLING, G. (1968). *J. Bact.*, **96**, 596.

KINGSBURY, D. T. (1966). *J. Bact.*, **91**, 1696.

KIRALY, K. (1973). W.H.O./V.D.T./R.E.S./G.O.N., 73, 81.

LUCAS, C. T., CHANDLER, F. L., MARTIN, J. E. and SCHMALE, J. D. (1971). *J. Amer. med. Ass.*, **216**, 1612.

MAELAND, J. A. (1968). *Acta path. microbiol. scand.*, **73**, 413.

MAELAND, J. A. (1969a). *Acta path. microbiol. scand.*, **76**, 484.

MAELAND, J. A. (1969b). *Acta path. micribool. scand.*, **77**, 505.

MAELAND, J. A. (1969c). *Acta path. microbiol. scand.*, **77**, 495.

MAELAND, J. A. and KRISTOFFERSEN, T. (1971). *Acta path. microbiol. scand.*, Section B., **79**, 226.

MAELAND, J. A., KRISTOFFERSEN, T. and HOFSTADT, T. (1971). *Acta path. microbiol. scand.*, Section B., **79**, 233.

MAELAND, J. A. and LARSEN, B. (1971). *Brit. J. vener. Dis.*, **47**, 269.

REYN, A. (1965). *Bull. Wld Hlth Org.*, **32**, 459.

REYN, A. (1969). *Bull Wld Hlth Org.*, **40**, 251.

SCHMALE, S. D., DANIELSSON, D. G., SMITH, J. F., LEE, L. and PEACOCK, W. L. (1969). *J. Bact.*, **99**, 469.

SCHOLTZ, W. (1900). *Arch. Derm. Syph.*, Bd. XLIX, 1–28.

SWANSON, J., KRAUS, S. J. and GOTSCHLICH, E. C. (1971). *J. exp. Med.*, **134**, 886.

SWANSON, J. (1973). *J. exp. Med.*, **137**, 571.

THONGTHAI, C. and SAWYER, W. D. (1973). *Infect. Immunity*, 7, 373.

TULLOCH, W. J. (1929). 'A System of Bacteriology in Relation to Medicine', vol. 2, p. 250. H.M.S.O.

WAITKINS, S. A. (1973). Ph.D Thesis, University of Sheffield.

WAITKINS, S. A. and FLYNN, J. (1973). *J. med. Microbiol.*, **6**, 399.

WARD, M. E., WATT, P. J. and GLYNN, A. A. (1970). *Nature, Lond.*, **227**, 382.

WARD, M. E. and WATT, P. J. (1971). *J. clin. Path.*, **24**, 122.

WARD, M. E. and GLYNN, A. A. (1972). *J. clin. Path.*, **25**, 56.

WARD, M. E., GLYNN, A. A. and WATT, P. J. (1972). *Brit. J. exp. Path.*, **53**, 289.

WARD, M. E. and WATT, P. J. (1972). *J. infect. Dis.*, **126**, 601.

WARD, M. E. and WATT, P. J. (1973) (unpublished).

WASSERMAN, A. (1898). *Z. Hyg. InfektKr.*, **27**, 298.

WATT, P. J. (1970). *J. med. Microbiol.*, **3**, 501.

WATT, P. J., WARD, M. E. and GLYNN, A. A. (1971). *Brit. J. vener. Dis.*, **47**, 448.

WATT, P. J., GLYNN, A. A. and WARD, M. E. (1972). *Nature New Biol.*, **236**, 186.

WEISTREICH, G. A. and BAKER, R. F. (1971). *J. gen. Microbiol.*, **65**, 167.

6 Therapy

R. S. Morton

Introduction

By the early 1960s it was becoming clear that cure rates with penicillin, and other antibiotics, in gonorrhoea were related to both dosage and the percentage of relatively resistant strains circulating locally within the population. In spite of this, drug trials have continued to appear which make no reference to this last aspect. Such reports can be of local interest only and have been largely ignored in this review.

In some reports, drugs under trial are compared with routine penicillin schedules of known failure rate.

The spiral of rising failure rates, followed by higher dosage schedules, followed by improved cure rates, followed by a repetition of the whole cycle has been going on for some 20 years. The single-dose treatment of gonorrhoea using aqueous procaine penicillin is now in some areas of Asia and the West Coast of the U.S.A. reaching tolerance level with single injections of 4·8 and even 6·4 mega units being in use. Knowledge of the mechanism of development of resistance is scanty. Willcox (1967) gave his views on the part played by under-treatment.

Increasingly throughout the world there is a growing tendency to base decisions regarding treatment schedules on observations of clinical failure rates together with confirmatory laboratory evidence of antibiotic resistance (see Table IV). This evidence may be of two kinds: (a) that the majority of 'failures' are indeed due to relatively resistant strains and (b) that the percentage of relatively resistant strains in the area is increasing with the passage of time. To a growing number of workers the need for regular monitoring and reviewing of resistance at say 3-monthly intervals has become an essential tool of control (Ronald et al, 1968). The lack of standardisation of sensitivity estimation methods can be overcome by use of three strains of recognised sensitivity obtainable from Dr. Alice Reyn at the W.H.O. Gonorrhoea Reference Laboratory, The Serum Institut, Amagar Boulevard, Copenhagen, Denmark. The organisms are lypholised and require to be reconstituted

Table IV. Sensitivity of the gonococcus to penicillin (per cent M.I.C. in mcg per ml) (reproduced from Willcox, R. R. (1972). Venereal diseases. *Med. Clin. North Amer.*, p. 1063).

Area	Authors	M.I.C. <0·06	M.I.C. 0·06–0·12	M.I.C. >0·12
United Kingdom	Lynn et al	65·0	18·5	16·5
London	Leigh et al	63·0	18·0	19·0
Norway	Gunderson et al	65·5	17·8	16·7
North America				
Canada	Amies	34·9	19·0	46·1
United States	Fishmaller et al	20·9	22·4	56·7
Australia	Hatos	22·0	6·8	71·2
Africa				
Uganda	Arya and Phillips	19·1	7·5	73·4
Far East				
Hawaii	Keys et al	14·5	11·6	73·9
Japan				
Philippines				

before use. The majority of workers define a less sensitive (or relatively resistant) strain as one requiring 0·125 i.u. or more of penicillin per ml for inhibition. How the information obtained in the laboratory can be used for the benefit of the individual patient, can improve general management in increasingly busy departments and be employed as an epidemiological tool for control has become obvious (Morton and Higson, 1966; Lomholt and Berg, 1966). There is growing consciousness that such measures can be employed in early warning systems, detecting and giving notice of the spread of relatively resistant strains from one part of the world to another. Application of the same measures could prevent gonorrhoea becoming an expensive disease. Results of a sample basic study are shown in Table V.

Oral treatment of gonorrhoea has its limitations. The tablets may not be taken as ordered or they may be shared with an undeclared consort. Single oral dose schedules have been used. The most satisfactory appears to be ampicillin combined with probenecid, which slows down kidney excretion of the antibiotic. Ampicillin is said to have the great advantage over all others in that it does not invite the emergence and spread of cross-resistance.

The use of intramuscular benzathine penicillin alone or in combination with other penicillins offers the gonococcus a 'tail' of low serum concentration likely to engender resistance (Lomholt and Berg, 1966). Failure rates such as the 12·5 per cent reported from Poland by Lejman et al (1965) and the 10·8–15·3 per cent failure rate reported by Staheli (1964) when using this form of penicillin daily are generally regarded as propagating the dissemination of partially resistant strains.

Table V. Singapore gonococci population—antibiotic sensitivity study. Sensitivities of 104 mixed strains of gonococci from Singapore—examined February–March 1970 at the W.H.O. Neisseria Centre Copenhagen (Dr. Alice Reyn) (reproduced from R. S. Morton, W.H.O./VDT/WPRO/70, 328)

Antibiotic	Method	Definition of resistance or lessened sensitivity	Sensitive	Moderately sensitive	Less sensitive	Resistant	% less sensitive or resistant	43 other Far East stains* % less sensitive or resistant
Penicillin	Plate dilution (four-fold dilution)	I.C.$_{50}$ 0·083 u/ml (0·053 mcg/ml) or less=less sensitive	14	—	90	—	87	90·7
Streptomycin	One plate 25 mcg/ml	I.C.$_{50}$ is 25 mcg/ml or more	33	—	—	71	70	79·1
Tetracycline	Plate dilution (four-fold dilution)	I.C.$_{50}$ is 1·13 mcg/ml or more	44	—	60	—	57	74·4
Spiramycin†	Plate dilution (four-fold dilution)	I.C.$_{50}$ is 1·13 mcg/ml or more	38	—	66	—	63	79·1
Rifampicin	Plate dilution (four-fold dilution)	I.C.$_{50}$ is 0·25 mcg/ml (arbitrary value)	41	—	63	—	60	Not done
Sulphathiazole	Disc diffusion	238 mcg/ml +++=sensitive ++=moderately sensitive +=less sensitive r=resistant	93	8	2	1	3	—
Chloramphenicol	Disc diffusion	50 mcg/ml	63	40	1	1	1	—
Kanamycin	Disc diffusion	50 mcg/ml	17	79	8	—	8	—
Nalidix acid	Disc diffusion	50 mcg/ml	104	—	—	—	Nil	—

* See Annex I 'Second W.P.R. Seminar on Venereal Disease', p. 57. Dr. Reyn of Copenhagen reports that Singapore strains are also marginally more sensitive than batch examined from Penang and Saigon.

† Erythomycin testing omitted as results known to correspond very closely to spiramycin findings.

There is a clear correlation between the above penicillin sensitivity determinations and the response/failure in the patients concerned.

It has now also become apparent that any schedule of treatment resulting in a failure rate of 5 per cent or more is a cause for concern. It should be reviewed as a matter of urgency.

The problem of classifying early recurrence after treatment is a perplexing one. Willcox (1964) has suggested that all recurrences in the first week after treatment should be arbitrarily classified as failure/relapse while those occurring after a week should be shown as re-infections. Hewitt (1969) discussed default from follow-up as a function of treatment. He suggested that defaulters should be included when estimating percentage failures.

Willcox (1970) gave a detailed survey of antibiotic therapy in South-east Asia. He listed the root causes of the problem of resistance. He included social and political turmoil, prostitution, poor contact-tracing, free sale of antibiotics, with self treatment and sub-curative dosage, and not least poor levels of diagnostic procedures. He saw gonorrhoea as likely to prove a costly burden to governments in South-east Asia if these problems failed to receive early attention.

Lee et al (1972) in the U.S.A. suggested topical prophylactics for females as a means of prevention of gonorrhoea. At the Second International V.D. Symposium in 1972, Greenberg of Ottawa reported on a trial of a preventive gonococcal vaccine. He claimed to be able to gain an antibody response in 90 per cent of those receiving three 1 ml injections at 14-day intervals. The vaccine was made using type 1 strains of gonococci (*Lancet*, 1972).

Penicillin—by mouth

The only oral penicillin which has been widely used in gonorrhoea has been the acid-resistant ampicillin. Although *in vitro* tests have shown it to be less active than benzyl penicillin against partially resistant strains, this has not been borne out by clinical experience. Willcox (1964) and Smith (1966) found it gave better results in treatment failures than did retreatment with procaine penicillin. Alergant (1965) working in Liverpool and using a single dose of 1 g claimed satisfactory results. Willcox (1964) working in London, used two doses of 1 g, each at 4–6 hours interval, and found it as good as 1·2 mega units of aqueous procaine penicillin in a single injection. Ampicillin has also been used in doses of 1 g orally, plus 600 000 units of aqueous procaine penicillin. intramuscularly. The failure rate was 3 per cent compared with 11·6 per cent when the same dose of procaine penicillin only was given (Alergant, 1965). All these treatments were completed at a single session and have advantages on all counts over divided dosage schedules lasting 36 hours (Marmell et al, 1964; Heineman and Vinikoff, 1965).

Gunderson et al (1969) contrasted a single 2 g dose of ampicillin given together with 1 g of probenecid, with a combination of injectable pencillins. He found the former superior. Groth and Hallquist (1970) had near identical results. All their strains were sensitive to 0·1 units of penicillin or less per ml. Eriksson (1970) in a well-designed trial used ampicillin in various dosage with and without probenecid, and also compared the results with those obtained using injectable penicillin. The best results were again obtained with ampicillin and probenecid. His percentage of less sensitive strains was 24·4. His trial included about 4 000 patients, both males and females. Kvale et al (1971) used a single dose of 3·5 g of ampicillin with probenecid in divided doses and had a 4 per cent failure rate. Bro-Jorgensen and Jensen (1971a) using 1 or 2 g of ampicillin with probenecid in 1 915 males and 921 females found only marginal differences in the failures between those with sensitive and those with less sensitive organisms. Those with less sensitive organisms comprised 30 per cent of the whole. Sullivan (1970), who treated 124 teenage girls with oral ampicillin in divided dosages, declared that such regimens were only useful in closed societies.

With its relative absence of side effects the single oral dose of ampicillin with probenecid has proved the most acceptable alternative to the single injection of penicillin.

Penicillin—by injection

Borring (1965) writing from Copenhagen found 23·2 per cent failures in 659 men treated for uncomplicated gonorrhoea with 300 000 units of aqueous procaine penicillin. The sensitivity levels of the organisms concerned matched the failures; nevertheless 55 patients were cured in spite of their organisms showing reduced sensitivity. On the strength of these observations 174 men were treated with 1·2 mega units of aqueous procaine penicillin combined with 1·0 mega units of sodium benzyl (crystalline) penicillin, daily for 3 days. There was 100 per cent cure rate. Krook and Juhlin (1965) using 900 000 units of aqueous procaine pencillin in Sweden had a 1·6 per cent failure rate in infections due to sensitive strains and a 56·3 per cent failure rate in infections caused by organisms with an I.C.^{50} of 0·5–2·5 i.u. per ml. Combined injection therapy, using 1·2 mega units of aqueous procaine penicillin with 1 mega unit of sodium benzyl penicillin, on one occasion gave a failure rate of 8·3 per cent. The authors expressed the view that to be effective the concentration of penicillin in whole blood should be at least 10 times the I.C.^{50} value of the strain concerned.

Lomholt and Berg (1966) working in Greenland found an overall failure rate to two penicillin schedules to be 28 per cent. One schedule employed a single injection of 600 000 units sodium benzyl penicillin, 600 000 units aqueous procaine penicillin and 1·2 mega units of benzathine penicillin. The other schedule employed a single injection of 1·2 mega units of aqueous procaine penicillin daily for 3 days. Penicillin sensitivity testing of 152 strains showed that 47 per cent of them were in the relatively resistant range. (There was complete resistance to streptomycin in 15 per cent and 9 per cent showed reduced sensitivity to tetracycline.) The authors believed that the 'tail' of low blood levels caused by the benzathine penicillin in the first schedule was dangerous, as it had promoted resistance in the organisms remaining in the uncured. On the strength of this combined therapeutic and laboratory evaluation, they treated 228 males and females with a single injection of 5 mega units of sodium benzyl (crystalline—water soluble) penicillin given intramuscularly in 8 ml of 0·5 per cent lignocaine (lidnocaine). The injection was preceded by half an hour with 1 g of probenecid orally. There was only one failure. Schmidt and Roholt (1965) first reported the use of this schedule and noted that it gave adequate blood levels for 8 hours, that is, sufficient to kill the most resistant strains then reported. Juhlin (1965) reported that 1·2 mega units of aqueous procaine penicillin combined with 1 mega unit of benzyl penicillin gave serum concentrations sufficient to cure infections due to strains with an I.C.[50] of 1·2–2·2 i.u. per ml.

Gjessing and Ödegaard (1966) compared penicillin alone and in combination with other antibiotics. In the first group of 500 men, 169 were infected with less sensitive strains and 50 of these (29·6 per cent) failed to respond to 600 000 units of aqueous procaine penicillin. In the second group of 500 men, 207 were infected with less sensitive strains and 15 (7 per cent) failed to respond to the same dosage of penicillin plus 1 g of ampicillin given orally at the same time. In a third group of 500 men, 256 were infected with less sensitive strains and 13 (5·1 per cent) failed to respond to the same dosage of penicillin by injection plus 0·5 or 0·75 g of chloramphenicol.

Wray (1965) looked for other causes of failure besides growing resistance. She noted that when the duration of symptoms and signs in men, at the time of treatment, was more than 6 or 7 days, that is by the time the posterior urethra became involved, the chances of failure doubled irrespective of the sensitivity of the organism. She expressed the view that such cases should receive double the routine dosage. The incidence of post-gonococcal non-specific urethritis was much the same in the failures as in the successes.

It is, however, the problems of development, measurement, control and reversal of resistance which pervade the literature in the second half of the 1960s. Thus Smith and Levey (1967) in Australia found 44 per cent of 104 strains to be relatively resistant. They attributed this development to inadequate dosage and inappropriate forms of penicillin. They expressed a preference for multiple dosage schedules using benzyl penicillin. Amies (1967) in Canada, reviewing a period of 8 years found 27 per cent of strains resistant to 0·3 units of penicillin per ml and 8 per cent to 1·0 units per ml. Such strains he judged to need 2·8 mega units of aqueous procaine penicillin for inhibition. Chako and Yogeswari (1966) writing from India report that in 1963–64 no less than 45·6 per cent of strains required more than 0·05 units per ml while in 1964–65 the percentage was 60·4. The response rate to treatment corresponded. They found a positive relationship of growing resistance between penicillin, streptomycin and chloramphenicol.

Ödegaard and Gjessing (1967) noted that growing resistance ceased in Greenland after the introduction of the 5 mega unit regimen (*vide supra*) and that since then better results have been obtained using streptomycin.

Warren (1968) writing from Southampton showed a significantly higher incidence of partially resistant strains isolated from patients infected abroad. Such patients he argued should be considered candidates for higher dosage than that used in the endogenously infected.

Holmes et al (1967) writing from the Far East showed that of 63 men treated with a single injection of 2·4 mega units of aqueous procaine penicillin, 18 (29 per cent) failed to respond. Of 14 of these failures treated with 4·8 mega units, three failed. Of 41 strains isolated and tested, 26 (63 per cent) were in the relative resistant range as defined by the author. In view of these findings the 2·4 mega regime was preceded by 1 g of probenecid and followed by 0·5 g of the drug at 6, 12 and 18 hours. There was only one clinical failure in the group so treated, although 77 per cent of the strain in the series were in the relatively resistant range.

The results of three penicillin regimens employed in London contrasts with this. Nicol et al (1968) found 37·3 per cent of 91 strains tested to be in the partially resistant range. Ten of these were among the 13 (14·2 per cent) clinical failures following 600 000 aqueous procaine penicillin. Morrison et al (1968) found an 8·5 per cent failure rate in the same area using 1·2 mega aqueous procaine penicillin and 5·8 per cent failures using 2·4 mega units of the same preparation. Leigh et al (1969) reported on the penicillin sensitivity of the strains dealt with at St. Mary's Hospital, London. Such dosages as these, used in London, are modest, compared with those in use in some parts of the world where on account of sheer bulk and consistency, dosages must be reaching the limits of injectability and acceptability. The advent of probenecid seems to offer a welcome extension to the useful life of the 'one-shot' penicillin regimen in gonorrhoea.

One of the most significant papers of 1969 was the report by Olsen and Lomholt (1969) from Greenland where the gonorrhoea morbidity rate was 10 000/100 000 population per annum. In 1963 some 80 per cent of local strains were showing reduced sensitivity. Failure rates with schedules then in use were running at 27 per cent. Improvement in both aspects had occurred due to re-thinking. An attempt was made to capitalise on this and to measure the improved cure rate and epidemiological advantage of using a "one shot" treatment regimen of 5 mega units of benzyl penicillin in 8 ml of 0·5 per cent lignocaine preceded by probenecid 1 g. A cure rate of 99 per cent was effected. At the beginning of the trial, which lasted nearly 2 years and involved 832 infected patients, 56 per cent of the gonococcal strains were showing reduced sensitivity. At the end of the trial only 19 per cent were in this category. The potential of this thinking and practice, for control of the deteriorating situation in the Western Pacific, was pressed in all its detail at the W.H.O. V.D. Control Seminar held in Manila in December 1968. The schedule mentioned is amongst the most effective control tools available.

Reyn (1969) in a review of sensitivity patterns in the Far East and South-east Asia noted that whereas in 1961 some 61 per cent of strains were less sensitive to penicillin this had deteriorated by 1967–68 to 90 per cent. Cross resistance was developing to a wide range of antibiotics. Alice Reyn contrasts this with evidence of some reversion of a similar trend in Northern Europe (vide supra, Olsen and Lomholt). She believed the improvement due to employment of more adequate dosage schedules. Similar responses to early warnings are indicated more widely than ever before.

Attempts have been successfully made elsewhere in the world. Maurer and Schneider (1969) reduced their 25 per cent failure rate with 2·4 mega units of aqueous procaine penicillin to 7·6 per cent by preceding the injection with probenecid orally. Lynn et al (1970), dealing with a gonococcal population where 35·1–37·3 per cent of strains were partially resistant, halved their failure rate to 6·2 per cent by increasing the procaine penicillin dosage from 600 000 units to 2·5 million units. Platts (1970a) in New Zealand had a 95 per cent cure rate with combined or fortified penicillin, ie 1 mega unit of benzyl plus 1·2 mega units of procaine.

The British Co-operative Clinical Group (1971) reviewed the treatment practices in 206 clinics run by 107 venereologists. Penicillin was the drug of first choice in all but two clinics. It was used alone in nearly 80 per cent. In the remainder it was reinforced by probenecid. Aqueous procaine penicillin, most popularly in doses of 1·2 mega units, was used by 54 per cent of venereologists while 44 per cent used it fortified by benzyl penicillin. Hilton (1971) who was one of the first to recommend and use probenecid, treated infected males with 1·2 mega units of penicillin aluminium monosterorate plus probenecid in divided doses from 1964–66 and had a failure rate of 2·1 per cent. From 1966–69 he used 1·2 mega units of aqueous procaine penicillin followed by 2·0 g of probenicid in four 6-hourly doses with a 6·8 per cent failure rate. He showed a relationship between failure and sensitivity. In the early part of the study 18·1 per cent of his strains were in the less sensitive range whereas later 31·7 per cent were so classified.

There is little in the literature regarding penicillin in complicated gonorrhoea. Bjornberg (1970) treated 36 cases of benign gonococcal sepsis (septicaemia) with 1 mega unit of benzyl penicillin plus 1·2 mega units of aqueous procaine penicillin daily from 5–7 days and claimed cure in all. Thatcher and Pettit (1971) recommended systemic and local pencillin for infantile gonococcal conjunctivitis. Bro-Jorgensen and Jensen (1971a) treated 921 females, of whom 37 per cent had rectal involvement, with ampicillin and probenecid and found the cure rate identical with the response rate in those without proctitis. Of all their strains 30 per cent were in the less sensitive range. Ericsson (1971a) found a fortified injectable penicillin (ie procaine with benzyl) less effective in rectal gonorrhoea than ampicillin. Between 23 and 27 per cent of his strains were in the less sensitive range. In a further paper (Ericsson 1971b), the serum levels obtained with ampicillin and probenecid were discussed in relation to the sensitivity of the strains. Bro-Jorgensen and Jensen (1971b), treating 13 men with gonococcal tonsillitis with ampicillin and probenecid, found five failures; although concomitant genito-urinary infection cleared. With Hallgren (1971) two cases of gonococcal tonsillitis failed to respond to ampicillin with probenecid but each was cured by a tetracycline, 250 mg, 6-hourly for 7 days.

Statham and Morton (1968) reported on seven women with endocervical gonorrhoea. All were wearing an intra-uterine contraceptive device (I.U.C.D.). Three had salpingitis, one developing it in spite of routine treatment. They recommended that in the presence of gonococcal infection the I.U.C.D. should be viewed as a foreign body and be removed before starting antibiotic treatment.

Cornelius et al (1971) found in eight patients an eight-fold variation in pencillin serum concentration after 2·4 mega units of aqueous procaine penicillin. They found average and peak concentrations to be higher in patients taking probenecid; but declared that biological variation in absorbing rates tend to mask its effect. They studied four groups of patients with 11 in each group and used 2·4 and 4·8 mega units of procaine penicillin with and without probenecid. Silver and Darling (1971) in north-west England found 50 per cent of the strains in the relatively resistant range, many of them in immigrants and locally born females under 21 years. These groups are known to form sexual liaisons. Failure and relapse could be correlated with relative resistance. The authors were thus able to correlate clinical, sociological and laboratory data on the emergence of resistance and consider these in terms of their control programme. Nielsen (1970) found no difference in sensitivity of organisms isolated from prostitutes and all others.

Nelson (1971) had failure rates of 8·2 per cent in 194 and 2·1 per cent in 140 in groups treated with single doses of 2·4 and 4·8 mega units of procaine penicillin.

Woodcock (1971) reappraised the effect of treatment on incubating syphilis. He used four approaches. His series was small. He comes to the tentative conclusion that penicillin used in gonorrhoea is more likely to cure syphilis than mask it.

A series of semi-synthetic penicillin compounds, which hydrolyse *in vivo* to form ampicillin, have been found to be no more efficacious than ampicillin itself. Amoxycillin (1-amino-*p*-hydroxy-benzyl penicillin) was used by Willcox (1972) in 281 males with gonorrhoea. Single 2 g doses gave a 9·5 per cent failure rate. This was not improved when the drug was given with probenecid. Smaller doses were less efficient and double dosage with 1·5 g per dose was only marginally superior. Amoxycillin therefore offers no advantages over ampicillin. Another derivative, pro-ampicillin hydrochloride was tried by Forström and Lassus (1972) with similar results. Alergant (1973) combined 1 g of amoxycillin orally with 1·2 mega units of aqueous procaine penicillin to gain a 99 per cent cure rate.

Streptomycin

The problem with this antibiotic in gonorrhoea has been the emergence of absolute resistance over nearly 30 years. In the first 20 years or so it rose to 25 per cent of strains in Denmark (Reyn, 1963). Since that time there have been reports from elsewhere such as 12 per cent in Sweden (Gastrin and Kallings, 1964); 12–16 per cent in Canada (Snell et al., 1963); 50 per cent in Turkey (Ang and Oner, 1965) and 15 per cent in Greenland (Lomholt and Berg, 1966). Some of these writers noted that many streptomycin-resistant strains were relatively resistant to penicillin. The average figure is about 50 per cent. The drug has fallen into disfavour as the second choice for gonorrhoea and few recent reports on its activity have been published.

Borring (1965) in Denmark treated 105 men with 1 g streptomycin hydrochloride daily for 3 days with a 79·8 per cent cure rate. There was a 95 per cent correlation between this and sensitivity (Reyn et al, 1969). Spitzer and Willcox (1968) and Evans (1966) have shown that the failure rate in male cases treated with a single injection of 1·0 g of streptomycin in London had changed steadily from 8·5 per cent in 1951 to 31·7 per cent in 1966. Arya and Phillips (1970) reporting from Uganda noted that diminished penicillin sensitivity was almost always associated with complete resistance to streptomycin and diminished resistance to tetracycline. The findings correlated with treatment failure rates. There have been similar cross-resistance reports from the Far East *eg* Morton (1970) in Singapore (see Table V).

Kanamycin

This antibiotic is effective and injectable. It has been available for over 10 years, and is generally used in a single 1 g regimen with excellent results (Wilkinson et al, 1967). Single injections of 2 g have been free from side effects. In one London series (Csonka and Murray, 1967), 31 cases were treated with no failures. In another (Hooton and Nicol, 1967), 186 patients were treated with six failures. McGill et al (1969) treated 100 women with 2 g, with between 5 and 9 per cent failures. Farrell (1969) secured a cure rate around 95 per cent. Fluker and Hewitt (1970) used a single 2 g regimen in 100 men with rectal gonorrhoea, and had 15·5 per cent failures as compared with 3 per cent in 35 males with gonorrhoeal urethritis. They suggested that a high diffusion gradient existed between blood stream and rectum. Their results in rectal cases compared with a 27·1 per cent failure rate using 1·8 mega units of aqueous procaine penicillin. Shapiro and Lentz (1970) in a series of 836 females had a cure rate of 91 per cent.

Garrod and Waterworth (1968) studying the combined action of drugs noted an additive effect with kanamycin and penicillin and kanamycin and sulphafurazole.

Kanamycin has therefore largely replaced streptomycin for patients sensitive to penicillin or in those where syphilis is suspected.

In view of its likeness to streptomycin the development of resistance is a possibility.

Spectinomycin (Actinospectacin, Trobicin)

This treponicidal antibiotic has been available since 1961. It has usually been given in a single injection. Tiedeman et al (1965) had a cure rate in excess of 90 per cent using 1·6 g. It has proved to be useful in cases of penicillin failure according to Willcox (1966).

Cornelius and Domesck (1970) treated 108 males and 28 females with 2 g of spectinomycin hydrochloride with 100 per cent cures. A 4 g regimen in 70 women gave only 95 per cent cures. Excellent results have been claimed by Platts (1970b) and Sadi and Maluli (1971). Reyn et al (1973) gave 2 g to 61 males and 4 g to 52 females. Of the 109 followed up only one failed to respond. The I.C.[50] values ranged from 2·2 to 12·6 μg/ml. Repeated isolates from the failure showed the organism to have resistance to more than 480 μg/ml of spectinomycin, yet be sensitive to penicillin, streptomycin and tetracycline. The authors see spectinomycin as a valuable alternative to penicillin.

Holder et al (1972) used the drug in 15 men with gonococcal proctitis. A single dose of 4 g cured 13.

Pederson et al (1972) reported trials with schedules of 2 g and 4 g of spectinomycin hydrochloride. Cure rates in men were 100 per cent and 96·6 per cent; and in women 95·7 per cent and 95·3 per cent respectively. The results were significantly better than those obtained with 2·4 and 4·8 mega units of aqueous procaine penicillin. Sensitivity studies were carried out. A similar study was reported by Duncan et al

(1972). Stratigos et al (1973) reported from Greece that a single 2 g dose gave excellent results. All 70 strains tested were inhibited by 30 μg discs. This is equivalent to a readily obtained blood concentration.

The tetracyclines

After the penicillins and streptomycin, drugs of this group have been the most widely used in gonorrhoea. Resistance has emerged but is partial only. Reyn (1963) studied 82 streptomycin-resistant strains and found 54 of them partially resistant to tetracycline. Thayer et al (1964) noted less sensitive strains in the U.S.A. while in Turkey, Ang and Oner (1965) gave the percentage of tetracycline resistant strains as 32·8. Lomholt and Berg (1966) reported 9 per cent from Greenland. The emergence of resistant strains means that misdiagnosing gonococcal urethritis as non-specific urethritis may come to light if the drug of choice used is a tetracycline given, say, as 250 mg, 6-hourly for 4 or 5 days.

Single or divided oral dosage regimens of several tetracyclines have been employed since the late 1940s. Cure rates have usually exceeded 80 per cent and have been as high as 97 per cent. Varying results have been reported using the newer tetracycline, demethylchlortetracycline or ledermycin. Vanderstoep et al (1964) had 11 per cent failures. Using a single oral dose of 1·2 g Willcox (1968) had 13 per cent failures. Using divided doses over several days Sokoloff (1965) claimed 100 per cent cures. Morton and Higson (1966) reported 14 per cent failures using methacycline or rondomycin in divided doses over 3 days. The sensitivity of organisms to both methacycline and penicillin was measured in this series. Enfors and Molin (1970) used 1·2 g in a single dose in 200 females with a cure rate of 77·8 per cent. Where rectal infection was present the cure rate was only 58·8 per cent. The results were much poorer than those in a control group treated with fortified penicillin. Bartunek (1971) had similar results in a series of female patients.

Smithurst (1970) used 5 and 10 g schedules of tetracycline over 5 days with a cure rate of 94·7 per cent, a response which matched that obtained in his area by 2·4 mega units of aqueous procaine penicillin preceded by probenecid. Johnson et al (1970) also reported on three regimes of tetracycline and compared their results with those obtained with penicillin plus probenecid and with a large single dose of ampicillin.

McLone et al (1968) treated 100 men with a single 1·5 g dose of tetracycline hydrochloride (sigmamycin). There were two failures out of 62 patients completing follow-up.

Willcox (1971) gave two doses each of 1·2 g of deteclo—a triple tetracycline compound. He had a failure rate of 9·6 per cent in the 89 patients who were followed up.

Mutchnick (1972) in the U.S.A. gave a single dose of 300 mg of doxycycline monohydrate (vibramycin) to 50 servicemen with gonorrhoea. The cure rate was under 80 per cent. According to Petzoldt (1972), doxycycline given to syphilitic rabbits, in doses to produce serum levels equivalent to those obtained after 300 mg in the human, does not mask syphilis. Baytch and Rankin (1971) had poor results with doxycycline. Lassus (1968) reported two single dose schedules of doxycycline 200 mg and 300 mg. The failure rates were 14 and 6 per cent respectively. Two of the nine failures had organisms with diminished sensitivity. Grey et al (1970) had a 12·7 per cent failure rate with 300 mg. Liden et al (1971) using the same dose had a 2·4 per cent failure rate in a group of 250 men and women. Masterton and Schofield (1971) and Moffett et al (1972) using the same single 300 mg dose had a failure rate of 6·4 and 5·5 per cent in males and females in Glasgow.

Erythromycin

Lyng (1963), like others in the 1950s, had only 65 per cent cure rates using 1·5 g in six divided doses. Martini et al (1968) using a single 2·5 g dose of erythromycin stearate claimed a cure rate of 91·5 per cent. Reyn and Bentzon (1969), reviewing the development of growing resistance and cross resistance, noted a worsening situation in regard to erythromycin. Smith and Osick (1969) using three regimens had cure rates varying from 52–72 per cent. In India, Moses et al (1971) found 50 per cent of 216 strains to have reduced sensitivity to erythromycin. These findings correlated with clinical failure to respond to the drug in 80–90 per cent of cases.

Chloramphenicol

Earlier reports of blood dyscrasias due to this antibiotic have discouraged its use in gonorrhoea in which condition it gave good results. As chloromycetin succinate in an injectable preparation of 1 g it gave a 95 per cent cure rate (Willcox, 1963). As a less effective synthetic—thiamphenicol—it has also proved useful (Riboldi, 1966).

Reyn and Bentzon (1968) noted growing resistance to chloramphenicol but this was not found by Bergman and Tarnvik (1970).

Spiramycin (Rovamycin)

Up to the early 1960s this drug had given good results in a single 4 g oral dose in London. In a single 2·5 g dose in France it gave a cure rate of 97·4 per cent. Clarke (1964) and Schmidt et al (1965) however averaged a 17 per cent failure rate. There was no correlation in this last trial between *in vitro* susceptibility to spiramycin and the failures. Heinke et al (1969) using a single dose of 2·5 g in 135 patients fared no better but by giving two doses at a 3-hour interval they secured a 94·8 per cent cure rate in 117 men and women.

In Czechoslovakia quantitative sensitivity tests on 321 strains seen during 1966, 1967 and 1968 were carried out using 10 antibacterials. Only small percentages were found to show any degree of resistance to spiramycin, erythromycin or tetracycline (Hejzlar et al, 1968).

Co-trimoxazole (Bactrim, Septrin)

This drug is a combination of trimethoprim and sulphamethoxazole; the first is a blocker of bacterial folic acid metabolism and the second a sulphonamide. The combination has a wider spectrum than the sulphonamides only and it is bactericidal. These points were shown by Csonka and Knight (1967). Sulphonamides alone (sulphatriad) cured between 31 and 33 per cent, whereas the new combination cured 89 to 93 per cent. Carrol and Nicol (1970) gave 400 mg daily for 5 days to 136 men and 51 women with cure rates of 95·5 and 93 per cent respectively in those attending for follow-up. Arya et al (1970) in Uganda increased their cure rate from 65 per cent on a 12-hour schedule to 96 per cent on a 48-hour schedule.

Philips et al (1970) reported on sensitivity to co-trimoxazole and compared the findings with 11 other antibacterials. Waugh (1971) had a 12·1 per cent failure rate with a 7-day course, the tablets being taken 12-hourly. Evans et al (1972) using a similar schedule, had an 18 per cent failure rate in a series of 101 men. Almost all the strains concerned with failure were relatively resistant to penicillin and completely resistant to streptomycin. Rodin and Seth (1972) used the drug in a variety of schedules and compared the overall recurrence rate (6·7 per cent), with that obtained using 1·2 mega units of aqueous procaine penicillin (8·8 per cent), and the same plus 2 g of probenecid (1·9 per cent). The recurrence rates are those pertaining at the end of one week's follow-up.

Svindland (1973) pointed out that co-trimoxazole had a special place in the treatment of seafarers with gonorrhoea, who may well have been exposed to syphilis also.

Cephalosporins

These antibiotics are similar in structure and action to penicillin. They have a spectrum-like ampicillin and are relatively resistant to a staphylococcal penicillinase. Cephaloridine (ceporin) must be given by injection but oral preparations, such as cephalexin capsules and tablets (ceporex, keflex), are available.

Oller (1967) using injections of 1 g and 2 g in two groups of men with gonorrhoea had 15·3 per cent failures in the first group of 72 and 5·2 per cent failures in the second of 116. McLone et al (1968) gave a single 2 g injection to 85 women. Of the 58 attending for follow-up eight (14 per cent) failed to respond. Jouhar and Fowler (1968) using a similar schedule in 234 women had a cure rate of 93·6 per cent. Keys et al (1969) in a series of 97 males cured 84 per cent with 2 g. This study was carried out in the U.S. Navy in the Far East. The authors compared their results unfavourably with those obtained using penicillin, ampicillin, and kanamycin. Pariser and Marino (1970), amongst other findings, had five patients who responded to 2 g of cephaloridine intramuscularly after failure with 4·8 mega units of aqueous procaine penicillin. Willcox (1971) tried the oral preparation cephalexin. He gave 2 g and after 6 hours a further 2 g. Of 102 patients 82 were followed with a 14·6 per cent failure rate. Ackman and Reid (1972) used cephalexin with much the same results.

Cave et al (1970) studied sensitivity and compared the results obtained with cephalosporin with the levels found with other anti-bacterials.

Rifampicin (Rifadin, Rimactone)

This bactericidal drug, which is effective by mouth, acts by interfering with bacterial nucleic acid metabolism. It may interfere with bilirubin clearance. Thrombo-cytopenia has been reported in association with prolonged use. The main indication for use has been tuberculosis.

Cobbold et al (1968) gave a single 900 mg dose of rifampicin to 103 men with gonorrhoea. They had a failure rate of 11·2 per cent in 89 attending for follow-up. Blood level concentrations at 2 and 24 hours were 27·2 and 1·64 mg/ml. The M.I.C. required was 0·02 mg/ml. Steenbergen (1971), using the same dosage in 50 men, had four failures. Panduro (1971), using the same schedule, had 13 per cent failures in men and 9 per cent in women. Malmborg et al (1971), with similar results, reported some gonococci partially and others completely resistant to rifampicin. Hopsu-Havu and Helander (1972), who had 15 per cent failures, noted that the drug had no treponicidal activity.

Arya et al (1971), reporting from Uganda, were concerned about the antibiotic inducing resistance in the tubercle bacillus.

Miscellaneous

Gentamicin sulphate (Sulmycin), in a single injection of 5 mg per kg body weight, was given to 62 patients with gonorrhoea with a 94 per cent success rate. Serum levels determined in five patients were well above M.I.C. values in 158 strains tested. Gentamicin is not treponicidal. Hantscheke and Mauss (1970) gave two doses each of 80 mg to 23 patients with satisfactory results.

Greenberg et al (1971), writing from Canada, gave preliminary results of the use of a preventive gonococcal vaccine. Kellog type 1 colonies were killed with thiomersol and left for partial autolysis to take place. Fifty-four volunteers were inoculated weekly for 3 weeks, after which their serum was tested for antibodies by bentonite flocculation and tissue culture inhibition. Of 43 subjects, orginally found to have flocculation tests negative, 31 developed rising antibody titres. In all but one the rise in titre was two-fold. Thirty-two of the 36 patients in whom the test was initially negative developed inhibitory antibodies. The results of the two tests failed to correlate but the authors claim that the clear development of antibody warrants trials of the prophylactic value of the method.

Willcox (1972) reconsidered the case for epidemiological or abortive treatment. He points out that the practice is not unusual in trichomoniasis and in non-gonococcal urethritis and he commends it for use in female contacts of gonorrhoea where smear results are negative. He makes it clear that indiscriminate treatment without adequate clinical and bacteriological examination is not advocated. Willcox sees epidemiological treatment, when used selectively, as a useful control tool.

Coda

There is no doubt that the geography of antibacterial resistance in gonorrhoea requires study to the point where confident early warning of the spread of resistant strains can be issued with regularity. The use of such reports should make for more scientific use of antibiotics. The regular monitoring involved calls for more than the one existing W.H.O.-approved gonorrhoea reference laboratory. This kind of lead appears to be an essential prerequisite if the unique part which modern therapy can play in gonorrhoea control is to reach its full potential, worldwide.

REFERENCES

ACKMAN, C. F. D. and REID, E. C. (1972). Canad. med. Ass. J., 106, 350.
ALERGANT, C. D. (1965). Proceedings of Symposium, Ciba.
ALERGANT, C. D. (1973). Brit. J. vener. Dis., 49, 274.
AMIES, C. R. (1967). Canad. med. Ass. J., 96, 33.
ANG, G. and ONER, A. (1965). Istanbul Univ. Tip. Fak. Med., 28, 251.
ARYA, O. P. and PHILLIPS, I. (1970). Brit. J. vener. Dis., 46, 149.
ARYA, O. P., PEARSON, C. H., RAO, S. K. and BLOWERS, R. (1970). Brit. J. vener. Dis. 46, 214.
ARYA, O. P., RAO, S. K. and NNOCHIRI, E. (1971). Brit. J. vener. Dis., 47, 184.
BARTUNEK, J. (1971). Med. Welt., 22, 504.
BAYTCH, H. and RANKIN, D. W. (1971). Brit. J. vener. Dis., 48, 129.
BERGMAN, S. and TARNVIK, A. (1970). Acta derm.-venereol., Stockh., 50, 317.
BJORNBERG, A. (1970). Acta derm.-venereol., Stockh., 50, 313.
BORRING, J. (1965). Brit. J. vener. Dis., 41, 193.
BRITISH CO-OPERATIVE CLINICAL GROUP (1971). Brit. J. vener. Dis., 47, 17.
BRO-JORGENSON, A. and JENSEN, T. (1971a). Brit. J. vener. Dis., 47, 443.

BRO-JORGENSON, A. and JENSEN, T. (1971b). *Brit. J. vener. Dis.*, **47**, 660.
CARROLL, B. R. T. and NICOL, C. S. (1970). *Brit. J. vener. Dis.*, **46**, 31.
CAVE, V. G., HURDLE, E. S. and CATELLI, A. R. (1970). *N.Y. J. Med.*, **70**, 844.
CHAKO, C. W. and YOGESWARI, L. (1966). *Indian J. med. Res.*, **54**, 823.
CLARKE, G. H. V. (1964). *Brit. J. vener. Dis.*, **40**, 122.
COBBOLD, R. I., MORRISON, G. D. and WILLCOX, R. R. (1968). *Brit. med., J.* **4**, 681.
CORNELIUS, C. E. III and DOMESCK, G. (1970). *Brit. J. vener. Dis.*, **46**, 212.
CORNELIUS, C. E. III, SCHROETER, A. L., LESTER, A. and MARTIN, J. E. JR. (1971). *Brit. J. vener. Dis.*, **47**, 359.
CSONKA, G. W. and MURRAY, M. (1967). *Postgrad. med. J. Suppl.*, 123.
CSONKA, G. W. and KNIGHT, G. T. (1967). *Brit. J. vener. Dis.*, **43**, 161.
DUNCAN, W. C., HOLDER, W. C. and KNOX, J. M. (1972). *Anti-microbiol. Agents Chemother.*, **1**, 210.
ERIKSSON, G. (1971a). *Acta derm-venereol., Stockh.*, **51**, 305.
ERIKSSON, G. (1971b). *Acta derm.-venereol., Stockh.*, **51**, 467.
ERIKSSON, G. (1970). *Acta derm-venereol. Stockh.*, **54**, 451.
ENFORS, W. and MOLIN, L. (1970). *Brit. J. vener. Dis.*, **46**, 209.
EVANS, A. J. (1966). *Brit. J. vener. Dis.*, **42**, 251.
EVANS, A. J., LUCAS, G. T. and HUMAN, R. P. (1972). *Brit. J. vener. Dis.*, **48**, 179.
FARRELL, I. (1969). *Brit. J. vener. Dis.*, **45**, 232.
FLUKER, J. L. and HEWITT, A. B. (1970). *Brit. J. vener. Dis.*, **46**, 454.
FOSTRÖM, L. and LASSUS, A. (1972). *Brit. J. vener. Dis.*, **48**, 510.
GARROD, L. D. and WATERWORTH, P. M. (1968). *Brit. J. vener. Dis.*, **44**, 75.
GASTRIN, B. and KALLINGS, L. O. (1964). *Acta derm.-venereol., Stockh.*, **44**, 286.
GJESSING, H. C. and ÖDEGAARD, K. (1966). *Brit. J, vener. Dis.*, **42**, 107.
GREENBERG, L., DIENNA, B. B., KENNY, C. P. and ZNAMIROWSKI, R. (1971). *Bull. W.H.O.*, **45**, 531.
GREY, R. C. F., PHILIPS, I. and NICOL, C. S. (1970). *Brit. J. vener. Dis.*, **46**, 401.
GROTH, O. and HALLQUIST, L. (1970). *Brit. J. vener. Dis.*, **46**, 21.
GUNDERSON, T., ÖDEGAARD, K. and GJESSING, H. C. (1969). *Brit. J. vener. Dis.*, **45**, 235.
HALLGREN, L. (1971). *Svenska Läk. Tiden.*, **68**, 569.
HANTSCHKE, D. and MAUSS, J. (1970). *Z. Haut-n. Gesch.-Kv.*, **15**, 407.
HEINEMAN, S. and VIMIKOF, R. (1965). *Med. Times.*, **93**, 290.
HEINKE, E., SCHALLER, K. F. and SCHIRREN, H. (1969). *Dtsch. med. Wschr.*, **94**, 1182.
HEJZLAR, M., VYMOLA, F., SEDMIDUBSKY, V., HEJKOVA, L. and WEBERSCHINKE, J. (1968). *Cesk. Derm.*, **43**, 179.
HEWITT, A. B. (1969). *Brit. J. vener. Dis.*, **45**, 40.
HILTON, A. L. (1971). *Brit. J. vener. Dis.*, **47**, 107.
HOLDER, W. R., ROBERTS, D. P., DUNCAN, W. C. and KNOX, J. M. (1972). *Brit. J. vener. Dis.*, **48**, 274.
HOLMES, K. K., JOHNSON, W. D. and LLOYD, T. M. (1967). *J. Amer. med. Ass.*, **202**, 461.
HOOTON, W. E. and NICOL, C. S. (1967). *Postgrad. med. J.*, **43**, Suppl. 68.
HOPSU-HAVU, V. K. and HELANDER, I. (1972). *Z. Haut. Gesch.-Kv.*, **47**, 441.
JOHNSON, D. W., KVALE, D. A., AFABLE, V. L., STEWART, S. D., HULVERSON, C. W. and HOLMES, K. K. (1970). *New Engl. J. Med.*, **283**, 1.
JOUHAR, A. J. and FOWLER, W. (1968). *Brit. J. vener. Dis.*, **44**, 223.
JUHLIN, L. (1965). *Acta derm.-venereol., Stockh.*, **45**, 231.
KEYS, T. F., HALVERSON, C. W. and CLARKE, E. J. JR. (1969). *J. Amer. med. Ass.*, **210**, 857.
KROOK, G. and JUHLIN, L. (1965). *Acta derm.-venereol., Stockh.*, **45**, 242.
KVALE, P. A., KEYS, T. F., JOHNSON, D. W. and HOLMES, K. K. (1971). *J. Amer. med. Ass.*, **215**, 1449.
LANCET, (1972). Editorial, **1**, 1109.

LASSUS, A. (1968). *Chemotherapy*, **13**, 366.

LEE, T. Y., UTIDJIAN, H. M. D., SINGH, B., CARPENTER, U. and CUTLER, J. C. (1972). *Brit. J. vener. Dis.*, **48**, 376.

LEIGH, D. A., LE FRANC, J. and TURNBULL, A. R (1969). *Brit. J. vener. Dis.*, **45**, 151.

LEJMAN, K., KOWARZ-SOKOLOWSKA, H., STADIŃSKI, A. and STARZYCKI, Z. (1965). *Przegl. derm.*, **52**, 105.

LIDEN, S., HAMMAR, H., HILLSTRÖM, L., WALLIN, J. and OHMAN, S. (1971). *Acta Derm.-venereol., Stockh.*, **51**, 221.

LOMHOLT, G. and BERG, O. (1966). *Brit. J. vener. Dis.*, **42**, 1.

LYNG, R. (1963). *Brit. J. vener. Dis.*, **39**, 236.

LYNN, R., NICOL, C. S., RIDLEY, M., RIMMER, D., SYMONDS, M. A. E. and WARREN, C. (1970). *Brit. J. vener. Dis.*, **46**, 404.

MALMBORG, A. S., MOLIN, L. and NYSTRÖM, B. (1971). *Chemotherapy*, **16**, 319.

MARMELL, M., JILLS, J.R., BROCON, C.D. and PRIGOT, A. (1964). *N.Y.J. Med.*, **64**, 985.

MARTINI, J., HALABI, J. and BORGONO, J. M. (1968). *Rev. med., Chile*, **96**, 525.

MASTERTON, G. and SCHOFIELD, C. B. S. (1971). *Brit. J. vener. Dis.*, **48**, 121.

MAURER, H. and SCHNEIDER, T. J. (1969). *J. Amer. med. Ass.*, **207**, 946.

McGILL, M. I., MOFFETT, M., MASTERTON, G. and SCHOFIELD, C. B. S. (1969). *Scot. med. J.*, **14**, 176.

McLONE, D. G., SCOTT, A. T., MACKEY, D. M. and HACKNEY, J. F., (1968). *Brit. J. vener. Dis.*, **44**, 218.

MOFFETT, M., McGILL, M. I., MASTERTON, G. and SCHOFIELD, C. B. S. (1972). *Brit. J. vener. Dis.*, **48**, 126.

MORRISON, D. G., COBBOLD, R. J. C., BOR, S., SPITZER, R. J., FOSTER, D. N. and WILLCOX, R. R. (1968). *Brit. J. vener. Dis.*, **44**, 319.

MORTON, R. S. and HIGSON, D. W. (1966). *Brit. J. vener. Dis.*, **42**, 175.

MORTON, R. S. (1970). W.H.O./WPRO/328/70 Assignment Report, Singapore 0012.

MOSES, J. M., DESAI, M. S., BHOSLE, C. B. and TRASI, M. S. (1971). *Brit. J. vener. Dis.*, **47**, 273.

MUTCHNICK, M. G. (1972). *Brit. J. vener. Dis.*, **48**, 381.

NELSON, M. (1971). *H.M.S.H.A. Hlth. Rep.*, **86**, 285.

NICOL, C. S., RIDLEY, M. and SYMONDS, M. A. E. (1968). *Brit. J. vener. Dis.*, **44**, 315.

NIELSEN, R. (1970). *Brit. J. vener. Dis.*, **46**, 153.

ÖDEGAARD, K. and GJESSING, H. C. (1967). *Brit. J. vener. Dis.*, **43**, 284.

OLLER, L. Z. (1967). *Brit. J. vener. Dis.*, **43**, 39.

OLSEN, G. A. and LOMHOLT, G. (1969). *Brit. J. vener. Dis.*, **45**, 144.

PANDURO, J. (1971). *Brit. J. vener. Dis.*, **47**, 440.

PARISER, H. and MARINO, A. F. (1970). *Sth. med. J.*, **63**, 384.

PEDERSEN, A. H. B., WIESNER, P. J., HOLMES, K. K., JOHNSON, C. J. and TURCK, M. (1972). *J. Amer. med. Ass.*, **220**, 205.

PETZOLDT, D. (1972). *Brit. J. vener. Dis.*, **48**, 514.

PHILIPS, I., RIMMER, D., RIDLEY, M., LYNN, R. and WARREN, C. (1970). *Lancet*, i, 263.

PLATTS, W. M. (1970a). *N.Z. med. J.*, **71**, 351.

PLATTS, W. M. (1970b). *Med. J. Aust.*, **2**, 500.

REYN, A. (1963). *Acta. derm.-venereol., Stockh.*, **43**, 383.

REYN, A. (1969). *Bull. W.H.O.*, **40**, 259.

REYN, A. and BENTZON, M. W. (1968). *Brit. J. vener. Dis.*, **44**, 140.

REYN, A. and BENTZON, M. W. (1969). *Brit. J. vener. Dis.*, **45**, 223.

REYN, A., SCHMIDT, H., TRIER, M. and BENTZON, M. W. (1969). W.H.O. Document VDT/RES/GON/72, 69.

REYN, A., SCHMIDT, H., TRIER, M. and BENTZON, M. W. (1973). *Brit. J. vener. Dis.*, **49**, 54.

RIBOLDI, A. (1966). *Minerva derm.*, **41**, 35.

RODIN, P. and SETH, A. D. (1972). *Brit. J. vener. Dis.*, **48**, 517.

RONALD, A. R., EBY, J. and SHERRIS, J. C. (1968). *Acta microbiol. Agents Chemother.*, **8**, 431.

SADI, A. and MALULI, A. M. (1971). *Rev. Bras. Pesquisas Med. Biol.*, **4**, 113.

SCHMIDT, H. NOIRDSON, A. M., REYN, A. and BENTZON, M. W. (1965). *Brit. J. vener. Dis.*, **41**, 120.

SCHMIDT, H. and ROHOLT, K. (1965). *Ugeskv. Laeg.*, **127**, 478.

SHAPIRO, L. H. and LENTZ, J. W. (1970). *Obstet. Gynec., N.Y.*, **35**, 794.

SILVER, P. S. and DARLING, W. M. (1971). *Brit. J. vener. Dis.*, **47**, 367.

SMITH, D. O. and OSICK, O. (1969). *Curr. Ther. Res.*, **11**, 1.

SMITH, D. O. and LEVEY, J. M. (1967). *Med. J. Aust.*, **1**, 849.

SMITH, E. B. (1966). *Milit. Med.*, **131**, 345.

SMITHURST, B. A. (1970). *Brit. J. vener. Dis.*, **46**, 398.

SNELL, E., MORRIS, D. A. and STRONG, J. (1963). *Canad. med. Ass. J.*, **89**, 601.

SOKOLOFF, B. (1965). *Clin. Pharmacol. Ther.*, **6**, 350.

SPITZER, R. J. and WILLCOX, R. R. (1968). *Acta derm-venereol., Stockh.*, **48**, 537.

STAHELI, L. T. (1964). *J. Amer. med. Ass.*, **190**, 854.

STATHAM, R. and MORTON, R. S. (1968). *Brit. med. J.* **4**, 623.

STRATIGOS, J. D., MARSELLOU-KINTI, O., KASSIMATIS, V. and DAIKUSC, K. (1973). *Brit. J. vener. Dis.*, **49**, 60.

STEENBERGEN, E. P. van (1971). *Brit. J. vener. Dis.*, **47**, 111.

SULLIVAN, J. F. (1970). *Med. J. Aust.*, **2**, 785.

SVINDLAND, H. B. (1973). *Brit. J. vener. Dis.*, **49**, 50.

THATCHER, R. W. and PETTIT, T. H. (1971). *J. Amer. med. Ass.*, **215**, 1494.

THAYER, J. D., SAMUELS, S. B., MARTIN, J. E. and LUCAS, T. B. (1964). *Anti-microbiol. Agents Chemother.*, Detroit, 433.

TIEDEMAN, J. H., HACKNEY, F. J. and PRICE, E. V. (1965). *Publ. Hlth Rep., Wash.*, **77**, 485.

VANDERSTOEP (1964). *Sth. med. J.*, **57**, 201.

WARREN, R. M. (1968). *Brit. J. vener. Dis.*, **44**, 80.

WAUGH, M. A. (1971). *Brit. J. vener. Dis.*, **47**, 34.

W.H.O., V.D. CONTROL SEMINAR, MANILA (1968). Western Pacific Office W.H.O., Manila, Philippines.

WILKINSON, A. E., RACE, J. W. and CURTIS, F. R. (1967). *Postgrad. med. J. Suppl.* **63**, 64.

WILLCOX, R. R. (1963). *Brit. J. vener. Dis.*, **39**, 160.

WILLCOX, R. R. (1964). *Brit. J. vener. Dis.*, **40**, 118.

WILLCOX, R. R. (1966). *Clin. med.*, **73**, 80.

WILLCOX, R. R. (1967). Report to V.C.H., Ibadan, Nigeria (unpublished).

WILLCOX, R. R. (1968). 'Antibiotic Treatment of V.D.', p. 123. Krager, Basle.

WILLCOX, R. R. (1970). *Brit. J. vener. Dis.*, **46**, 217.

WILLCOX, R. R. (1971). *Brit. J. vener. Dis.*, **47**, 31.

WILLCOX, R. R. (1972). *Brit. J. vener. Dis.*, **48**, 504.

WILLCOX, R. R. (1972). W.H.O. Document WHO/VDT/72, 381.

WOODCOCK, K. R. (1971). *Brit. J. vener. Dis.*, **47**, 95.

WRAY, P. M. (1965). *Brit. J. vener. Dis.*, **41**, 117.

Part 2
Syphilis

7 Epidemiological and Social Aspects

J. R. W. Harris

EPIDEMIOLOGY

As transmission in venereal syphilis is dependent on mucous membrane contact, the momentum of the spread of infection at any instant in time is a function of local human behaviour patterns and environmental factors. The quality of the local control, treatment and community health education will modify the transmission rate. With national and international travel the prevalence of infection in any area will be directly dependent on the incidences in adjacent areas and to a lesser extent on the incidence of early infection in remote areas. Thus the epidemiology of syphilis on a global basis is dependent on myriads of local, social and behavioural patterns, which are moulded by the quality of the diagnostic, therapeutic, educational and control facilities available.

It would be unwise, therefore, to study any particular country and attempt to draw general conclusions from the statistics of that area. At the same time it is impossible to consider all areas. Therefore it is proposed to compare and contrast the patterns in rich and poor communities in developed and developing countries.

It is relevant to remember at the outset that there has been a general recession in the incidence of venereal syphilis during the last hundred years (Idsøe and Guthe, 1967). There have always been periodic recrudescences of the disease in times of war and the recent increases in the annual incidences of early syphilis apparently commenced around 1956 to 1959. While information from the developed countries is available there are many countries in the world which have been unable to publish any statistics at all for the last decade. Thus trends in the developing countries can only be inferred from the reports available. Although epidemiology, control and health education are interdependent, this section will deal exclusively with the distribution of venereal syphilis as there are separate sections on control and health education.

In the U.S.A. the incidence of infectious syphilis in 1963 was 11·7 per

100 000 population per year, and by 1971 the incidence was 11·5 per 100 000 per year (Lucas, 1972). This is in spite of a most intensive programme of control in a country with a buoyant economy and a high level of education. Brown (1964) proposed that syphilis could be eradicated from the U.S.A. by 1972 if 30 per cent of newly infected persons were treated before the disease was transmitted. He did however note that this would not be possible unless the family physicians co-operated with the control programme and reported the cases as they were diagnosed. As can be seen from the statistics the control programme failed. The reasons for this failure are as follows. Private physicians treated 82·8 per cent of all cases of primary and secondary syphilis in the U.S.A. (Brown, 1971), yet only 12 per cent of the cases of infectious syphilis were reported to the government authorities to allow control procedures. Control, health education of the public and adequate therapeutic facilities have been limited by the relative lack of co-operation of the private physicians. Syphilis is still epidemic in the U.S.A. at the present time (Webster, 1970).

In the United Kingdom in 1963 the rate of infectious syphilis was approximately 2·48 per 100 000 and in 1972 it was 3·48 per 100 000 (Chief Medical Officer of Health, 1973). Here the majority of patients are treated in venereology units and only a small number are treated in private. Thus contact tracing and control methods can be readily applied and the momentum of spread of the disease is controlled.

In October 1968, the seminar which was attended by delegates from 25 countries on the American continent, concluded that infectious syphilis was on the increase in most developing countries. The debatable value of statistics from these countries was clearly illustrated when the incidences in El Salvador and Gautemala were compared. The prevalence of infectious syphilis in El Salvador was 70·2 per 100 000 per year while in Guatemala it was only 3·5 per 100 000 per year (Llopis, 1972). From Chile, Coria Ricotti et al (1969) concurred with the seminar view while Dogliotti (1972), noted that in 1971 a total of 2 132 patients were treated for primary and secondary syphilis in Baragwanath Hospital, Johannesburg. This gives a minimal incidence in that community of 211 per 100 000 per year. Rhodes and Anderson (1970) have described the explosive onset of sexually transmitted syphilis in New Guinea among a population which had lost its immunity, previously acquired from endemic yaws. One doctor saw over 100 cases in 3 months (Smith, 1971). Larsson and Larsson (1970) reported an estimated incidence of 3·2 per cent for congenital syphilis from Addis Ababa. Krishina and Panjabi (1972) noted in their series that syphilis occurred in 2·42 per cent of pregnancies. Obviously prevalences of congenital syphilis, such as these, are related to high incidences of infectious syphilis in the respective communities. Vukotich (1968), Parry (1968), and Edington and Gilles (1969) have observed that cardiovascular syphilis and neurosyphilis are still frequently found in many parts of the developing world. This is to be expected since antibiotic usage is low in these populations and is coupled with inadequate or non-existent medical and contact tracing services.

Morton (1971) estimated that the syphilis infection rate in Singapore during 1969 was 72 per 100 000 per year. Yet Singapore would be regarded by most people as a rich developing country which has had opportunities to develop much better control than many other countries in the developing world. If the rate in such a country is as high as this, it is likely that infectious and indeed late syphilis, for many years to come, will be prevalent in many corners of the globe.

REFERENCES

BROWN, W. J. (1964). *J. Amer. med. Ass.*, **190**, 35.
BROWN, W. J. (1971). *J. infect. Dis.*, **124**, 428.
CHIEF MEDICAL OFFICER OF HEALTH AND SOCIAL SECURITY (1973). *Brit. J. vener. Dis.*, **49**, 89.
CORIA RICOTTI, A., CASANUEVA ESCOBAR, V. and CAPMOS MENCHACA, D. (1969). *Rev. Chil. Pediat.*, **40**, 425.
DOGLIOTTI, M. (1972). Personal communication.
EDINGTON, G. M. and GILLES, M. H. (1969). 'Pathology in the Tropics', p. 516. Arnold, London.
IDSØE, O. and GUTHE, T. (1967). *Brit. J. vener. Dis.*, **43**, 227.
KRISHINA, U. and PANJABI, J. (1972). *Bombay Hosp. J.*, **14**, 32.
LARSSON, Y. and LARSSON, U. (1970). *Ethiop. med. J.*, **8**, 163.
LLOPIS, A. (1971). *Bol. Ofic. Sanit. Panamer.*, **70**, 26.
LUCAS, J. B. (1972). *Med. Clin. N. Amer.*, **56**, 5, 1073.
MORTON, R. S. (1971). *Brit. J. vener. Dis.*, **47**, 48.
PARRY, E. H. O. (1968). *Ethiop. med. J.*, **6**, 103.
RHODES, F. A. and ANDERSON, S. E. J. (1970). *Papua New Guinea med. J.*, **13**, 49.
SMITH, D. (1971). Personal communication.
VUKOTICH, D. (1968). *Ehtiop. med. J.*, **6**, 125.
WEBSTER, B. (1970). *Brit. J. vener. Dis.*, **46**, 406.

SOCIAL ASPECTS

The increasing incidence of infectious syphilis in the developed world during the last decade is a reflection of the social and environmental patterns in those countries. Changes in the organism itself and adjustments in the method of control appear only to modify the momentum. The developing countries, in many cases, show very high prevalence rates for infectious and late syphilis. Here the social and environmental patterns are different, control is poor or non-existent, health education is impeded by illiteracy and there are many competing priorities for the very limited human and economic resources available. Obviously many countries are between the extremes and an attempt will be made to discuss the spectrum.

In the developed world the widespread use of antibiotics during the last 30 years has undoubtedly, reduced the incidence of late and latent syphilis (Idsøe et al, 1972). Tertiary syphilis would appear to be restricted to the geriatric population in many instances (Krishman and Lomax, 1970), The increase in population has not generally been such that an enormous rise in the number of susceptibles has occurred. There has been a great acceleration of population mobility with industrialisation, urbanisation, migration of industrial workers both between and within countries (Willcox, 1970), and occupational and recreational travel (Sencer, 1969). Particularly high rates of syphilis have traditionally occurred among sailors (Schofield, 1964; Guthe and Idsøe, 1964) and soldiers (Greenberg, 1972). Today airline personnel, international journalists and television crews, entertainers and their entourage and holidaymakers continue to transfer syphilis across international frontiers (Willcox, 1972). This multiplies the potential for promiscuity and ensures that transfer of infection is a reality even on an international scale. Thus the problem of syphilis is an international one, modified at national or indeed regional level by local environmental and social factors.

In Western society there have been marked changes in social pattern during the last decade. Promiscuity is encouraged by increasing emphasis on sex in the mass media. Social acceptance of promiscuity is helped by a decline in influences which previously restrained it, and there is a reduced fear of sexually transmitted disease. The attitude of society in general to the homosexual has altered, although individual attitudes may not have changed much.

Certainly in developed countries the most important factor in the transmission of syphilis today is the promiscuous homosexual (Lancet, 1964). Idsøe and Guthe (1967) have reviewed the relationship between homosexuality and infectious syphilis during the early and mid-sixties. The pattern has changed little since then, except that the part played by the homosexual has probably increased. In the West London unit for sexually transmitted diseases 82 per cent of the infectious syphilis during the years 1968–71 was homosexually transmitted (Fluker, 1972). The problem is particularly one of large cities where young male homosexuals congregate (Hermans and de Cock, 1963). The homosexual is frequently bisexual and also has heterosexual contacts (Neser and Parrish, 1969). Because of the transient nature of many of the sexual encounters contact tracing is difficult. The important statistic is not the number of contacts who have attended but the number who have been untraceable (Harris et al, 1972). Even today some of the homosexual patients are still blissfully unaware of the high risk of infection with syphilis which accompanies promiscuous homosexual behaviour.

In some countries, such as the U.S.A., a major contributory factor in the failure to reduce the incidence of infectious syphilis has been the professional ignorance of the medical profession. With the advent of the post-penicillin era, a wave of complacency settled over the medical profession. As syphilis was no longer a problem, it was relegated to a minor position. Today the teaching of venereal diseases occupies little or no time in medical school curricula (Webster, 1972). The doctors who have graduated from medical school during the last 20 years have little or no knowledge of the diagnosis and management of sexually transmitted disease. Yet it is generally accepted that these doctors are treating over 80 per cent of the patients with syphilis in the U.S.A. (Webster, 1970).

In developing countries the success of the yaws eradication programme has resulted in millions of individuals becoming susceptible to infection with *T. pallidum* (see section on *Endemic Treptonematoses* (Guthe et al, 1972). The problems of urbanisation, population movement and limited medical resources are illustrated by the high rates of early syphilis reported by Larsson and Larsson (1970) and Dogliotti (1971, 1972) in Ethiopia and Johannesburg. In developing countries contact tracing is very difficult (Onifade and Osoba, 1972). Obviously Western control methods are not applicable to poor developing countries. On the other hand rich developing countries such as Singapore can adopt Western-style control successfully (Morton, 1970).

The social factors present in each continent and country differ greatly. Only prolonged study of the prevalence of disease and the precipitating social and environmental factors can direct management and control along successful lines.

REFERENCES

DOGLIOTTI, M. (1971). *S. Afr. med. J.*, **45**, 8.
DOGLIOTTI, M. (1972). Personal communications.
FLUKER, J. L. (1972). *Practioner*, **209**, 605.
GREENBERG, J. H. (1972). *Med. Clin. N. Amer.*, **56**, 5, 1087.
GUTHE, T. and IDSØE, O. (1964). *T. Norsk. Laegeforen*, **84**, 1262.
GUTHE, T., RIDET, J., VORST, F., D'COSTA, J. and GRAB, B. (1972). *Bull. Wld Hlth Org.*, **46**, 1.
HARRIS, J. R. W., MAHONY, J. D. H., HOLLAND, J. and McCANN, J. S. (1972). *J. Irish med. Ass.*, **65**, 62.
HERMANS, E. M. and DE COCK, P. (1963). *Dermatologica*, **127**, 278.
IDSØE, O., GUTHE, T. and WILLCOX, R. R. (1972). *Bull. Wld Hlth Org.*, **47**, Suppl. 13.
IDSØE, O. and GUTHE, T. (1967). *Brit. J. vener. Dis.*, **43**, 227.
KRISHMAN, M. U. and LOMAX, W. (1970). *Geront. Clin., Basel*, **12**, 76.
Lancet (1964). **1**, 481.
LARSSON, Y. and LARSSON, U. (1970). *Ethiop. med. J.*, **8**, 163.
MORTON, R. S. (1970). *Singapore med. J.*, **11**, 214.
NESER, W. B. and PARRISH, H. M. (1969). *Sth. med. J.*, **62**, 177.
ONIFADE, A. and OSOBA, A. O. (1972). *J. trop. Med. Hyg.*, **75**, 213.
SCHOFIELD, C. B.S. (1964). *Acta derm.-venereol., Stockh.*, **44**, 445.
SENCER, D. J. (1969). *Amer. J. publ. Hlth*, **18**, 341.

WEBSTER, B. (1972). *Med. Clin. N. Amer.*, **56**, 5, 1101.
WEBSTER, B. (1970). *Brit. J. vener. Dis.*, **46**, 406.
WILLCOX, R. R. (1970). *Brit. J. vener. Dis.*, **46**, 412.
WILLCOX, R. R. (1972). *Med. Clin. N. Amer.*, **56**, 5, 1057.

8 Clinical Aspects

J. R. W. Harris

PRIMARY SYPHILIS

During the last 10 years the introduction of improved serological and fluorescent techniques have facilitated the diagnosis of syphilitic infection at the primary stage. At the same time there has been a reappraisal of the clinical variations of the primary inoculation lesion, and of the importance in the developed countries of the extragenital primary. Paradoxically, the excellence of the eradication programme against the endemic treponematoses has facilitated the spread of venereal syphilis in developing countries (W.H.O., 1970). All the technical advances of the last decade in the diagnosis of primary syphilis are for socio-economic reasons inapplicable to such countries. Indeed, areas of the world are unable to avail themselves of the diagnostic methods in use in developed countries 30 years ago.

For many years a diagnostic dilemma has occurred when the patient presents with a seronegative primary to a medical unit lacking expertise in dark ground microscopy. The introduction of the FTA-ABS test (Bradford et al, 1965) ,with its high degree of specificity and its increased sensitivity, in relation to other tests in primary syphilis, has improved the situation. Nevertheless, as patients with early primary lesions can still have negative FTA-ABS serology, several groups of workers have developed and evaluated a fluorescent method for detection of *T. pallidum* in specimens taken from primary syphilitic lesions. Gardner and Robson (1968) believed that this method would be applicable to a country such as Australia, which had a limited number of units with sufficient experience in dark ground microscopy, and yet had an excellent postal service. Jue et al (1967) from Berkeley, California, and Wilkinson and Cowell (1971) in London compared this direct fluorescent method with dark field examination and found that both methods show good agreement. Kellogg (1970) expressed reservations, but Danielsson et al (1970) applied the technique using one-step inhibition and staining and found it satisfactory. This method would appear to be of value in those countries which have a relatively low incidence of syphilis and a reliable postal service. It would also be valuable on board ship as a retrospective diagnosis could be made when the patient attends the venereology unit at the next port. In a seronegative oral primary this would seem to be the diagnostic method of choice.

In 1965 there were several publications from Italy enthusing over the value of an intradermal treponema colour test. Cottini and Lazzaro (1965) and Cocuzza and Randazzo (1965) felt that this method had a high degree of specificity and sensitivity, and that it was frequently positive in the pre-serological primary stage. The test involved the intradermal inoculation of killed Nichols treponemata after previous intravenous administration of Evans blue dye. A positive result was recorded when a coloured spot appeared at the site of inoculation. The test was based on the assumption that a humoral antibody is bound in the skin early in the pre-serological stage of treponemal infection. However, this test has not come into wide usage, and there have been no further reports regarding its use in subsequent years.

The epidemiological trend in the developed countries that syphilis is common among the promiscuous homosexual, has led to many reports of primary syphilis of the oral and anorectal regions. The diagnostic difficulties encountered are obvious. Many of the anorectal lesions are painful, and atypical in appearance (Samenius, 1968); others are insignificant and pass unnoticed (Smith, 1965); the interpretation of the dark ground microscopy of specimens from the oral lesions is extremely difficult (Vincenti, 1971).

Gastin and Ossandon (1965) reported 13 cases where primary chancre of the cervix had been initially diagnosed as carcinoma, and Rossi et al (1967) emphasised the pseudoneoplastic clinical aspects of primary syphilis in this site. When one considers that infectious syphilis is not the prerogative of the young, the importance of reiteration of this established fact is obvious. Certainly, Young and Sun (1965) found that over an 8-year period at St. Luke's Hospital, New York, 5·2 per cent of patients with early syphilis were over 60 years old.

Dogliotti (1971), from Baragwanath Hospital, Johannesburg, described a number of Bantu patients with atypical primary chancres who had an associated suppurative inguinal lymphadenopathy. Coltiu and Forsea (1971) described two patients with a similar syndrome. Lejman and Bogdaszewska-Czabanowska (1964) stressed the diagnostic difficulties when the primary lesion is secondarily infected with pyogenic organisms and they also reported in 1969 secondary infection with fuso spirochaetal organisms (Lejman and Bogdaszewska-Czobanawska, 1969).

These reports refresh the basic concept that many primary *T. pallidum* inoculation lesions do not conform to the classical Hunterian description, and should stimulate us to review the value of retaining such a terminology as *Typical Primary Chancre* in the clinical management of sexually transmitted diseases in the modern era.

SECONDARY SYPHILIS

The study of secondary syphilis during the last decade has been promoted by the concurrent developments in immunology and electron microscopy. There has been a greater appreciation of the nature and degree of renal and hepatic involvement, while from Japan the improvements in gastric endoscopy and gastric photography have validated the involvement of the gastric mucosa at this stage of infection. The concept of locomotor system manifestations in secondary syphilis has been re-evaluated, and there is still some controversy as to the degree of invasion of the central nervous system at this point in the disease process. As might be expected from the multifocal and uncommon manifestations of infectious syphilis there have been numerous reports of atypical and uncommon clinical entities. These isolated case histories, while of undoubted interest, will not be included unless they demonstrate a clinical maxim which might be of diagnostic value.

Brophy et al (1964) and Falls et al (1965) reported the occurrence of the nephrotic syndrome in secondary syphilis and presented the electron microscopic findings on renal biopsy, before and after treatment. They observed swelling of the endothelial cells with electron dense deposits adjacent to either side of the basement membrane and noted fusion of the epithelial foot processes. The abnormalities returned to normal following adequate antibiotic therapy. These findings closely resemble those noted by Kaplan et al (1972) in the glomerulopathy of congenital syphilis. Braunstein et al (1970) from Boston, described their histological findings on a renal biopsy from a patient with the nephrotic syndrome during the course of secondary syphilis. They were similar to those already mentioned with the addition of perivascular mononuclear infiltration and mesangial cell proliferation. Braunstein et al demonstrated that the electron dense deposits were IgG but were unable to detect complement deposition in the same site. On the basis of this, they postulated that the renal pathology suggested an immune deposit disease (see Figs. 15 and 16.

Bhorade et al (1971) were able, using immunofluorescent techniques, to demonstrate the presence of these complement deposits (BIC globulin) on electron microscopy. Two years later Kaplan et al (1972) came to the same conclusion regarding the nephrotic syndrome found in congenital syphilis. Hellier et al (1971) described the occurrence of the nephrotic syndrome in acquired secondary syphilis from Southampton.

McCracken et al (1969) reported the association of the nephrotic syndrome and acute hepatitis in a patient with secondary syphilis and referred to the paper of Zellerman and Norcross (1967) who discussed

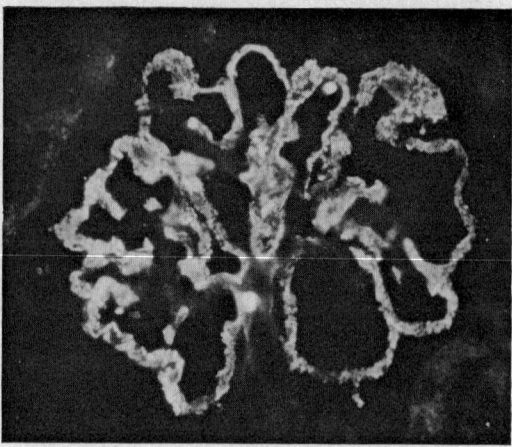

Fig. 15. *Case 2.* Immunofluorescence with anti-IgG (× 137) showing deposits within and along the epithelial aspect of the glomerular basement membrane. (From a paper by J. Wigglelinkhiuzen and others *Arch. Dis. Childh.* (1973). 48, 375. Reproduced by courtesy of the authors and the Editor of the Journal.)

a patient suffering from syphilitic hepatitis. A liver biopsy from this patient showed chronic inflammation and regenerative nodules. The response of the patient to antibiotic therapy was dramatic. Albertazzi et al (1970) considered a similar case and discussed the diagnostic difficulty of distinguishing this condition from virus hepatitis since there can be great similarity between the clinical and histopathological pictures of the two forms. This view was not shared by Lee et al (1971) and Baker et al (1971) who reported cases of patients presenting with hepatic tenderness, jaundice and skin rashes pathogenic of secondary syphilis. They found gross elevation of alkaline phosphatase levels to more than 10 times normal and maintained that this was a disproportionate increase in relation to the transaminase rise. Also the histological picture of the liver biopsy from the patient reported by Baker et al (1971) was not like that found in virus hepatitis. The predominant features were of several necrotic areas extending from portal triads to central veins. In these areas there was moderate lymphocytic and histiocytic infiltrations. The portal tracts were oedematous and there was no cholestasis. A similar histological picture was described by Sobel and Wolf (1972). The fact that Australian antigen was not present in these patients, and that the response to antibiotic therapy was so marked, was felt to weigh strongly in favour of active syphilitic hepatitis being a distinct entity.

Sherlock (1971) while admitting that gross elevations of alkaline phosphatase of this nature were unusual in viral hepatitis, and that the

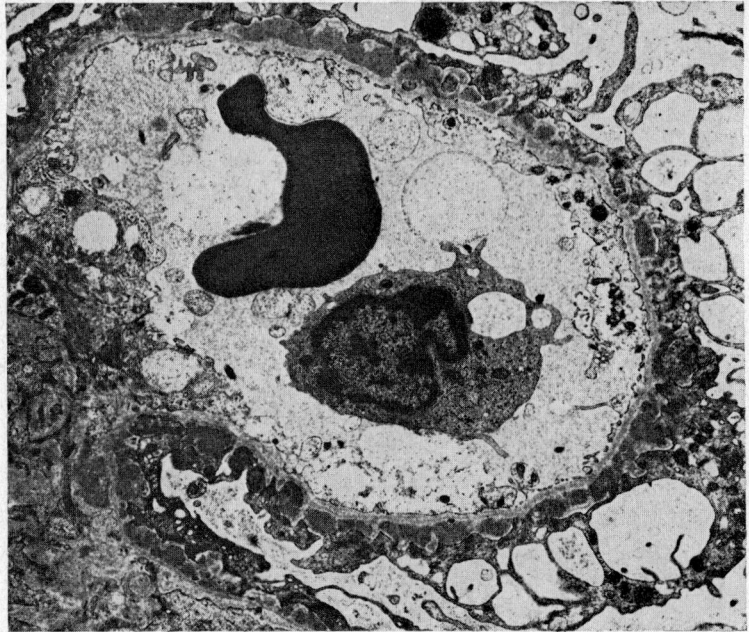

FIG. 16. *Case 3, first biopsy*. Electron micrograph of glomerular capillary containing polymorphonuclear leucocyte and an erythrocyte. There are numerous electron-dense subepithelial deposits along the basement membrane. The epithelial foot processes are fused and there is much vacuolation of the epithelial cell cytoplasm (×4 800). (From a paper by J. Wigglelinkhiuzen and others (1973). *Arch. Dis. Childh.*, 48, 375. Reproduced by courtesy of the authors and the Editor of the journal.)

hepatic histology did not resemble that of viral hepatitis, still felt that the evidence for an active hepatitis in the secondary stage was poor. However, many would feel that this view is overcautious, especially when one considers the findings of Karmi et al (1969) from Bristol, where they found that of 49 patients with liver cirrhosis six had syphilis, and several of these had never had previous intravenous therapy or clinical jaundice. It is relevant to note that many patients have jaundice associated with involvement of another system. The patient described by McCracken et al (1969) had nephrosis, the patient reported by Sobel and Wolf (1972) had uveitis, and Parker (1972) related the case of a patient with jaundice, perceptive nerve deafness and papilloedema. In the other cases referred to above the cutaneous signs of secondary syphilis either were or had been present prior to diagnosis. From this one might say that any patient with hepatitis, who exhibits multisystem disease and is found on biochemical testing to have a disproportionate increase of alkaline phosphatase in relation to transaminase rise may well be suffering from syphilitic hepatitis.

Yamaguchi et al (1969) documented two cases with gastric lesions during secondary syphilis. The patients presented with sudden onset of extreme epigastric pain and post-prandial recurrent vomiting. The pain was so severe that the initial differential diagnosis in each case was peptic ulceration or acute pancreatitis. Biochemical analysis of gastric aspiration showed decreased quantity and hypoacidity. Radiologically a concentric stricture was seen in the pylorus in one patient, and in the other a large shallow ulcer was visualised. On endoscopy the mucosa over and around the concentric stricture was tinged dark red and appeared polypoid. The other patient's mucosa was interrupted by a number of ulcerative lesions of various sizes with a yellowish white exudate on the ulcer bases. Gastric biopsy revealed the presence of plasma and eosinophilic infiltrates corresponding with the histological appearance of biopsy material from the skin and vaginal lesions. The gastric ulceration in the second patient was diminishing in size before commencement of antibiotic therapy, and the gastric secretion and hypoacidity returned to normal following treatment. A similar clinical picture has been reported by Mitchell and Bralow (1964) from Philadelphia in a young women with secondary syphilis.

Macfaul and Catterall (1971) reported the detrimental effect of corticosteroid therapy alone on choroido-retinitis due to secondary syphilis. They speculated that the exacerbation in uveitis and choroido-retinitis was precipitated by corticosteroid therapy suppressing local immunity. The intra-ocular manifestations responded rapidly when antisyphilitic treatment was given to the patient. This is a very important concept as corticosteroid therapy is used in the treatment of the nephrotic syndrome and hepatitis. Thus delayed diagnosis of the true syphilitic aetiology of the patient's illness, coupled with inappropriate corticosteroid administration, may well lead to a deterioration in the patient's condition.

Sarkany (1965) reported polyarthralgia with lytic changes in the right sterno-clavicular joint in a young woman with secondary syphilis. Datta (1965) in a review of 300 patients with secondary syphilis emphasised that 18 of them had predominant locomotor manifestations with arthralgia and bone tenderness. Beardwell and Jacobs (1969) reaffirmed that generalised arthralgia can be a presenting feature and Kahn et al (1970) reported four patients with inflammatory articular involvement associated with secondary syphilis. In two of their patients the subacute febrile polyarthritis suggested rheumatic fever. Waugh (1972) also drew attention to bone pain as a presenting feature of secondary syphilis.

An interesting paper by Spangler et al (1964) highlights an explanation for the occurrence of negative serology in secondary syphilis. They concluded that the negative serological result in five patients with secondary syphilis was due to excessive reagin in the serum producing the prozone phenomenon which could be abolished on dilution of the serum. This may explain the report by Roitburd (1968) describing two cases of seronegativity in secondary syphilis. However, if the patient has the 'malignant' form of the disease then the serology will also be negative. Two such cases were described by Cripps and Curtis (1969) and Degos et al (1970).

Certain aspects of the reticulo-endothelial involvement in secondary syphilis have received attention. Yarrington and Jensen (1967) and Goffinet et al (1970) felt that on occasions the lymphadenopathy of infectious syphilis can be indistinguishable clinically from that commonly associated with reticuloses or carcinomatous deposits. Hartsock et al (1970) in a report from the U.S. Armed Forces Institute of Pathology describe nine cases in which a node biopsy had been taken from those who complained of localised painful lymphadenopathy. Histological examination showed evidence of syphilitic infection in these patients. Wright (1969) documented a patient who had noticed pain in the cervical and inguinal lymph nodes following alcohol ingestion. This phenomenon has been previously recognised in Hodgkin's disease and the reticuloses, but has not been reported before or since in relation to syphilitic infection.

The documentation of unusual sites of condylomata lata such as the toeweb (Minikin et al, 1967), the external ear (Jarvis and Kuschke, 1968), the face (Lal, 1971), and the axilla (Rhodes and Anderson, 1970) can be explained by variations in climate and hygiene which result in the cutaneous areas in question being sufficiently moist to promote the development of condylomata. These papers do, however, underline the importance of a meticulous clinical examination.

Chambers et al (1969) observed that fresh blood and its components, eg platelet concentrates, can transmit syphilis despite the donor being non-reactive on routine serological testing. Their patient presented with secondary syphilis following such a transfusion.

The literature of the last 10 years contains seven cases of perceptive deafness during the course of infectious syphilis. One of these was a patient with meningovascular syphilis recorded by Wetherill et al (1965). The other six patients described by Alergant (1965), Schneider and Bolte (1972) and Willcox and Goodwin (1971), developed sudden impairment of hearing which deteriorated in several instances during the first few days of treatment. Despite adequate antibiotic therapy several patients had residual permanent eighth nerve damage. The value of steroid therapy will be considered in the section on treatment later in the chapter. All the patients had abnormal C.S.F.s and whatever views one might have on the advisability or necessity for routine C.S.F.

examination in the secondary stage of syphilis, there can be no doubt that it is essential in any patient with hearing loss.

Mikhail and Chapel (1969) discussed a patient with the rare cutaneous follicular papulopustular manifestation of early syphilis and demonstrated the frequent association of this type of lesion with abnormal C.S.F. findings. At this stage it would therefore be relevant to consider the vexed question of routine C.S.F. examination in secondary syphilis.

Following the work of Jefferiss (1963) there was a considerable body of opinion that routine examination of the C.S.F. in a patient with secondary syphilis should be abandoned. The work of Fernando (1965, 1968) in Ceylon substantiated this argument. He examined a total of 231 C.S.F.s and found that only three revealed any abnormality. In all three this was a minimal elevation of cell count. Datta (1968) investigated 70 patients with secondary syphilis and found that four of them had an abnormal C.S.F. However, there was no mention of the presence or absence of red blood cells in these C.S.F.s and he found no correlation between the degree of abnormality and the severity of the rash in the secondary stage. Oxelius et al (1969) reported a patient with secondary syphilis who had definite damage to the blood-brain barrier. This was shown by the presence of macro-globulin in the C.S.F. detectable by gel diffusion. This macro-globulin is not present in normal C.S.F. The situation, therefore, would appear that examination of the C.S.F. using the parameters which have been in use for the last 30 years, will usually show no evidence of involvement of the central nervous system in secondary syphilis. Nevertheless, this system is occasionally involved when the blood-brain barrier has been damaged. The problem is that we may not be using sensitive enough methods to establish the presence of such damage, and the assumption that such damage has not occurred may be premature.

LATENT SYPHILIS

Idsøe et al (1972) have established that the prognosis is very good in treated early latent and late latent syphilis. They admit that the differentiation between early and late latency is arbitrary in many cases. Nevertheless, using the present tests of cure the results would appear to be excellent.

However, there is evidence that permanent neurological damage can occur during the secondary stage of syphilis (Willcox and Goodwin, 1971; Schneider and Bolte, 1972). The observations of Oxelius et al (1969) substantiate this. The prospective study of Hooshmand et al (1972) indicates that the methods primarily used to assess C.S.F. (leucocyte count, total protein levels, etc) are not sensitive enough. It is difficult to distinguish relapse from re-infection. Considering these facts and the limitations of our knowledge of the interaction between host and T. pallidum, latent syphilis requires further study.

Several of the more recent serological tests may, ultimately, prove of value in the management of latent syphilis. The cardiolipin F antibody, detected by Wright et al (1970), is found mainly in early syphilis. The FTA-IgM-ABS test of O'Neill and Nicol (1972), when fully evaluated, may prove a valuable indicator of disease activity.

VISCERAL SYPHILIS

In 1969 Karmi and his co-workers re-evaluated the relationship between cirrhosis and syphilitic infection. They summarised the results of ten series of patients with cirrhosis in the recent literature and came to the conclusion that 10–20 per cent of the patients with cirrhosis might well have syphilis. However as the great bulk of the clinical material on which the series were based had in fact presented prior to the advent of antibiotic therapy they studied 49 patients with cirrhosis and found that six of the men in the series had syphilis. Harris et al (1973) studied 49 patients with chronic liver disease in Belfast and noted that four of their male patients had syphilis. Therefore it would appear that in the United Kingdom a significant proportion of male patients with cirrhosis may well have syphilis. It is not yet clear whether the cirrhosis is part of the syphilitic disease process or whether it is a clinical association.

CARDIOVASCULAR SYPHILIS

The incidence of cardiovascular syphilis in the developed countries has decreased during the antibiotic era. It is not surprising that the vast majority of publications on cardiovascular syphilis during the last 10 years have referred to the disease among the elderly in the developed world, while from certain developing countries a completely different picture emerges. Thus the great advances in cardiovascular surgery during the last decade have limited application in our society, while in the developing countries economics prevent the use of such techniques.

Several important clinical facts have been established. In Tokyo Sakamoto et al (1968) have emphasised that the maximal intensity of the murmur associated with syphilitic aortic incompetence is frequently along the right border of the sternum in the third and fourth interspaces. They investigated 801 patients with aortic incompetence, of whom 58, ie 7·1 per cent, had the maximal intensity located in the third and fourth interspaces. They then found that 54 of the total patients had syphilis, and 27, ie 50 per cent, of these were in the group with maximal intensity located to the right of the sternum. This fact is explained by Harvey et al (1963), who showed that those patients with diseases of the aortic root will have maximum radiation of the murmur down the right side of the sternum, while patients with isolated aortic incompetence will have radiation of the murmur down the left side of the sternum.

There has been some controversy as to the association of calcification of the ascending aorta with cardiovascular syphilis. Baumgartner et al (1970) and Cohen (1970) reported patients who exhibited such calcification but did not have cardiovascular syphilis. Vukotich and Giel (1970) in their series of 27 patients from Addis Ababa found calcification in the ascending aorta in only one patient. Since poor Ethiopians rarely exhibit atherosclerosis they felt that the absence of calcification might be related to this. Furthermore they found no evidence to confirm the principle that manual labour was an aetiological factor in the development of cardiovascular syphilis. In Ethiopia it is the women who tend to carry out the manual labour and yet there were 23 males in their series of 27 patients.

Friedman (1969) indicated that dissecting aneurysm and calcification of the aortic ring and valves may supervene in luetic aortitis, and Kallichurun (1969), while discussing heart failure among the Bantu in Durban, insisted that sub-acute bacterial endocarditis may frequently complicate syphilitic aortic valve lesions. Beckerling et al (1969), also from Durban, stated that left ventricular aneurysm was often of syphilitic aetiology in the African patient. Masterson (1965) in reporting a case of cardiovascular syphilis drew attention to the association with generalised amyloid disease. Schneider and Spitz (1968) from Cincinnatti reviewed 16 patients with unruptured aortic sinus aneurysms and found that eight were of syphilitic aetiology. Suarez and De Suarez (1969) from Caracas indicted syphilis as being associated with the aneurysms of the sinus of Valsalva, although they admitted that there was a possibility of concomitant syphilitic infection in these two patients. Aortic incompetence occurring as a complication of congenital syphilis was reported in a patient by White (1965) and cardiovascular syphilis in a 20-year-old male by Hiltenbrand et al (1967).

Beck et al (1965) described how syphilitic obstruction of the coronary ostia had been successfully treated by endarterectomy in two patients at Groote Schuur Hospital. A year later Schire et al (1966) outlined the clinical factors which they considered important in the diagnosis of coronary ostial disease. If the patient was a young man with angina pectoris or if the angina was disproportionate in the presence of aortic incompetence, then ostial stenosis should be excluded. Similarly if aortic incompetence was present or the ascending aorta was dilated or calcified, then ostial stenosis should be considered. Frater and Jordan (1968) reported the first case of successful surgical treatment of this condition from New York. Michaud et al (1970), on the basis of their five patients, felt that as the survivors had immediate and lasting relief from the anginal syndrome the results were among the best in direct coronary surgery. The frequency of ostial obstruction in association with syphilitic aortitis was reviewed by Datey and Kelkar (1969) in Bombay. Fifty-one of their 200 cases of syphilitic aortitis had coronary ostial stenosis.

NEUROSYPHILIS

It is apparent that the diagnosis of neurosyphilis becomes more difficult. The classical text-book descriptions of tabes dorsalis and general paralysis of the insane (G.P.I.) are becoming rare in the developed world (Koffman, 1956). There is an increasing awareness by clinicians that neurosyphilis today has a wide variety of symptomatology and clinical presentation (Wetherill et al, 1965; Joffe et al, 1968). Widespread use of antibiotics and psychoactive drugs may be responsible for fractionating psychiatric, neurological and serological components of neurosyphilis (Gowardman, 1970). Reliance on clinical and laboratory parameters established in the pre-antibiotic era is outmoded (Mahony et al, 1972). It must be assumed that in an antibiotic environment many patients will inadvertently receive some antibiotic therapy prior to presentation to the clinician. The methods and results of treatment of neurosyphilis have remained controversial and enigmatic (Hooshmand et al, 1972). An attempt therefore will be made to discuss neurosyphilis as a spectrum of disease.

The incidence of neurosyphilis cannot be accurately assessed. It would appear to be decreasing in the developed world during the last decade. In many developing countries with improved medical diagnostic facilities there has been an apparent increase in prevalence. From Senegal (Heraut et al, 1971) and Jamaica (Burke, 1972) have come reports of high rates of neurosyphilis. Yet from Ethiopia, Vukotich and Giel (1970) comment on the low rate of neurosyphilis relative to other forms of early and late syphilis in Addis Ababa. Ashcroft et al (1967) referred to the difficulties of diagnosis of neurosyphilis among populations whose level of sero-reactors was high. Cosnett (1965) described acute encephalitic forms of neurosyphilis among young Zulus whose C.S.F. examination was unhelpful but whose therapeutic response to pencillin was remarkable.

Retrospective studies in psychiatric hospitals in the United Kingdom by Dewhurst (1969a) indicated that depression and dementia are the most common presentations of neurosyphilis. Dawson-Butterworth and Heathcote (1970) observed that the dementia initially responded well to treatment but dementia almost always occurred later. They attempted to differentiate between the patient's pre-and post-treatment condition and their state after many years in a mental hospital. This ambitious project dealt with only 45 patients, many of whom had been living in a large mental hospital for several years. Dementia and confusion were the most common features in their series. There was a high prevalence of ataxia and dysarthria many years after treatment. Gowardman (1970) feels that schizophrenic-form reactions in vulnerable personalities can also be a presenting feature. Shalickova and Hatulay (1971) maintain that schizophrenic-form reaction is common in neurosyphilis of congenital origin. Grandiose delusions can still occur as the main mental aberration but their prevalence is low (Dewhurst, 1969).

Scala and Fucci (1970) feel that treatment improves the duration but not the quality of life. They admit to a preponderance of elderly patients in their series and also admit that senility can alter the prognosis. Wilner and Brody (1968) in their review of 100 patients noted that progression of the disease had occurred in 31 despite treatment. However, in all of these series, some of the patients had been treated with fever therapy alone and others had had fever therapy with penicillin. Hence it is difficult to draw conclusions on the prognosis of neurophilis using modern methods of therapy. Several workers did speculate that the neurosyphilitic process might lead to increased susceptibility to other neurological diseases.

Serre et al (1970) advocated laminectomy in tabetic spinal arthropathy to relieve root pain and improve the motor and sensory function of the lower limbs. They discussed the clinical and symptomatic differentiation between compression of the spinal cord in the vertebral canal and root compression in the intervertebral foramen or in the canal at the level of the cauda equina. Their review of 57 cases, described in the literature, over a 24-year period showed the relative frequency of the various compression syndromes. Johns reported two further cases in 1970 and McNeel and Ehni (1969) disputed the views of Serre et al that surgical intervention was always advisable. Passerini and Vaghi (1966) noted that 4 per cent of the patients with syphilitic cord involvement had spinal arthropathy. Hooshmand et al (1972) reported nine patients with neurosyphilis who had symptoms of cervical spondylosis. Five of these had minimal or no changes on X-ray of the cervical spine. Six of the nine cases underwent myelography which showed irregular filling of the cervical canal and multiple 'moth-eaten' filling defects in the cervical region not necessarily limited to the vertebral interspaces. In four patients, treated with penicillin, there was partial improvement. The value of myelography in distinguishing between compression due to arthropathy and pachymeningitis is obvious.

Harper et al (1967) advocated the use of specific serological tests in the investigation of patients with neurogenic bladders and stated that neurosyphilis remains a definite clinical problem in urology in the U.S.A. Dawson-Butterworth and Heathcote (1970) were of the opinion that neurogenic bladder had become an uncommon accompaniment of neurosyphilis in the United Kingdom. The autonomic neuropathy was investigated by Courtney Evans et al (1971). They found that some patients with autonomic denervation are unable to adjust their respiratory system in response to hypoxia.

Dewhurst (1968), Dawson-Butterworth and Heathcote (1970) and Hooshmand et al (1972) all indicate that a small number of patients with neurosyphilis deteriorate clinically in spite of therapy with adequate dosages of penicillin. It is difficult to establish whether the progression is due to prolonged activity of the syphilitic process or to the secondary effects of irreversible brain damage. Since the work of Collart et al (1962) there has been increasing evidence, in cases of late syphilis, of the persistence of treponeme-like forms in tissues and intraocular and cerebrospinal fluids. The identity of these treponemal forms and the evidence for their continued virulence is still under debate (Smith, 1969). Gager et al (1968) and Ch'ien et al (1970) feel that the continued presence of these forms indicates the need for further high dosage antibiotic therapy. However, Rice et al (1970) felt that until the possible significance of such treponeme-like forms could be assessed there is no necessity to alter methods 'of treatment of early syphilis. The possible significance of treponeme-like forms has been reviewed (Willcox, 1964; Lancet, 1968; Turner et al, 1969; W.H.O. 1970; Sparling, 1971; Dunlop, 1972).

Milich (1968) has been concerned that neurosyphilis can occur among patients who have completed adequate treatment for early infectious syphilis. Tumasheva and Garmatyuk (1968) believe that anti-syphilitic treatment is capable of preventing auto-immunisation only if given early in the course of infection. On the basis of their studies, on the detection of anti-brain antibiodies in the C.S.F., they feel that from the onset of relapsing secondary syphilis auto-immunisation occurs.

An excellent prospective study of neurosyphilis, from the Medical College of Virginia, was published in 1972 by Hooshmand and his co-workers. From July 1965 until July 1970 they evaluated 251 patients who were diagnosed as having neurosyphilis. Their diagnostic criteria were as follows:

1. positive blood FTA-ABS and ophthalmic or neurological findings suggestive of neurosyphilis;
2. positive blood and C.S.F. FTA–ABS with abnormal blood cell counts in C.S.F. (more than five white blood cells per mm^3 with no evidence of bacterial or viral menengitis);
3. blood and C.S.F. FTA–ABS in patients with progressive neurological symptoms in whom other aetiological factors had been ruled out.

In this last group the diagnosis was not considered to be compatible with neurosyphilis unless the C.S.F. showed an increase in leucocyte count for a temporary period of only a few weeks after penicillin therapy had been started, or unless there had been a considerable improvement in the patient's symptoms following penicillin therapy.

Treatment involved a minimum of 20 mega i.u. of penicillin G procaine penicillin over at least 3 weeks.

Adult seizure disorder was one of the most outstanding symptoms of the disease and occurred in 24·2 per cent of the patients in this series. Ophthalmic symptoms, dizziness and confusion associated with a cerebrovascular accident were the other common presentations. Almost half of the patients presented with unrelated symptoms and the diagnosis was made as an incidental finding. Some abnormality on neurological examination was seen in 75·8 per cent of the patients. Sensory dysfunction consisted mainly of posterior column loss. Reflex changes were the most frequent clinical finding. Almost half the patients had ophthalmic signs, of which papillary changes were the most common. Only a few cases exhibited psychiatric disorders. The authors were most impressed by the fact that the great majority of cases no longer had the classical picture of neurosyphilis but tended to present in an atypical fashion.

The diagnostic criteria utilised by Hooshmand et al (1972) will undoubtedly become widely used. The lack of value of the non-treponemal tests needs to be emphasised. Fulford and Brostoff (1972) reported six patients with signs and symptoms of a neurological disorder resembling multiple sclerosis associated with chronic biological false positive Wassermann serology. Gowardman (1970) and Dewhurst (1968) both remarked that a negative serological or C.S.F. non-treponemal test did not exclude the diagnosis of neurosyphilis. Hooshmand and his colleagues (1972) were of the same opinion. These latter workers feel that the serological results of specific tests must be considered in the context of the other clinical and laboratory findings. Dewhurst (1969b) noted that many untreated patients with neurosyphilitic psychoses had low C.S.F. leucocyte counts and low total protein levels. Grahmann (1969) showed the limitations of the Lange curve in his review of 24,000 samples of C.S.F. The paralytic curve was found in 436 cases of whom only 143 were suffering from neurosyphilis. Scalla and Fucci (1970) observed that C.S.F. leucocyte counts and protein levels were frequently normal in the presence of neurosyphilis. Hooshmand et al (1972) found that only 26 of 212 patients whom they deemed to have active neurosyphilis had more than 10 leucocytes per mm^2 and 39 had less than five leucocytes per mm^3. Similarly 61·2 per cent of their patients had total C.S.F. protein levels less than 45 mg per 100 ml (within normal limits). Thus reliance on non-specific serological and C.S.F. tests, C.S.F. total protein levels and C.S.F. leucocyte counts in an antibiotic era is unjustified.

Mattern et al (1965) found in their investigation of 35 patients with neurosyphilis that there was a marked increase in C.S.F. immunoglobulins in these patients. The increase in IgG was most marked but C.S.F. IgA and IgM were also raised in a large proportion of the patients. Oxelius et al (1969) who continued these investigations showed that after treatment of the neurosyphilis the IgG level in the C.S.F. decreased slowly while the IgM fell rapidly. They felt that there was evidence of local production of IgG and IgM. Schmidt et al (1970) found similar increase in IgG and also noted that an increase in albumin indicated severe damage to the blood-brain barrier. Hooshmand et al (1972) investigated 99 patients with neurosyphilis and found abnormal levels of γ globulin in 67. From these studies it is obvious that an estimation of total C.S.F. γ-globulin and an immunophoresis of γ-globulin will be valuable in assessing the activity of neurosyphilis.

SYPHILIS AND THE EYE

The persistence of treponeme-like forms in late syphilis, despite apparently adequate penicillin therapy, has already been discussed in this chapter. The subject has been extensively reviewed (Turner et al, 1969; Dunlop, 1972). These forms were first reported in animals and man by Collart et al (1962) and confirmed in man by Boncinelli and his associates (1966). Smith et al (1967), Goldman and Girard (1967) and Christman et al (1968) found treponemes in the aqueous humour of patients with late syphilis who had had large doses of penicillin. Treponeme-like forms have also been found in iritis associated with secondary syphilis by MacFaul and Catterall (1971), and Schmidt and Goldschmidt (1972). Smith and his co-workers from Miami, initially used Krajian silver stain and later, fluorescent antibody techniques (see Fig. 19) to demonstrate the treponemes in aqueous humour, ocular tissue and temporal artery biopsies (Smith et al, 1967; Smith, 1969; Montenegro

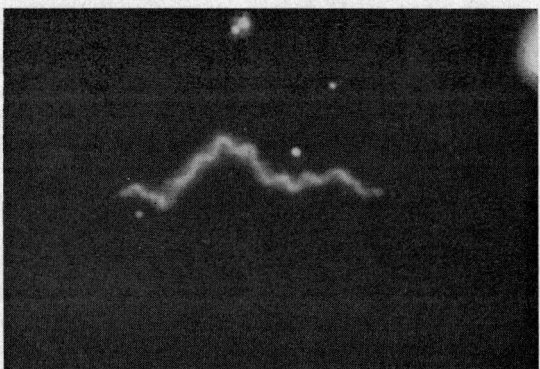

Fig. 19. Another spirochaete which stained with FA stain from the aqueous humour of Case 171. Note the perfect morphology of these organisms. (From a paper by J. Lawton Smith and others (1971), Brit. J. vener. Dis., 47, 226. Reproduced by permission of Dr. J. Lawton Smith and the Editor of the British Journal of Venereal Diseases.)

et al, 1969). They emphasised the diagnostic value of the FTA–ABS (Smith and Taylor, 1965). However, this test is not infallible and although it has a high specificity, false positive reactions have been observed in patients with anti-nuclear factor, alcoholic cirrhosis, rheumatoid factor and lymphosarcoma (Jokinen and Lasuss, 1972; Hooshmand et al, 1972; Harris et al, 1974; Mackay et al, 1969).

Wilkinson (1968) reported that glass filaments could resemble treponemes. Montenegro et al (1969) reviewed the Miami material and agreed that on occasions the treponeme-like forms were artefacts (glass shavings, etch marks, curled strands from lysed red cells, bacterial flagella, water marks due to the absorption of fluorescent antibody stain or dried protein), but that others were incontrovertible treponemes. Golden and Thompson (1969) proposed that the spiral organisms seen by numerous competent observers were frequently treponemes but not *T. pallidum*. Hanson (1970) observed that spirochaetes of one form or another had been found in most flesh-eating animals.

Despite this confusion it was agreed that antibiotic levels in the eye and C.S.F. were demonstrably lower than in the serum. Shorr et al (1969) studied the levels of erythromycin reaching the aqueous humour and Goldman (1970) noted that ampicillin entered the anterior chamber. Boyle et al (1970) felt that significant treponemacidal concentration of cephalexin could be obtained in aqueous humour after doses of 1–3 g. These levels persisted for 12 hours with a peak between 2 and 4 hours.

The fundamental questions posed by this research are whether the treponeme-like forms found after treatment of syphilis are *T. pallidum* and if so whether they are virulent, avirulent or of low virulence. In some cases at least, the treponeme-like forms found after treatment are *T. pallidum* (Dunlop, 1972). Several studies suggested a relationship between treponeme-like forms and active manifestations of syphilis (Agarwal, 1960; Whitfield and Wirostko, 1970). However, subsequent work at Moorfield's Eye Hospital, London, has shown no correlation between activity of the syphilitic process and the presence of treponeme-like forms (Dunlop, 1972).

The situation at present seems to be that in a few patients the persisting organisms are *T. pallidum*. The significance of these organisms to the patient is uncertain. There is insufficient evidence, at this stage, that the presence of treponeme-like forms indicates the need for further anti-syphilitic treatment, if the patient has already been adequately treated.

Certain aspects of ophthalmic syphilis have been discussed under the heading of congenital syphilis.

CONGENITAL SYPHILIS

It has been a long-established fact that the clinical diagnosis of congenital syphilis in the first weeks of life presents many difficulties.

The clinical manifestations frequently do not occur at the time of birth but tend to appear during the first few weeks or months of life. When this is considered in the context of developed countries whose medical profession had decreasing clinical acquaintance with the disease, it is easy to understand the increasing emphasis placed on serological diagnosis. At the same time improved diagnostic facilities in developing countries have demonstrated an apparently widening clinical spectrum of the disease and underline its importance in those areas.

Aiuti et al (1967) reported that the newborn infant with congenital syphilis had the ability to respond to antigenic stimulation. The bone-marrow of their patient showed plasmoblasts and mature plasma cells. Serological studies showed the presence of high levels of IgM in the neonates blood—280 mg per cent for the baby, and 80 mg per cent for the mother. As IgM levels in the premature and full-term baby rarely exceed 15 mg per 100 ml (Fogel et al, 1969) this was positive proof of an active intrauterine immunological response by the foetus to the spiro-chaetal organisms. Scotti and Logan (1968) from Atlanta, reported the initial results of their work in demonstrating the presence of this specific IgM antibody in the sera of newborn infants, using an indirect fluores-cent antibody technique. Their initial conclusions were that the test was specific for congenital syphilis in the newborn, and was non-reactive in the case of passive transfer of maternal syphilitic antibody, whereas other tests such as the VDRL and the FTA–ABS might well be positive. The following year they published a much larger series which indicated the limitations of the technique (Scotti et al, 1969). The test was positive in 18 infants with congenital syphilis and negative in 107 who had positive serological FTA–ABS but were regarded as having reagin spill over. However, it was negative on serum testing from a further 16 infants, several of whom later developed congenital syphilis. They concluded that a positive result indicated the presence of congenital syphilis but that a negative result did not exclude the diagnosis. Alford et al (1969) indicated that this Igm fluorescent treponemal antibody technique was superior to all other serological or clinical methods in evaluating the presence of congenital syphilis, whether specific antibody production was initiated in utero or post-natally. Mamunes et al (1970) in their evaluation of the test found similar results to those above and also showed that while the total IgM was not a reliable indicator of the presence of activity, the IgM fluorescent treponemal antibody test could detect considerably less than 1 mg per 100 ml of anti-treponemal IgM antibody.

While there is undoubtedly agreement as to the great value of this technique, its occasional limitation was shown by Ackerman (1969) who reported from California the occurrence of a fatal case of congenital syphilis with extremely severe but localised skin manifestations. The serum of this infant showed an apparent absence of IgM, although the

VDRL titre was two tubes dilution higher than VDRL titre on the mother's serum. Sepetjian et al (1970) found that sera from three infants gave positive results to the fluorescent IgM test and yet the seropositivity was believed to be due to reagin spill over as these infants were not considered to have congenital syphilis. They suggested that spill over of IgM might occur due to degenerative changes in the placenta in the pregnancy and that the test was not entirely specific for congenital syphilis, but might be of value in its exclusion. However, if this is suspected the coeruloplasmic concentration in the serum of mother and child should be determined. Comparison of the two concentrations may ascertain whether leakage has occurred. The coeruloplasmin concentration in the serum of pregnant women is four to six times that of normal adults, and that of normal infants is only half that of adults (W.H.O. Scientific Group, 1970). Despite these last two reports one cannot but emphasise the great value of this technique in the diagnosis of congenital syphilis. Unfortunately its sophistication and expense render it for the present at least, inapplicable in those developing countries which have a high incidence of congenital syphilis and where the need for such a test is so great.

In countries which carry out routine antenatal serological testing, the only mothers who may have infants affected by congenital syphilis are those who fail to attend for antenatal care or acquire syphilis after the first trimester. The occurrence of congenital syphilis in the infant of a seronegative mother has received attention during the last 10 years. Bethonod et al (1965) reported several such cases in Lyons and reiterated the views of Woody and his colleagues (1964) that there should be two serological examinations in each pregnancy; the first when the patient presents at the antenatal clinic and the second during the last trimester. Hallock and Tunnessen (1968) reported a similar episode in Philadelphia in 1968 as did Tinkler (1968) in Bristol. Al Salihi et al (1971) recommended that attention should be focused on high risk patients and in these individuals serological testing should be repeated at the beginning of the third trimester and again at the time of admission for labour and delivery. While these are undoubtedly counsels of perfection, it seems unlikely that repeat tests will be introduced as a routine. Nevertheless, in a country with enough resources and a significant syphilitic infection rate, the proposals of Al Salihi and his colleagues should receive consideration. The case reported by Tinkler (1968) is quite fascinating in that the maternal serology was negative on testing during pregnancy using the CWR, PPR, and RPCFT tests. The infant was diagnosed at the age of 16 months as a congenital syphilitic and the mother again had serological tests. The maternal TPI and RPCFT were both negative and the FTA-ABS was reported as showing a low titre of anti-treponemal antibody. The mother re-attended 13 months later and the same serological tests were all strongly positive.

The reports from developing countries in recent years of numbers of infants with congenital syphilis, underline the paradox of having excellent diagnostic and therapeutic paediatric units in the presence of inadequate or unsuitable antenatal screening. Consideration of these reports indicates that in this environment, congenital syphilis continues to present and behave in the manner documented in the pre-antibiotic era. Certain facts in recent publications are, however, worthy of mention The findings of Larsson and Larsson (1970) in Addis Ababa that 15·5 per cent of I 408 pregnant women were seropositive on VDRL testing, substantiate the contention of Schaller (1968) that in a community with endemic and acquired treponematoses, antenatal serological testing becomes a dubious clinical tool. Again Larsson and Larsson (1970) were unable to follow up 74 of these seropositive mothers, thus showing the difficulty of applying repeated examinations as a diagnostic aid. They found that mucocutaneous lesions dominated the clinical picture in the 30 infants who were found to have congenital syphilis. This was in contrast to the report from Kapala by Bwibo (1971) who described 21 cases of congenital syphilis where swelling of the extremities with pseudoparalysis was the common mode of presentation. This apparent discrepancy in clinical presentation is easily explained if one assumes that the patients in Ethiopia were being seen at an earlier stage of the disease process. A disease such as congenital syphilis which has a wide clinical spectrum, altering with the passage of time, can present with apparent variations dependent on the age at which the infant is examined.

The renal, haematological and radiological manifestations of early congenital syphilis have been studied during the past few years. Following reports from Merlini and Gusmano (1956) and Pollner (1966) of single cases of the nephrotic syndrome in young infants with congenital syphilis, came the investigations of McDonald et al (1971) from Cape Town. This survey of very young infants with the nephrotic syndrome showed that in six of ten patients reviewed congenital syphilis was the aetiological factor, and in that area syphilis is the commonest cause of the nephrotic syndrome in infants less than 1 year old. There was an excellent response to penicillin therapy and in view of this the authors suggested that congenital syphilis should be considered in all young infants with the nephrotic syndrome, as the response to the antibiotic therapy was so impressive. Hill et al (1972) and Kaplan et al (1972) carried out immunopathological studies on renal tissue obtained by biopsy from young infants with the nephrotic syndrome of syphilitic aetiology. Their findings suggested strongly that the renal lesions of congenital syphilis had an immune pathogenesis, in which an antigen–antibody complex is deposited on the basement membrane of the glomerulus. Wigglelinkhiuzen and his colleagues (see fig 15, p. 100) and Kaplan et al found that the antibody present in this complex was IgG.

Hill et al demonstrated the presence of IgG, IgA and IgM. Unsuccessful attempts were made, using direct fluorescent technique with fluorescent labelled rabbit anti-*T. pallidum* globulin, to find *T. pallidum* antigens in the kidney.

Frieman and Super (1966) demonstrated that syphilis was the most common cause of thrombocytopenia and bleeding, during the first few weeks of life, among Bantu babies in Baragwanath Hospital. They described 15 cases and felt that in view of the severe complications which may attend bleeding and cathesis, early diagnosis was essential; of four patients where there was a delay in diagnosis only one lived. Nevertheless, with prompt diagnosis and treatment the response to antibiotic therapy was excellent. Apart from the thrombocytopenia 10 of the infants had severe anaemia and six were jaundiced. Juhlian (1968) in reporting a similar case from Uppsala emphasised that treatment needed to be continued for some time, as the expected increase in the thrombocyte count only appeared on the seventeenth day of therapy. Baggio et al (1969) found that this coagulation disturbance was associated with macroglobulinaemia. The finding of macroglobulinaemia in the absence of thrombocytopenia had been reported in 1966 by two independent groups of workers (Francois et al, 1966; Marchi et al, 1966). Macroglobulinaemia was found in association with crytoglobulinaemia by Marchi and De Pra (1968). Leucoerythroblastic anaemia was found in eight infants aged under 6 months (Suggit and Lovric, 1968).

There have been two excellent papers on the radiological diagnosis of congenital syphilis. The first by Cremin and Fisher (1970), from the University of Cape Town, is a review of 102 patients aged under 6 months. The authors feel that the changes are due to growth disturbance, incomplete bone formation and collapse at the growing ends of bones. In view of the dystrophic, rather than the inflammatory origin of the lesions, they suggest that the nomenclature be reviewed. Forty-nine of their patients demonstrated metaphyseal changes with porosity occurring under the dense zone. Similar changes may be seen in congenital rubella and prematurity. The other metaphyseal changes which occur can also be found in congenital cytomegalovirus infection. They felt that the dystrophic type of osteitis was indistinguishable from congenital rubella. Coblentz et al (1970) from the University of Southern California reported the radiological findings in eight neonates with congenital syphilis. They believe that radiological evidence of congenital syphilis can be present frequently, in spite of negative reaction to reagin tests. Their view is that the abnormalities are of inflammatory origin. They feel that the changes in the diaphyses of the long bones are identical to those of neonatal pyogenic septicaemia and that pathological fractures are a feature of the metaphyseal disturbance. This concept of pathological fractures mimicking the 'Battered Baby syndrome' was referred to in a case report by Fisher et al (1972).

Eighth nerve involvement and interstitial keratitis have progressed relatively unimpeded with the advent of penicillin. The use of topical corticosteroid for interstitial keratitis in the mid-fifties and systemic steroids for eighth nerve involvement in the early sixties have improved the situation. Goldman and Girard (1967) reported the persistence of treponemes in the aqueous humour of two patients with interstitial keratitis. These two patients were treated with antibiotics in dosage levels which would previously have been regarded as curative. Goldman had carried out part of this work at the University of Miami under the directorship of J. L. Smith. During the next 3 years Smith and his co-workers produced many papers relating to both congenital and acquired syphilis. The hypothesis was that penicillin penetrates poorly into the aqueous humour. In order to achieve adequate therapeutic penicillin levels in the aqueous humour large dosages of penicillin would have to be given. Goldman (1970) noted that ampicillin entered the anterior chamber of the eye and recommended that this antibiotic be used in combination with probenecid. Smith and his co-workers, using Krajian Dieterle silver stains, maintained that *T. pallidum* could be demonstrated in eyes affected by interstitial keratitis (Montenegro et al, 1969; Smith, 1969). Immunofluorescent studies indicated that some of the treponemes found in the eye in late syphilis might well be T. pallidum (Goldman and Girard, 1968). Wilkinson (1968) stated that forms resembling treponemes might be artefacts such as glass spirals or filaments. Montenegro et al (1969) reviewed the work of their group and agreed that some of the findings, previously reported as treponemes, were artefacts although others were apparently treponemes. Rice et al (1970) investigated a number of patients with congenital syphilis. In their discussion of selected cases they describe two patients with previously treated congenital syphilis, from whose eyes treponeme-like forms were obtained. They felt that some of the forms seen were *T. pallidum* (see Fig. 20). However, if this were so, there is no evidence that current therapeutic regimens for early syphilis should be altered (Dunlop, 1972).

Britten and Palmer (1964) discussed the relation between inactive interstitial keratitis and glaucoma. In their study of 174 eyes exhibiting inactive interstitial keratitis two patients were found to have advanced glaucoma. They were considered in conjunction with seven other patients with known glaucoma and inactive interstitial keratitis. The importance of regular surveillance of such patients is implied as glaucoma develops insidiously.

Karmondy and Schuknecht (1966) analysed the symptomatology and clinical findings of 47 patients with eighth nerve involvement due to congenital syphilis. They found that the patients fell into two distinct groups. Those affected early in childhood developed profound bilateral deafness of sudden onset accompanied by minimal vestibular dysfunc-

5

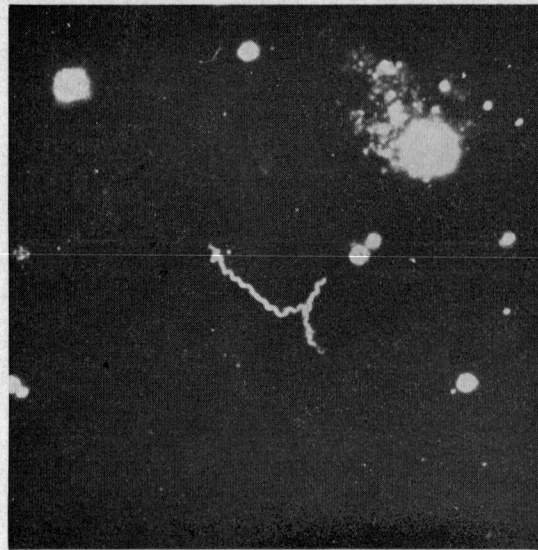

Fig. 20. Treponeme-like forms in aqueous humour from Mr. Q.D. (Case 1). × 630, enlarged × 7. (From a paper by N. S. C. Rice and others (1970). *Brit. J. vener. Dis.*, 46, 1. Reproduced by kind permission of the authors and the Editor of the *British Journal of Venereal Diseases*.)

tion. The patients affected at a later stage presented a picture otologically indistinguishable from Ménière's syndrome. Further research has been concerned with the second group.

Morrison (1969) used prednisone in the treatment of 22 patients with congenital syphilitic eighth nerve involvement who had previously received anti-treponemal therapy without effect. Ten patients showed definite hearing improvement. The author felt that an adequate response should occur within 4 weeks if there was going to be any response at all. Treatment commenced with 30 mg prednisone daily for 1 week and continued at 25 mg prednisone daily for a further 3 weeks. In the absence of any response the drug was withdrawn as rapidly as possible. However, if there had been improvement treatment was continued over the next 5 months with prednisone in gradually diminishing doses.

Certain workers felt that treponemes might be present in the inner ear in this condition and to achieve adequate therapeutic penicillin levels in the endolymph large doses of the drug should be given (Kerr et al, 1970). Kerr and his co-workers used prednisone 30 mg daily for 10 days in conjunction with ampicillin 6 g daily for 4 weeks. Using this regimen three patients showed a satisfactory response. Kerr et al (1973) elaborated on their initial communication, and on the basis of their management of 25 cases outlined the criteria for selection of those patients who might be expected to benefit from the treatment. They felt that any patient who had had profound deafness with complete loss of speech discrimination, for a period of over 6 months, had suffered irreparable damage and could not hope to benefit from treatment. As the underlying problem is one of word discrimination, the patients were evaluated and monitored using a speech discrimination test. This test was based on a number of lists of 25 monosyllables, presented to the test ear (the other ear being masked) at 40–45 dB above the average air conduction thresholds for 500, 1 000 and 2 000 Hz. The number of words repeated correctly was then expressed as a percentage. During treatment definite improvements in speech discrimination could be measured with this method and were in close agreement with the patient's subjective impression. At the same time pure tone audiograms would show little or no change, thus underlining the lack of value of the pure tone audiogram as a monitoring aid in the management of this condition. They have recently utilised ACTH 40 units weekly in these cases where response might be expected but where the results obtained with the prednisone/ampicillin regimen were not entirely satisfactory. They believe that if one ear is profoundly affected and the other exhibits progressive deafness the ACTH should be given indefinitely. The accompanying tinnitus and vertigo usually decreased as speech discrimination improved; the additon of anti-vertiginous drugs were helpful on occasions. The authors believe that as speech discrimination features prominently in the disease process the anatomical site involved is in relation to the auditory nerve, in either the spiral or Rosenthal's canal instead of the organ of Corti. While they admit that no treponemes have been recovered from the endolymph they point out that Mack et al (1969) found what they believed to be *T pallidum* in the enchondral bone of the labyrinthine canal.

REFERENCES

ACKERMAN, B. D. (1969). *J. Pediat.*, **74**, 459.

AGARWAL, L. P. (1960). *Documenta Ophthalmologica*, **14**, 97.

AIUTI, F., SERRA, G. B., TURBESSI, G., UNGARI, S. and ORZALESI, M. (1967). *G. Mal. Infett. Parassit.*, **19**, 332.

AL SALIHI, F. L., CURRAN, J. P. and SHTEIR, O. A. (1971). *J. Pediat.*, **78**, 121.

ALBERTAZZI, A., STRANI, G. F. and SARTORIS S. (1970). *G. Ital. Dermatol.*, **45**, 440.

ALERGANT, C. D. (1965). *Brit. J. vener. Dis.*, **41**, 300.

ALFORD, C. A., POLT, S. S., CASSADY, G. E., STRAUMFORD, J. V. and REMINGTON, J. S. (1969). *New Engl. J. Med.*, **280**, 1086.

ASHCROFT, M. T., MIALL, W. E. and STANDARD, K. L. (1967). *Brit. J. vener. Dis.*, **43**, 96.

BAKER, A. L., KAPLAN, M. M., WOLFE, H. J. and McGOWAN, J. A. (1971). *New Engl. J. Med.*, **284**, 1422.

BAGGIO, P., DRIGO, P. and REALDI, G. (1969). *Quad. Sclavo. Diagn. clin. Lab.*, **5**, 151.

BAUMGARTNER, B. R., WENGER, N. K., LANTZ, M. A. and NORINS, L. C. (1970). *Brit. J. vener. Dis.*, **46**, 386.

BEARDWELL, A. and JACOBS, J. H. (1969). *Proc. Roy. Soc. Med.*, **62**, 197.

BECK, W., BARNARD, C. N. and SCHRIRE, V. (1965). *Brit. Heart. J.*, **27**, 911.

BECKERLING, C. H., GIBB, B. H., HAUGHTON, H. G. H. and LE ROUX, B. T. (1969). *Thorax*, **24**, 173.

BETHENOD, M., NIVELOSS, J., HARTEMAN, E. and PICOUD, J. (1965). *J. Med., Lyon*, **46**, 1086.

BHORADE, M. S., CARAG, H. B. and LEE, H. J., (1971). *J. Amer. med. Ass.*, **216**, 1159.

BOISSIERE, H. (1967). *Concours méd.*, **89**, 7207.

BONCINELLI, U., VACCAR,, R., PINCELLI, L. and LANCELLOTTI, M. (1966). *G. ital. Derm.*, **107**, 1.

BOYLE, G. L., HEIN, H. F. and LEOPOLD, I. H. (1970). *Amer. J. Ophthal.*, **69**, 868.

BRAUNSTEIN, G. D., LEWIS, E. J., GALVAWEK, E. G., HAMILTON, A. and BELL, W. R. (1970). *Amer. J. Med.*, **48**, 643.

BRADFORD, L. L., BODILY, H. L., KETTERER, W. A., PUFFER, J., THOMAS, J. E. and TUFFANELLI, D. L. (1965). *Pub. Hlth Rep., Wash.*, **80**, 797.

BRITTEN, H. J. A. and PALMER, C. A. L. (1964). *Brit. J. Ophthal.*, **48**, 181.

BROPHY, E. M., ASHWORTH, C. T., ARIAS, M. and REYNOLDS, I. (1964). *Obstet. Gynec.*, **24**, 930.

BURKE, A. W. (1972). *Brit. J. vener., Dis.*, **48**, 249.

BWIBO, N. O. (1971). *E. Afr. med. J.*, **48**, 185.

CHAMBERS, R. W., FOLEY, H. T. and SCHMIDT, P. J. (1969). *Transfusion, Basel*, **9**, 32.

CH'IEN, L., HATHWAY, B. M. and ISRAEL, C. W. (1970). *J. Neurol. Neurosurg. Psychiat.*, **33**, 376.

CHRISTMAN, E. H., HAMILTON, R. W., HEATON, C. L. and HOFFMEYER, I. M. (1968). *Arch. Ophthal.*, **80**, 303.

COBLENTZ, D. R., CIMINI, R., MIKITY, V. G. and ROSEN, R. (1970). *J. Amer. med. Ass.*, **212**, 1061.

COCUZZA, C. and RANDAZZO, S. D. (1965). *Minerva derm.*, **40**, 357.

COHEN, J. A. (1970). *J. Amer. med. Ass.*, **214**, 375.

COLLART, P., BOREL, L. J. and DUREL, P. (1962). *Ann. Inst. Pasteur*, **102**, 596.

COLTOIU, A. and FORSEA, D. (1971). *Derm.-vener., Buc.*, **16**, 267.

COSNETT, J. E. (1965). *Cent. Afr. J. Med.*, **11**, 103.

COTTINI, G. B. and LAZZARO, C. (1965). *G. ital., Derm.*, **106**, 77.

COURTNEY EVANS, R. J., BENSON, M. K. and HUGHES, D. T. D. (1971). *Brit. med. J.*, i, 530.

CREMIN, B. J. and FISHER, R. M. (1970). *Brit. J. Radiol.*, **43**, 333.

CRIPPS, D. J. and CURTIS, A. C. (1969). *Arch. Derm.*, **100**, 122.

DANIELSSON, D., JOHANNISSON, G. and HEDERSTEDT, B. (1970). *Acta path. microbiol. scand.*, **78**, 267.

DATTA, A. K. (1965). *Indian J. Derm. Venereol.*, **31**, 108.

DATTA, A. K. (1968). *Indian J. Derm. Venereol.*, **34**, 18.

DATEY, K. K. and KELKAR, P. N. (1969). *Indian Heart J.*, **21**, 253.

DAWSON BUTTERWORTH, K. and HEATHCOTE, P. R. M. (1970). *Brit. J. vener. Dis.*, **46**, 295.

DEGOS, R., TOURAINE, R., COLLART, P., DANIEL, F. and AUDEBERT, G. (1970). *Bull. Soc. fr. Derm. Syph.*, **77**, 10.

DEWHURST, K. (1968). *J. Neurol. Neurosurg. Psychiat.*, **31**, 496.

DEWHURST, K. (1969a). *Brit. J. Psychiat.*, **115**, 31.

DEWHURST, K. (1969b). *Acta neurol. scand.*, **45**, 119.

DOGLIOTTI, M. (1971). *S. Afr. med. J.*, **45**, 8.

DUNLOP, E. M. C. (1972). *Brit. med. J.*, ii, 577.

FALLS, W. F., FORD, K. L., ASHWORTH, C. J. and CARTER, N. W. (1965). *Ann. intern. Med.*, **63**, 1047.

FERNANDO, W. L. (1965). *Brit. J. vener. Dis.*, **41**, 168.

FERNANDO, W. L. (1968). *Brit. J. vener. Dis.*, **44**, 134.

FISHER, R. H., KAPLAN, J. and HOLDER, J. C. (1972). *clin. Pediat.*, **II**, 305.
FIUMARA, N. J. and LESSELL, S. (1970). *Arch. Derm.*, **102**, 78.
FOGEL, B. J., TAMER, A. M. and FAJACO, R. M. (1969). *J. Floa. med. Ass.*, **56**, 777.
FRANCOIS, R., GERMAIN, D., RACLE, P. and MOREAU, P. (1966). *Pediatrie*, **21**, 47.
FRATER, R. W. M. and JORDAN, A. (1968). *Ann. thorac. Surg.*, **6**, 463.
FREIMAN, I. and SUPER, M. (1966). *Arch. Dis. Childh.*, **41**, 87.
FRIEDMAN, B. (1969). *W. Virginia Med. J.*, **65**, 65.
FULFORD, K. W. M. and BROSTOFF, J. (1972). *Brit. J. vener. Dis.*, **48**, 483.
GAGER, W. E., ISRAEL, C. W. and SMITH, J. L. (1968). *Brit. J. vener. Dis.*, **44**, 277.
GARDNER, H. F. and ROBSON, J. H. (1968). *J. clin. Path.*, **21**, 276.
GASTIN, L. and OSSANDON, M. (1965). *Rev. Chile Obstet. Ginec.*, **30**, 95.
GOFFINET, D. R., HOYT, C. and ELTRINGHAM, J. R. (1970). *Calif. Med.*, **112**, 22.
GOLDEN, B. and THOMPSON, H. S. (1969). *Survey Ophthal.*, **14**, 716.
GOLDMAN, J. N. (1970). *Trans. Amer. Acad. Ophthal. Oto-laryng.*, **74**, 509.
GOLDMAN, J. N. and GIRARD, K. F. (1967). *Arch. Ophthal.*, **78**, 47.
GOLDMAN, J. N. and GIRARD, K. F. (1968). *Arch. Ophthal.*, **79**, 716.
GOWARDMAN, M. G. (1970). *N. Z. Med. J.*, **71**, 178.
GRAHMANN, H. (1969). *Nervenarzt*, **40**, 92.
HALLOCK, J. and TUNNESSEN, W. W. (1968). *Obstet. Gynec., N.Y.*, **32**, 336.
HANSON, A. W. (1970). *Brit. J. vener. Dis.*, **46**, 303.
HARPER, J. M., POLITANO, V. A. and SCHWARCZ, B. (1967). *J. Urol.*, **97**, 862.
HARRIS, J. R. W., McCANN, V. J., KENNEDY, J. and FULTON, T. T. (1974). *Acta derm.venereol., Stockh.* (In press).
HARRIS, J. R. W., McCANN, V. J., KENNEDY, J., MAHONY, J. D. H. and FULTON, T. T. (1973). *Brit. J. vener. Dis.* (In press).
HARTSOCK, R. J., HALLING, L. W. and KING, F. M. (1970). *Amer. J. clin. Path.*, **53**, 304.
HARVEY, W. P., CORRADO, M. and PERLOFF, J. K. (1963). *Amer. J. med. Sci.*, **245**, 533.
HELLIER, M. D., WEBSTER, A. D. B. and EISINGER, A. J. M. F. (1971). *Brit. med. J.*, iv, 404.
HERAUT, L., ZWINGELSTEIN, J., AYATS, H. et al (1971). *Bull. Soc. Med. Afr. Noir. Lang. Franc.*, **16**, 190.
HILL, L. L., SINGER, D. E., FALLETTA, J. and STASNEY, R. (1972). *Pediatrics*, **49**, 260.
HILTENBRAND, C., MERLEN, J. F. and COTTEN, L. (1967). *Arch. Mal. Coeur*, **60**, 1041.
HOOSHMAND, H., ESCOBAR, M. R. and KOPF, S. W. (1972). *J. Amer. med. Ass.*, **219**, 726.
IDSØE, O., GUTHE, T. and WILLCOX, R. R. (1972). *Bull. Wld Hlth Org.*, **47**, Suppl. 13 and 20.
JARVIS, J. F. and KUSCHKE, E. R. H. (1968). *J. Laryng.*, **82**, 157.
JEFFERISS, F. J. G. (1963). *Brit. J. vener. Dis.*, **39**, 139.
JOFFE, R., BLACK, M. M. and FLOYD, M. (1968). *Brit. med. J.*, i, 211.
JOHNS, D. (1970). *J. Bone Jt Surg., Edin.*, **52**, 724.
JOKINEN, E. J., LASSUS, A. and LINDER, E. (1969). *Ann. clin. Res.*, **I**, 77.
JUE, R., PUFFER, J., WOOD, R. M., SCHOCHET, G., SMARTT, W. H. and KETTERER, W. A. (1967). *Amer. J. clin. Path.*, **47**, 809.
JUHLIN, L. (1968). *Acta derm.-venereol., Stockh.*, **48**, 166.
KAHN, M. F., BAILLER, F., AMOUROUX, J. and DE SEZE, S. (1970). *Rev. Rhum.*, **37**, 431.
KALLICHURUN, S. (1969). *S. Afr. med. J.*, **43**, 250.
KAPLAN, B. S., WIGGLESWORTH, F. W., MARKS, M. I. and DRUMMOND, K. N. (1972). *J. Pediat.*, **81**, 1154.
KARMONDY, C. S. and SCHUKNECHT, H. F. (1966). *Arch. Otolaryng.*, **83**, 18.
KARMI, G., THIRKETTLE, J. L. and READ, A. E. A. (1969). *Postgrad. med. J.*, **45**, 675.
KELLOGG, D. S. (1970). *Hlth lab. Sci.*, **7**, 34.
KELLOGG, D. S. and DEACON, W. E. (1964). *Proc. Soc. exp. Biol.*, **115**, 963.

KERR, A. G., SMYTH, G. D. and LANDAU, H. D. (1970). *Arch. Otolaryng* **91**, 474.
KERR, A. G., SMYTH, G. D. L. and CINNAMOND, M. J. (1973). *J. Lar. Otology*, **87**, I.
KOFFMANN, O. (1956). *Canad. med. Ass.*, **74**, 807.
LAL, S. (1970). *Indian. J. Derm. Venereol.*, **36**, 201.
LANCET (1968). ii, 718.
LARSSON, Y. and LARSSON, U. (1970). *Ethiop. med. J.*, **8**, 163.
LEE, R. V., THORNTON, G. F. and CONN, H. O. (1971). *New Engl. J. Med.*, **284**, 1423.
LEJMAN, K. and BODASZEWSKA-CZABANOWSKA, J. (1964). *Przegl. derm.*, **51**, 539.
LEJMAN, K. and BOGDASZEWSKA-CZABANOWSKA, J. (1969). *Brit. J. vener. Dis.*, **45**, 313.
MACFAUL, P. A. and Catterall, R. D. (1971). *Brit. J. vener. Dis.*, **47**, 159.
MACKAY, D. M., PRICE, E. V., KNOX, J. M. and SCOTTI, A. (1969). *J. Amer. med. Ass.*, **207**, 1683.
MCCRACKEN, J. D., HALL, W. H. and PIERCE, H. I. (1969). *Milit. Med.*, **134**, 682.
MCDONALD, R., WIGGELINKHUIZEN, J. and KASCHULA, R. O. C. (1971). *Amer. J. Dis. Child.*, **122**, 507.
MCNEEL, D. P. and EHNI, G. (1969). *J. Neurosurg.*, **30**, 55.
MAHONY, J. D. H., HARRIS, J. R. W., MCCANN, J. S., KENNEDY, J. and DOUGHAN, H. J. (1972). *Acta derm.-venereol. Stockh.*, **52**, 71.
MAMUNES, P., CAVE, V. C., BUDELL, J. W., ANDERSON, A. J. and STEWARD, R. E. (1970). *Amer. J. Dis. Child.*, **120**, 17.
MARCHI, A. G. and DE PRA, A. (1968). *G. Mal. Infett. Parassit.*, **20**, 249.
MARCHI, A. G., TAMBUSSI, A. M. and FAMULARO, L. (1966). *Minerva Pediat.*, **18**, 1155.
MASTERSON, G. (1965). *Brit. J. vener. Dis.*, **41**, 181.
MATTERN, P., SANDOR, G., PILLOT, J. and LOBEZ, D. (1965). *Ann. Inst. Pasteur*, Suppl. 120.
MERLINI, M. and GUSMANO, R. (1966). *Aggiorn. Pediat.*, **17**, 489.
MICHAUD, P., TERMET, H. and CHASSINOLLE, J. (1970). *Arch. Mal. Coeur*, **63**, 674.
MIKHAIL, G. R. and CHAPEL, T. A. (1969). *Arch. Derm.*, **100**, 471.
MILICH, M. V. (1968). *Soviet Med.*, **31**, 94.
MINIKIN, W., LANDY, S. E. and COHEN, H. J. (1967). *Arch. Derm.*, **95**, 217.
MITCHELL, R. M. and BRALOW, S. P. S. (1964). *Ann. intern. Med.*, **61**, 933.
MONTENEGRO, E. N. R, ISRAEL, C. W., NICOL, W. G. and SMITH, J. L. (1969). *Amer. J. Ophthal.*, **67**, 335.
MORRISON, A. W. (1969). *Proc. roy. Soc. Med.*, **62**, 959.
O'NEILL, P. and NICOL, C. S. (1972). *Brit. J. vener. Dis.*, **48**, 460.
OXELIUS, V. A., RORSMAN, H. and LAURELL, A. B. (1969). *Brit. J. vener. Dis.*, **45**, 121.
PARKER, J. D. (1972). *Brit. J. veneer. Dis.*, **48**, 32.
PASSERINI, A. and VAGHI, M. A. (1966). *Radiol. Med.*, **52**, 23.
POLLNER, P. (1966). *J. Amer. med. Ass.*, **198**, 263.
RHODES, F. A. and ANDERSON, S. E. J. (1970). *Papua New Guinea med. J.*, **13**, 49.
RICE, N. S. C., DUNLOP, E. M. C., JONES, B. R., HARE, M. J., KING, A. J., RODIN, P., MUSHIN, A. and WILKINSON, A. E. (1970). *Brit. J. vener. Dis.*, **46**, I.
ROITBURD, M. F. (1968). *Vestn. Derm. Vener.*, **42**, 82.
ROSSI, D., CARGIULO, F. and D'ALGESSIO, E. S. (1967). *Riv. ital. Ginec.*, **51**, 480.
RYAN, S. J., NELL, E. E. and HARDY, P. H. (1972). *Amer. J. Ophthal.*, **73**, 250.
SAKAMOTO, T., KAWAI, N., UOZUMI, Z., YAMADA, T., INDOUE, K., CHANG, S. Y. and UEDA, H. (1968). *Jap. Jeart. J.*, **9**, 117.
SAMENIUS, B. (1968). *Dis. Colon Rect.*, **II**, 462.
SARKANY, I. (1965). *Proc. roy. Soc. Med.*, **58**, 620.
SCALLA, A. and FUCCI, A. (1970). *Osped. Psichiat.*, **38**, 108.
SCHALLER, K. F. (1968). *Z. Haut.-u. Geschl.K-r.*, **43**, 17.
SCHMIDT, H., DEIN, E. and RASMUSSEN, E. B. (1970). *Brit. J. vener. Dis.*, **46**, 135.
SCHMIDT, H. and GOLDSCHMIDT, E. (1972). *Brit. J. vener. Dis.*, **48**, 400.
SCHNEIDER, S. and BOLTE, B. (1972). *Med. Welt.*, Stuttg., **23**, 319.

SCHNEIDER, H. J. and SPITZ, H. B. (1968). *Dis. Chest.*, **53**, 340.
SCHIRE, V., BARNARD, C. N. and BECK, W. (1966). *S. Afr. med. J.*, **40**, 553.
SCOTTI, A. T. and LOGAN, L. (1968). *J. Pediat.*, **73**, 242.
SCOTTI, A., LOGAN, L. and CALDWELL, J. G. (1969). *J. Pediat.*, **75**, 1129.
SEPETJIAN, M., MONIER, J. C., NIVELON, J. L., THIVOLET, J. and TISSOT GUERRZA, F. (1970). *Brit. J. vener. Dis.*, **46**, 18.
SERRE, H., GROS, C., SIMON, L., BRAUMELOU, H. and LAMBOLEY, C. (1970). *Rev. Rhum.*, **37**, 525.
SHALICKOVA, O. and HATULAY, K. (1971). *Ces. Psychiat.*, **67**, 260.
SHERLOCK, S. (1971). *New Engl. J. Med.*, **284**, 1437.
SHORR, N., MACK, L. W. and SMITH, J. L. (1969). *Brit. J. Ophthal.*, **53**, 331.
SMITH, D. (1965). *Dis. Colon Rectum*, **8**, 57.
SMITH, J. L. and TAYLOR, W. H. (1965). *Amer. J. Ophthal.*, **60**, 653.
SMITH, J. L. and ISRAEL, G. W. (1967). *Arch. Ophthal.*, **77**, 474.
SMITH, J. L., ISRAEL, C. W. and HARNER, R. E. (1967). *Arch. Ophthal.*, **78**, 284.
SMITH, J. L. (1969). *Trans. Amer. Acad. Ophthal. Otolaryng.*, **73**, 1113.
SOBEL, H. J. and WOLF, E. H. (1972). *Arch. Path.*, **93**, 565.
SPANGLER, A. S., JACKSON, J. H., FIUAMRA, N. J. and WARTHIN, T. A. (1964). *J. Amer. med. Ass.*, **189**, 87.
SPARLING, P. F. (1971). *New Engl. J. Med.*, **284**, 642.
SUAREZ, J. A. and DE SUAREZ, C. (1969). *Arch. Inst. Cardiol. Mex.*, **39**, 323.
SUGGIT, R. I. C. and LOVRIC, V. A. (1968). *Med. J. Aust.*, i, 760.
TINKLER, A. E. (1968). *Brit. J. vener. Dis.*, **44**, 136.
TUMASHEVA, N. I. and GARMATYUK, G. K. (1968). *Vestn. Derm. Vener.*, **42**, 43.
TURNER, T. B., HARDY, P. H. and NEWMAN, B. (1969). *Brit. J. vener. Dis.*, **45**, 183.
VINCENTI, N. H. (1971). *J. Laryng.*, **85**, 869.
VUKOTICH, D. and GIEL, R. (1970). *Trop. Geog. Med.*, **22**, 45.
WAUGH, M. A. (1972). *Brit. med. J.*, i, 803.
WETHERILL, J. H., WEBB, H. E. and CATTERALL, R. D. (1965). *Brit. med. J.*, i, 1157.
WHITE, R. J. (1965). *Brit. J. vener. Dis.*, **41**, 149.
WHITFIELD, R. and WIROSTKO, E. (1970). *Arch. Ophthal.*, **84**, 12.
W.H.O. SCIENTIFIC GROUP, TREPONEMATOSES RESEARCH (1970). *Wld Hlth Org. techn. Rep. Ser.*, Geneva, **455**,
WIGGLELINKHIUZEN, J., KASCHULA, R. O. and UYS, C. J. *Arch. Dis. Chrld.*, **48**, 375.
WILLCOX, R. R. and GOODWIN, P. G. (1971). *Brit. J. vener. Dis.*, **47**, 401.
WILLCOX, R. R. (1964). *Brit. J. vener. Dis.*, **40**, 90.
WILLCOX, R. R. (1971). *Abst. Hyg.*, **46**, 930.
WILKINSON, A. E. and COWELL, L. P. (1971). *Brit. J. vener. Dis.*, **47**, 252.
WILKINSON, A. E. (1968). *Trans. ophthal. Soc. U.K.*, **88**, 251.
WILNER, E. and BRODY, J. A. (1968). *Lancet*, ii, 1370.
WOODY, N. C., SISTRUNK, W. F. and PLATON, R. V. (1964). *J. Pediat.*, **64**, 63.
WRIGHT, D. J. M. (1969). *Postgrad. med. J.*, **45**, 191.
WRIGHT, D. J. M., DONIAH, D., LESSOF, M. H., TURK, J. L., GRIMBLE, A. S. and CATTERALL, R. D. (1970). *Lancet*, i, 740.
YAMAGUCHI, T. et al. (1969). *Stomach Invest.*, Tokyo, **4**, 619.
YARRINGTON, C. T. and JENSEN, O. C. (1967). *Otolaryng.*, Chicago, **86**, 113.
YOUNG, A. W. and SUN, A. P. (1965). *J. Amer. geriat. Soc.*, **13**, 462.
ZELLERMANN, H. E. and NORCROSS, J. W. (1967). *Lahey clin. Found. Bull.*, **16**, 255.

9 Non-venereal Treponematoses

J. R. W. Harris

ENDEMIC TREPONEMATOSES

In the course of various national and international programmes to eradicate the non-venereal treponematoses at least 160 million people had been examined, and 50 million treated by 1969. These campaigns were based on initial treatment surveys followed by periodic surveillance surveys to assess progress. The prevalence of infectious yaws lesions had been reduced to a fraction of the original figure and in Bosnia the rate of infectious lesions in endemic syphilis has been reduced to nil. In the areas where active transmission still occurs further treatment programmes will be necessary. In some regions, such as Western Samoa and Northern Nigeria, children born after the eradication campaign were found to have sero-positive treponemal tests, although no evidence of active clinical lesions was observed. Again the prevalence of high antibody levels suggests that the potential for infectious relapse may also have a predictive value (Guthe et al, 1972).

The eradication programme for endemic treponematoses has unfortunately resulted in many millions of individuals becoming susceptible to infection with *T. pallidum*. The occurrence of venereal syphilis has been reported in rural areas of New Guinea (Rhodes and Anderson, 1970), Western Samoa and Thailand (Guthe et al 1972), where yaws was previously endemic. In other countries where the eradication of endemic treponematoses has not been complete sexually transmitted syphilis co-exists with the endemic infection. In these situations the endemic infection will more frequently occur in rural areas and the sexually transmitted infection in the urban areas. This has been reported by Du Toit (1969) from the Karoo, by Schaller (1968) in Ethiopia and by Kooy (1970) in Surinam. The clinical implications of these facts are obvious as it will frequently be difficult to differentiate between the sexually acquired and endemic infections if the patient exhibits few clinical signs. The situation is further confused as the clinical demarcations between yaws and syphilis were re-evaluated by Smith et al (1971)

124

who demonostrated that contrary to previous opinions late yaws can produce neuro-ophthalmological abnormalities. This was a most impressive research study undertaken with the full co-operation of Dr. Rafael Medina, who has an international reputation as a clinician dealing with non-venereal treponematoses.

The problem of diagnosis of sexually transmitted syphilis in patients who originate from areas where endemic treponematoses were prevalent, occurs all over the world. As a result of population movement almost all clinicians have been confronted at one time or another with this situation. The clinical difficulties have been documented in the United Kingdom by Wray (1966) and Lanigan-O'Keefe et al (1967); in France by van Wymeersch and Drumel (1968) and Neil and Gentilini (1970); and in New Zealand by Fischman and Mundt (1971). The difficulties of evaluating serological techniques among such patients is discussed by Garner et al (1970).

There has been much interest in the high titre sero-reactivity in child sero-reactors (Guthe and Idsøe, 1968) as this indicates a recrudescence potential. When this is considered in conjunction with the presence of treponeme-like forms in human host tissues (Collart et al, 1962) it is obvious that there is much not yet understood about the host/agent relationship and the effect of antibiotic treatment on this relationship. The discovery of treponemes in the lymph nodes of wild African baboons whose serum was reactive in the TPI but not the VDRL tests, and who did not have clinical disease has added to the speculation (Fribourg-Blanc et al, 1966). These studies, indicating alteration in the disease pattern of the treponeme as a result of antibiotic treatment, may be applicable to the disease pattern of sexually transmitted syphilis in the years to come.

REFERENCES

COLLART, P., BOREL, L. J. and DUREL, P. (1962). *Ann. Inst. Pasteur*, **102**, 596.

DU TOIT, J. A. (1969). *S. Afr. med. J.*, **43**, 355.

FISCHMAN, A. and MUNDT, H. (1971). *Brit. J. vener. Dis.*, **47**, 91.

FRIBOURG-BLANC, A., NIEL, G. and MOLLART, H. H. (1966). *Bull. Soc. Path. exot.*, **59**, 54.

GARNER, M. F., BLACKHOUSE, J. L., COOK, C. A. and ROEDER, P. J. (1970). *Brit. J. vener. Dis.*, **46**, 284.

GUTHE, T. and IDSØE, O. (1968). *Brit. J. vener. Dis.*, **44**, 35.

GUTHE, T., RIDET, J., VORST, F., D'COSTA, J. and GRAB, B. (1972). *Bull. Wld. Hlth. Org.*, **46**, 1.

KOOY, P. (1970). *Trop. Geog. Med.*, **22**, 172.

LANIGAN-O'KEEFE, F. M., HOLMES, J. G. and HILL, D. (1967). *Brit. J. Derm.*, **79**, 325.

NIEL, G. and GENTILINI, M. (1970). *Bull. Soc. Path. extot.*, **63**, 180.

RHODES, F. A. and ANDERSON, S. E. J. (1970). *Papua New Guinea med. J.*, **13**, 49.

SCHALLER, K. F. (1968). *Z. Haut.-u. Gesch.-Kr.*, **43**, 17.

SMITH, J. L., DAVID, N. J., INDIGN, S., ISRAEL, C. W., LEVINE, B. M., JUSTICE, J.,

McCRARY, J. A., MEDINA, R., PAEZ, P., SANTANA, E., SARKAR, M., SCHATZ, N. J., SPITZER, M. L., SPITZER, W. O. and WALTER, E. K. (1971). *Brit. J. vener. Dis.*, **47**, 226.

W. H. O. TECH. REP. SER. (1970). **455**, 48.

WRAY, P. M. (1966). *Brit. J. vener. Dis.*, **42**, 25.

WYMEERSCH, H. van and Drumel, G. (1968). *Presse med.*, **76**, 1774.

10 Syphilis Serology

A. E. Wilkinson

Introduction

The introduction of the Treponemal Immobilisation (TPI) test in 1949 heralded a revolution in the serological diagnosis of syphilis because it provided a truly specific test for the first time. This led to a reappraisal of the classical tests for anti-lipoidal antibody (reagin) and to recognition of their function as screening rather than as diagnostic procedures. In the period reviewed, 1964–72, the main advances have been the introduction of simpler specific tests for treponemal disease, based on *Treponema pallidum* as antigen and using immunofluorescence or haemagglutination techniques for the detection of antibody. Newer tests for reagin have also been described and adapted for automated procedures. It is recognised that a variety of antibodies, both non-specific and anti-treponemal, are produced during infection with *T. pallidum* and other pathogenic treponemes. These, with the tests used to detect them are summarised in Table VI. None of these tests will

Table VI. Types of antibody produced during treponemal infection

Type of antibody	Test
Anti-lipoidal (reagin)	Complement fixation: WR
	Flocculation: VDRL, Kahn
	Rapid plasma reagin
	Automated reagin
Cardiolipin F	Immunofluorescence
Group-reactive anti-treponemal	Reiter protein complement-fixation test
	Reiter agglutination
	Reiter latex test
Specific anti-treponemal	Treponemal Immobilisation Test
	Fluorescent treponemal antibody tests
	Treponemal haemagglutination test

distinguish syphilis from infections with the other pathogenic treponemes, although these infections produce different patterns of response
in experimental animals (Paris-Hamelin et al, 1968).

TESTS FOR ANTI-LIPOIDAL ANTIBODY (REAGIN)

The VDRL slide test has won general acceptance as a test of high
sensitivity. Garner and Grantham (1968) have emphasised the importance of minimal 'rough' reactions which are usually disregarded. These
were seen in 514 out of 61 000 routine sera and TPI tests on them proved
to be positive in 189; almost two-thirds of these patients were not
known to have syphilis. VDRL antigen suspended in choline chloride
has been used to test plasma or unheated serum. Traces of metallic
impurities, such as copper, may make the antigen unstable. Portnoy
and Garson (1960) and Portnoy et al (1961) added a chelating agent
(EDTA) to this antigen for the Unheated Serum Reagin (USR) test;
antigen suspensions so prepared are thought to remain stable for 6
months when stored at 3–10°C. A further modification is the Rapid
Plasma Reagin (Circle) card (RPR) test (Portnoy, 1963, 1965). In this,
finely divided carbon particles are added to USR test antigen; results
can be read by the naked eye instead of microscopically as in the
VDRL and USR tests. The test is performed with disposable equipment
on plastic cards marked in circular areas and results are read after 8
minutes rotation. Evaluations of this test, usually in parallel with the
VDRL slide test, have been reported by Portnoy et al (1962), Falcone
et al (1964), Buck and Mayer (1964), Brown et al (1964), Tio (1970) and
Walker (1971). The RPR card test is rather more sensitive than the
VDRL slide test. In the evaluation of its performance on 203 sera with
negative TPI and FTA-ABS tests which had given biological false
positive (BFP) reactions, Garner and Backhouse (1972) found the
RPR reactive on 156 and the VDRL on 189; as these had been selected
on the basis of reactivity in the WR or VDRL tests, this disparity may
not be valid. They found the RPR test more specific than the VDRL in
tests on 255 sera from patients with lepromatous leprosy who had
negative treponemal tests; in this group the VDRL test was reactive in
24 but the RPR test in only 12. This confirms an earlier report by
Portnoy et al (1962). Because of its simplicity, stability of the antigen
and the use of disposable equipment, the RPR card test is a suitable
screening test for use both in the laboratory and in field surveys.

Automation of screening tests. The need to process very large numbers of
sera in laboratories such as those serving blood transfusion centres has
led to the development of truly automated tests as distinct from the use
of mechanical aids for the dispensing of reagents. Pugh and Gaze
(1965), Gaillon et al (1966) and Wagstaff et al (1969) have reported on

the use of the continuous flow Auto-Analyser equipment for carrying out a Wassermann reaction. Glenn and Turnbull (1971) have used a discrete system (the 'Bioanalyst') for this and reported fairly satisfactory results, although the automated method appeared less sensitive than manually performed tests on the same specimens.

In the Automated Reagin Test (ART) (McGrew et al, 1968), RPR card test antigen is used in Auto-Analyser equipment. Uninactivated serum or plasma and antigen are sampled automatically, passed through mixing and settling coils and the reactants deposited on a moving strip of filter paper. Positive results are shown by clumping of the carbon marker particles, while negative sera give a uniform grey streak. Evaluations have shown it to compare favourably with the manually performed VDRL test (Stevens and Stroebel, 1970; Cate et al, 1971; West et al, 1971; Wilkinson et al, 1972). About 100 specimens can be tested qualitatively per hour. Unlike most flocculation tests, prozones are very uncommon with this technique, which is an added advantage for a screening test. Lockyer (1970) has described the use of the same apparatus with a modified Laughlen antigen but this would not seem to offer any advantage, except in cost, over the cardiolipin RPR antigen.

Comparative sensitivity of tests for reagin antibody. Dandoy (1967) found the Kolmer WR slightly more sensitive than the VDRL test in primary syphilis but the two tests showed almost identical reactivity in secondary and early latent syphilis. Garner (1968) tested sera from 156 patients with primary syphilis and found the VDRL reactive in 76·9 per cent and a cardiolipin WR in 73·7 per cent. Wende et al (1971) found the VDRL reactive in 73·3 per cent of 322 cases of primary syphilis. Lassus et al (1970) studied the rate of reversal of tests for reagin and antibody in patients with early syphilis in whom the duration of infection was known. If treatment was given within 3 months of infection, rapid reversal occurred in most cases. Those treated more than 3 months after infection showed little change in their serological reactions and even a year after treatment the VDRL and Kolmer WR were still reactive in over half the patients. They consider the tests for reagin to be better indicators of the success of treatment than the treponemal tests. Atypical patterns of serological reactivity in Ugandan Africans with syphilis have been reported by Massawe and others (1972). They found that 12 per cent of patients with confirmed secondary syphilis had negative VDRL tests or tests reactive only at a very low titre. In 40 patients with general paralysis the VDRL test was negative in 21. Fischman and Mundt (1971) found that sera from immigrants from the Pacific Islands to New Zealand, who were thought to have yaws, reacted more strongly with a crude tissue extract WR antigen than with a cardiolipin WR antigen or with the VDRL test; the reverse was true of sera from patients with syphilis.

Cardiolipin F antibody. This was detected by Wright and others (1970) by an immunofluorescence technique. It produces diffuse staining of the cytoplasm of the distal tubules and to a lesser degree the proximal tubules in sections of rat kidney. It can be absorbed from the serum with VDRL antigen or cardiolipin, thus differing from cardiolipin M antibody found in primary biliary cirrhosis and in the sera of BFP reactors. It may be either IgG or IgM in nature and was found mainly in early syphilis, in 7 of 34 sera from primary syphilis, 20 of 21 secondary and 12 of 26 early latent syphilis. It is not completely specific for syphilis as it was found in the sera of two patients with very high titred chronic BFP reactions. It is suggested that its presence in latent syphilis may suggest that the infection is fairly recent.

GROUP ANTI-TREPONEMAL ANTIBODY

The Reiter protein complement-fixation test. Antigen for this test is prepared by precipitating an ultrasonicate of Reiter treponemes with 70 per cent saturated ammonium sulphate. This is a crude material, and Cannefax (1963) found that commercial antigens contained a considerable proportion of serologically inactive protein and carbohydrate. Some purification of the protein was possible by fractionation on DEAE cellulose or by high speed centrifugation. Bekker et al (1966) stress that for optimal sensitivity, undiluted serum should be tested in the RPCF test, which should be done quantitatively, as prozones may occur. When antigen was heated to destroy its protein content, positive reactions were still found in 0·96 per cent of 6 000 sera from healthy donors and in 10·9 per cent of 477 syphilitic sera. These reactions are thought to be due to an antibody reacting with a lipopolysaccharide impurity in the crude antigen. Similar findings were reported by Pillot and Dupouey (1964). Pillot et al (1965) found this antibody in the sera of 0·05 to 0·5 per cent of normal individuals and consider that the antigen concerned is situated in the treponemal sheath. Förström et al (1969) found 0·36 per cent false positive reactions in the RPCF test among 22 048 sera examined. Of these 79 sera, the reactions were transient in 49 and lasted for 6 months or more in 23, in seven the duration was not known. In 43 sera some tests for reagin were also positive. Ten patients had lupus erythematosus and two rheumatoid arthritis. Most of these patients had evidence of some infectious disease.

The antibody causing false positive reactions in the RPCF test is distinct from that causing BFP reactions in tests for reagin, and it is rare for the two antibodies to be present together. The RPCF test is most useful when used as a screening test in conjunction with a sensitive test for reagin; the combination has a higher detection rate than either test used alone. Morris (1968) screened 35 912 antenatal sera with RPCF, WR and VDRL tests; 48 sera were reactive with one or more tests and the specificity confirmed by TPI or FTA tests; of these 48, the RPCF was the only test positive on 13 sera. Salo et al (1967), using a quantitative test, found that it became positive in the primary stage before the TPI test; titres were maximal in the secondary stage and usually rather low in late symptomatic and latent syphilis. The antibody persists for long periods after treatment; Putkonen et al (1963) found the test positive in 54 of 57 patients treated for neurosyphilis less than 9 years previously, and in 46 of 50 in whom a longer period had elapsed. For an evaluation of the test on over 30 000 sera and a review of the literature the monograph by Förström (1967) should be consulted.

Fischman (1964) described the use of latex particles sensitised with Reiter protein antigen for an agglutination test; he found 92 per cent agreement with the RPCF test on 388 sera, but noted that not all batches of Reiter protein antigen were suitable for use. Carpenter et al (1966) coated latex particles with both Reiter protein and cardiolipin antigens for use as a screening test. Engelbrecht and Denis (1970) sensitised tanned formolised sheep erythrocytes with an ultrasonicate of Reiter treponemes. As the antigen aged, haemagglutination by normal sera developed; this could be avoided by using bis-diazobenzidine as a coupling agent. This method was tested in parallel with classical tests and the FTA-200 test on 50 syphilitic and seven BFP sera and gave satisfactory results. The sensitised cells could be lyophilised.

Banffer (1972) used counter-current electrophoresis to detect precipitating antibody in syphilitic sera against a lysate of Reiter treponemes as antigen. Positive reactions were found in 161 of 162 sera which were positive in the RPCF test but in none of 100 sera from blood donors which gave negative tests for reagin. This technique has the advantage that it can be used with anti-complementary sera.

SPECIFIC TREPONEMAL TESTS

Treponemal immobilisation test

The reputation of the TPI test as the most specific test available for the detection of treponemal disease has not been challenged, and recent developments have been concerned with modifications of technique to enhance the speed and sensitivity of the reaction. Metzger (1965) added lysozyme to the reaction mixture at a concentration of 200 μg/ml and provided anaerobic conditions by covering the contents of the tubes with a layer of liquid paraffin 1·5 cm in depth instead of incubating in the usual N_2/CO_2 atmosphere. Results could be read after 6 hours incubation so that the test could be completed in a working day and this method gave very close agreement with the standard method in tests on 612 specimens. Other simplified methods for performing the test have been described by Ovcinnikov (1965) and Weberschinka and

Kittnar (1966). The sensitivity of the TPI test is affected by the amount of complement present in the reaction mixtures. Müller and Segerling (1970) compared the haemolytic and immobilising activity of the serum of eight species. Human, pig and monkey sera were actively haemolytic but contained a heat-labile factor which immobilised unsensitized treponemes in the presence of guinea-pig complement. This factor was not found in sera from the rabbit, horse, goat, sheep, rat or cow. Rabbit serum had haemolytic activity but no immobilising action against sensitised treponemes in the presence of complement; the reverse was true of horse serum. Serum from the other four species had neither haemolytic nor immobilising activity.

Some centres, particularly in Scandinavia, have had difficulty in carrying out TPI tests because many rabbits inoculated with the Nichols strain of *T. pallidum* developed fever and 30 to 50 per cent died within a few days (Gudjonsson and Skog, 1970). Surviving animals did not develop fever when re-inoculated. The lethal agent was not retained by a Seitz filter and could be demonstrated in pleural fluid and lung tissue as well as in the testes. It produced a cytopathic effect on rabbit kidney cells and may be virus III, a member of the herpes group (Gudjonsson et al, 1970). Guinea-pigs, mice and hamsters are not susceptible to it. Frequent passage through rabbits of *T. pallidum* contaminated with this agent appears to provide the conditions for it to multiply and kill the animals; this effect is probably enhanced by treatment with cortisone to increase the yield of treponemes. An infected strain of *T. pallidum* can be purified by passage through hamsters (which are not susceptible to the agent) and thence back to rabbits (Jensen, 1971). Gudjonssen et al (1972) were able to separate *T. pallidum* from the agent by transferring popliteal nodes from rabbits which had survived infection for 3 months to healthy animals. Suspension of *T. pallidum* can be stored in liquid nitrogen in the presence of 10 per cent dimethyl sulphoxide for a year and gave satisfactory results in the TPI test (Hardy and Nell, 1972).

The presence of treponemicidal agents in sera may lessen the survival of *T. pallidum* under the conditions of the TPI test. Wilkinson et al (1967) found that this also occurred with metronidazole; a concentration of 5·2 μg/ml immobilised 50 per cent of the treponemes after 18 hours incubation. They found that treatment of a patient with a primary chancre with 200 μg metronidazole three times daily for 7 days did not affect the lesion, which still contained treponemes. Davies (1967) has reported the healing of secondary lesions after much higher daily doses (4 g) of metronidazole.

The TPI test has a high sensitivity in latent and late syphilis although it is accepted that it may be found negative in a minority of patients with disease of long standing, such as burnt-out tabetics and congenital syphilitics in middle life. Treatment given in late latent or late symptomatic syphilis is not thought to produce disappearance of immobilising antibody but results reported by Atwood et al (1968) question this view. They re-examined 67 patients treated for late latent or late symptomatic syphilis in 1950–52, all of whom originally had positive TPI tests, and found that seven had become TPI-negative although the FTA-ABS test was still reactive in six of these seven patients.

The specificity of the TPI test has been accepted as absolute although this is a big claim for any biological test. Julian et al (1963) injected goats with a homogenate of normal rabbit testes and found that the animals developed immobilising antibody at a low titre, although in one animal this reached 1 in 64. Immobilising activity could be removed by absorption of the goat sera with the testicular antigen but not from sera of patients thought on clinical grounds to be BFP reactors but whose TPI tests were positive. Immunisation of chickens, rabbits or guinea-pigs with testicular antigen did not lead to the production of immobilising antibody. These observations have not been satisfactorily explained. Frenk (1972) found seven sera out of 22 000 tested which gave repeatedly positive TPI tests although the patients concerned had no history or clinical evidence suggesting syphilis and FTA tests at a dilution of 1 in 20 were negative. In five of the patients the positivity of the TPI test declined with time, two becoming negative. These observations are thought to suggest that the TPI test may very rarely give false positive results and to emphasise the value of the FTA test as a confirmatory procedure.

Fluorescent treponemal antibody test

Indirect fluorescence tests with a film of a dried suspension of *T. pallidum* as antigen have proved to be a sensitive means of detecting anti-treponemal antibodies. Most normal, non-syphilitic sera contain globulins which react with *T. pallidum* at a titre rarely exceeding 1 in 50. *T. pallidum* shares common antigens with many cultivable or commensal treponemes (Deacon and Hunter, 1962; Meyer and Hunter, 1967), and these natural antibodies are thought to be produced in response to the normal treponemal flora of the body. In the FTA-200 test, serum is tested at a dilution of 1 in 200 to avoid reactions due to group-reactive antibody in normal sera. Colombani and Ripault (1964) found an overall agreement between the TPI test and an FTA test at a serum dilution of 1 in 100 of 87·26 per cent on 3 156 sera. The FTA-100 test was more sensitive than the TPI test in early syphilis but not in late syphilis. They compared the FTA test on undiluted cerebrospinal fluid with the TPI on 411 specimens and found the FTA procedure to be more sensitive. They claimed that activity of the disease process could be assessed by a comparison of the serum and spinal fluid FTA titres. Niel and Fribourg-Blanc (1965) have emphasised the value of FTA tests performed quantitatitvely. In a comparative study with the TPI test on 5 169 sera and 365 spinal fluids, they found FTA tires of 300–2 700 in early syphilis, 2 700–72 000 in the secondary stage and 1 350–4 000 in latency. High titres (4 000–10 800) were found in active late syphilis, but when the disease was not progressive, titres were much lower. Wilkinson and Rayner (1966) found 89·5 per cent agreement between the FTA-200 and the TPI test on 3 862 sera. They showed the presence of two antibodies in syphilitic sera, a group-reactive antibody which was removed by absorption of sera with intact Reiter treponemes, and antibody specific for *T. pallidum* which remained after absorption. Except in early syphilis, the group reactive antibody was the major component; this is probably due to infection taking place in a host already immunologically primed to produce group antibody in response to the commensal flora; infection with *T. pallidum*, which also contains group antigens, boosts the production of group antibody as well as leading to the production of antibody specific for *T. pallidum*.

A method for removal of group anti-treponemal antibody from sera before testing was first described by Hunter et al (1964). They first used sonicated Reiter treponemes for this, later this was replaced by a heated and concentrated culture filtrate of Reiter treponemes. Sera were diluted 1 in 5 in this reagent (sorbent) and then applied to the fixed film of treponemes as in the original FTA procedure. This absorbed fluorescent treponemal antibody (FTA-ABS) test has been widely used, and its performance has been reported by Knox et al (1966); Deacon et al (1966); Tuffanelli et al (1967); Wood et al (1967); Harner et al (1968); Johnston and Wilkinson (1968); Garner et al (1968); Hunter et al (1968); Mackey et al (1969) and Förström and Lassus (1969). These reports show that the FTA-ABS test has a high sensitivity at all stages of syphilis, including the primary stage, in which it is the most sensitive test now available. Antibody is still detectable after treatment as is found with other specific treponemal tests, such as the TPI and TPHA tests. The results of the test are illustrated in Table VII.

The FTA-ABS procedure has been found to be both more sensitive and more specific than the original FTA-200 test (Bradford et al, 1965; Johnston and Wilkinson, 1968) and has superseded the latter test in most laboratories. It has a high specificity; in studies on presumed normal sera Deacon et al (1966) found three reactive in 383 tested, Knox et al (1966) none in 301 and Johnston and Wilkinson (1968) none in tests on 107 sera from blood donors. Goldman and Lantz (1971) found three sera from 250 nuns which gave reactive FTA-ABS tests, TPI tests were negative on two of these and doubtful on one; a further five sera gave borderline FTA-ABS results. Mackey et al (1969) have also evaluated the specificity of the test.

The sorbent used to neutralise the effect of group-reactive anti-treponemal antibody in sera is prepared from a heated and concentrated culture filtrate of Reiter treponemes; its preparation and standardisation

Table VII. Comparative sensitivity of VDRL, TPI and FTA-ABS
tests on syphilitic sera (data of Deacon et al, 1966)

Diagnostic category	Treatment	Sera	VDRL Slide	TPI	FTA-ABS
			Per cent reactive		
Primary	Untreated	103	75·7	53·4	86·4
Secondary	Untreated	121	100·0	98·3	99·2
Latent or unspecified	Untreated	587	73·3	96·9	96·1
Late (CV, CNS or congenital)	Untreated	30	70·0	93·0	100·0
Primary	Treated	88	79·5	58·0	84·1
Secondary	Treated	149	94·0	90·6	99·3
Latent or unspecified	Treated	367	75·2	88·0	93·5
Late (CV, CNS or congenital)	Treated	87	79·0	92·0	93·0

have been described by Stout et al (1967). Reports by Cannefax et al
(1968), Wilkinson and Ferguson (1968), Rathlev (1968) and Hardy
and Nell (1972) have cast considerable doubt on the specificity of
sorbent as an immunological reagent. Some of the medium constituents
themselves have sorbing activity. The high osmolarity of sorbent
depresses IgG antibodies more than those of the IgM class. Although
sorbent does contain antigenic material which reacts in gel diffusion
tests or by complement fixation with antisera against Reiter treponemes,
no reactivity against syphilitic sera was detectable by these methods
(Wilkinson and Wiseman, 1971; Hardy and Nell, 1972). Dilution of
syphilitic sera 1 in 5 in sorbent under the conditions of the FTA-ABS
test may not remove all group-reactive antibody as is shown by the
ability of such absorbed sera to give fluorescence with Reiter treponemes
as antigen. This may not be of much importance in strongly positive
sera with a high titre, but in weakly reactive sera or sera in which the
FTA-ABS test is the only test positive and with no clinical evidence to
support the diagnosis, it is important to know that fluorescence is due to
specific antibody. Wilkinson and Wiseman (1971) have suggested that
in these circumstances the test should be repeated with an ultrasonicate
of Reiter treponemes as the sorbing agent; the absorbed serum should be
tested against both T. pallidum and Reiter treponemes as antigens and
results accepted as positive only if there is definite fluorescence with
T. pallidum and no fluorescence with Reiter treponemes, indicating
complete removal of group-antibody reactive with the latter antigen.
Group reactive anti-treponemal antibody is probably a mixture of
antibodies produced in response to antigens in commensal oral and
genital treponemes, some common to various species, and shared with
T. pallidum and others which are species-specific. Király et al (1967)

have produced evidence suggesting the presence of three shared antigens. Tringali and Cox (1970) found that FTA-ABS sorbent removed reactivity with *T. pallidum* from only two of 17 immune sera raised against various cultivable treponemes; reactivity with *T. pallidum* was abolished in all 17 sera after treatment with intact or ultrasonically disintegrated Reiter treponemes.

False positive FTA results have been reported with some sera containing anti-nuclear factor (Nebblett et al, 1966; Jokinen et al, 1969), but Bradford et al (1967) did not confirm this. If the treponemes used as an antigen are contaminated with antibody from the rabbit from which they are harvested, sera containing rheumatoid factor may give a false positive result (Wilkinson and Rayner, 1966). An atypical beaded staining of treponemes has been found with sera from patients with lupus erythematosus (Kraus et al, 1970a, b). Some of these sera gave homogeneous staining similar to that given by syphilitic sera; IgG antibody was responsible for these, but the beaded type of reaction was associated with IgG, IgM or IgA. These reactions are thought to be due to an anti-DNA antibody and can be abolished by treatment of the sera with DNA or nucleoprotein or by treatment of the treponemal antigen with DNA-ase (Kraus et al, 1971). A probable false positive FTA-ABS test in association with pregnancy has been reported by Buchanan and Haserick (1970). Possible false positive FTA-200 and FTA-ABS tests have been described in sera from diabetics by Hughes et al (1970).

IgM FTA tests in the diagnosis of neonatal syphilis. Scotti and Logan (1968) reported that FTA-ABS tests with a conjugate specific for IgM antibody were positive in three babies with darkground positive lesions of congenital syphilis but were negative in 10 infants born to seropositive mothers and in six normal babies whose mothers had negative serological tests for syphilis. IgM antibody does not pass the intact placenta, whereas IgG antibody can pass this barrier because of its smaller molecule. The presence of specific IgM anti-treponemal antibody is thought to indicate active production of antibody due to infection of the baby, IgG antibody may be due to passive transfer from the mother. These observations were confirmed on larger series of cases by Alford et al (1969); Scotti et al (1969); Armenio and Cecil (1970); Mamunes et al (1970); Kipnis et al (1971); and Johnston (1972a), although reservations have been expressed by Sepetjian et al (1970). Serial tests are necessary because some babies may show a delayed onset, the IgM-FTA test being negative at birth but becoming positive after an interval of several weeks.

FTA tests on cerebro-spinal fluid

Ripault and Colombani (1964) tested 302 specimens of cerebro-spinal fluid from patients with syphilis by the FTA test; 186 were reactive at dilutions of neat to 1 in 800 but only 162 gave reactive TPI tests. The FTA test was positive in 97 per cent of their patients with neuro-syphilis. Comparison of the FTA titres in the C.S.F. and serum is thought to be valuable; a C.S.F. titre 1/100 that of the serum suggests neural involvement; when the disease is active, this ratio may approach 1/10. Mattern et al (1965), tested C.S.F. from 35 patients with neuro-syphilis. FTA tests were positive at titres of 4–2 048 in all with an anti-IgG conjugate, but tests with conjugates specific for IgM and IgA were consistently negative. Oxelius et al (1969) have reported on the immunoglobulin levels in the C.S.F. in syphilis; α_2-macroglobulin was not detectable by gel diffusion in normal C.S.F. but was found in neurosyphilis, its estimation was thought to be of help in the assessment of activity.

The FTA-ABS test is thought to give reliable results on C.S.F. (Garner and Backhouse, 1971; Mahoney et al, 1972; Wilkinson, 1973). Tests on undiluted and unabsorbed C.S.F. were found more sensitive than FTA-ABS tests by Escobar et al (1970). Duncan et al (1972) examined 361 specimens from patients with syphilis including 38 with neurosyphilis; the unabsorbed FTA test was reactive in 20·9 per cent, the FTA-ABS in 9·4 per cent and the VDRL test in 3·6 per cent. 31 'normal' fluids gave negative results with all the tests. These workers advocate the testing of undiluted and unabsorbed C.S.F. as a provisional method. Anti-treponemal antibodies have been shown to develop in the C.S.F. of chimpanzees after infection with *T. pallidum*; this is thought to be due to local production and not leakage from the serum (Duncan and Kuhn, 1972).

Other immunofluorescence methods for the detection of anti-treponemal antibody

Matuhasi and Usui (1966) have shown that fixation of complement by syphilitic serum and *T. pallidum* can be detected by the use of guinea-pig serum labelled with fluorescein isothiocyanate; tests per-formed by this method showed a good general agreement with the indirect FTA test. The ability of syphilitic sera to block the staining of *T. pallidum* by a fluorescein-conjugated anti-serum was reported by Ruczkowska (1965) and Ruczkowska and Kiersnicka (1968). This FTA-inhibition test was found to be as sensitive and specific as the TPI or FTA-100 tests on a series of 1 500 sera and 100 cerebrospinal fluids. Wilkinson (1967) modified the technique by absorbing the conjugated anti-serum with Reiter treponemes to make it more specific for *T. pallidum*. He found an overall agreement with the TPI test of 91·2 per cent on 409 sera and that the inhibition procedure was more specific than the FTA-200 test; the major disadvantage was the difficulty of assessing slight degrees of inhibition by sera with a low content of antibody.

Technical advances in immunofluorescence methods

Automated equipment for the processing and staining of slides in the FTA-ABS test was described by Lewis et al (1970). Results are read visually but evaluations have shown a fair agreement with those of the manually performed test (Coffee et al, 1970; Hornstein et al, 1971; Coffee et al, 1971; Birry et al, 1972). O'Neill et al (1970) have described the use of a mechanised diluter for reagents; up to 22 sera can be tested on one teflon-coated multispot slide and 120 tests can be set up in 45 minutes. This facilitates the use of the FTA-ABS test on a wide scale as a screening procedure. Kasatiya and Birry (1972) advocate the use of incident light for reading immunoflorescence tests because of the speed and ease of reading and the greater intensity of fluorescence. The introduction of interference filters for use with a halogen quartz illuminator (Rygaard and Olsen, 1971) has also simplified fluorescence microscopy.

Roberts et al (1968a) studied the stability of reagents used in the FTA-ABS test on storage at different temperatures. Treponeme suspensions fixed on slides with acetone or 10 per cent methanol were stable for 5 months at $-20°C$ or $4°C$. Conjugates stored at $-20°C$ or $-60°C$ showed little deterioration after 4 to 6 months. Lyophilised sorbent was stable. The same authors (1968b) investigated non-specific background staining and considered this to due to be β-lipoprotein and albumen from the serum. It could be considerably reduced by treatment of the slides after incubation with the patient's serum with a 1 : 30 dilution of 2·5 per cent trypsin in buffered saline, pH 7·2. A medium for lyophilisation of *T. pallidum* for use in the FTA-ABS test has been developed by Hunter et al (1971; on reconstitution, the treponemes have a good morphology, stain well, and preserve their reactivity on fixed slides when stored at $-20°C$. Methods for determining the optimum titre of the conjugate were studied by Hardy and Nell (1971). Determination of the 'plateau end point' is advocated because this is independant of the titre of the positive serum used in standardisation. Immunochemical properties of commercially prepared conjugates for use in the FTA-ABS test have been compared by Hunter et al (1972).

Immunofluorescence methods for the detection of *T. pallidum*

Mothershed and Bullard (1968) and See (1972) have described methods of preparation and conjugation of specific antisera against *T. pallidum* The techniques used have been reviewed by Kellogg and Mothershed (1969) and Miller (1971). Comparisons of the immunofluorescence method with conventional darkground examination for the detection of *T. pallidum* in early syphilitic lesions (Jue et al, 1967; Garner, 1967;

Garner and Robson, 1968; Kellogg, 1970; Wilkinson and Cowell, 1971) have shown a good agreement. The IF technique has the advantage that specimens can be posted to a laboratory for examination and that it facilitates the examination of material in which treponemes other than *T. pallidum* may be present, as for example in lesions of the mouth.

Considerable loss of treponemes occurs during the staining and washing of specimens containing small numbers of organisms, as in spinal fluid and aqueous humour, but Chandler and Cannefax (1969) found them easier to demonstrate by FA staining than by darkground examination. The risk of treponemes becoming detached from one slide and settling on another during the staining and washing procedures was shown by Elsas (1972). Direct and indirect FA techniques give comparable results, but the specificity of the absorbed syphilitic serum must be ensured (Elsas, 1971). Separation of treponemes from fluids containing them by filtration through a Millipore membrane and their staining in situ on the membrane has been described by Chandler (1969); incident illumination has to be used to detect them.

Treponemal agglutination and haemagglutination tests

Suspensions of virulent *T. pallidum* when first prepared are inagglutinable by syphilitic serum but became agglutinable on storage or heating. Difficulties in the preparation of suspensions of a standardised agglutinability have hindered the use of agglutination as a diagnostic method. Metzger and Podwinska (1965) showed that lysozyme shortened the period of non-reactivity but that hyaluronidase had no effect. Proteolytic enzymes (trypsin, papain) had no effect on freshly prepared suspensions but enhanced agglutinability at a late stage, presumably after removal of the surface layer by the action of lysozyme. Electron microscopy showed that the development of agglutinability after exposure to lysozyme or trypsin was associated with morphological changes, bundles of fibrils becoming apparent (Metzger and Podwinska, 1966). Antibodies against cardiolipin and against heat-labile and heat-stable antigens in *T. pallidum* produce agglutination. The presence of incomplete agglutinins in syphilitic sera has been demonstrated; these are thought to be distinct from specific complete agglutinins. A test for their detection has been described by Podwinska and Metzger (1971); the results on 524 sera showed complete agreement with those of the TPI test.

Haemagglutination techniques have been based on the work of Rathlev (1967) who sensitised formolised tanned sheep erythrocytes with an ultrasonicate of Nicols strain *T. pallidum* purified by differential centrifugation (Rathlev and Pfau 1965). Three hundred sera were tested by this haemagglutination method which was found to have a specificity and sensitivity similar to the TPI and FTA-200 tests. The method was modified by Tomizawa and Kasamatsu (1966); interfering heterophil and group anti-treponemal antibodies were removed from sera before testing. Evaluations of this method in its original form or as a micro-method have been reported by Tomizawa et al (1969); Uete et al (1971); Paris-Hamelin et al (1970); Tringali (1970); Lc Clair (1971); Dixon et al (1972); Garner et al (1972a, b) and Johnston (1972b). Automated methods for performing the test quantitatively were described by Cox et al (1969) and have been evaluated by Logan and Cox (1970), Cox et al (1971) and Coffee et al (1972). Sequeira and Eldridge (1973) have described a simplified method with tanned chicken erythrocytes and unabsorbed sera which they claim is both sensitive and very specific.

Comparisons with the TPI and FTA-ABS tests in the reports cited have shown that the TPHA test has a high sensitivity at all stages of the disease except in primary syphilis in which it is less sensitive than the FTA-ABS test. Quantitative tests are easy to preform and give reproducible results. Johnston (1972b) found titres in both untreated and treated secondary and early latent syphilis greater than those in late syphilis; because of the overlap in the range of titres in treated and untreated groups, quantitation was thought to be of limited value as a means of following the course of the disease. Once present, TPHA antibody persists for many years and treatment seems to have little effect on it. The test has a good specificity, although false positive results figure in most of the published series. Johnston (1972b) tested 400 sera with positive tests for reagin which were thought to be BFP reactions because both TPI and FTA-ABS tests were negative; nine gave positive TPHA tests. Garner et al (1973) have reported 11·3 per cent positive TPHA tests in 267 sera from presumed BFP reactors with negative TPI and FTA-ABS tests. In tests on 267 sera from patients with lepromatous leprosy from an area where yaws was unknown, 26 BFP reactions were found, as judged by negative TPI and FTA-ABS tests. TPHA tests were positive on three of these sera. These reports suggest that when tests for reagin and the TPHA test are positive in a patient with no clinical evidence or history of syphilis, verification by the TPI or FTA-ABS test is desirable.

ANTIBODIES IN SYPHILIS
IMMUNOLOGICAL STUDIES

Serum immunoglobulin levels in syphilis

Onisk (1965) examined sera from 39 patients with untreated early syphilis by immunoelectrophoresis and filter paper electrophoresis. An early increase in IgM was noted and might precede reactivity of serological tests. IgG increased during the secondary stage and predominated in latency. Delhanty and Catterall (1969) compared the serum immunoglobulin levels of 55 patients with syphilis with those of a control group of healthy clinic patients. Although many syphilitic patients had levels within the normal range the mean IgG and IgM levels were greater than those of the control series in primary, secondary and latent syphilis, mean IgA levels were significantly raised in secondary syphilis, but not in the other groups. Laurell et al (1968) found high IgM levels in three of eight sera from patients with early syphilis and in all of seven sera from patients with late syphilis. In contrast, no increase in IgM was found in sera from 10 treated patients, five of whom had late syphilis; it is suggested that estimation of IgM levels may be of use in assessing activity in late syphilis. A decrease in IgM levels in late and treated syphilis was reported by Heitmann (1972) who also observed that IgA was increased in the later stages of syphilis and also in the sera of patients with BFP reactions. Serum protein, IgG and IgM levels in syphilitic sera were found to be significantly greater than in control sera by Hrncir et al (1972).

Immunoglobulin class of antibodies in syphilitic sera

Aho (1967) studied reactivity in the Kolmer WR and VDRL test in 50 syphilitic sera fractionated by ultracentrifugation and chromatography on DEAE cellulose. In primary syphilis, titres were higher in the 19S than in the 7S fractions and in some sera reactivity was confined to the 19S fractions. In secondary and early latent syphilis titres were higher in the 7S fractions; in late syphilis titres were often higher in the 19S fractions, but these last sera were selected because they had a high VDRL titre. A preponderance of 19S anti-lipoidal antibody was found in elderly patients with syphilis (Aho 1968). Julian et al (1969) fractionated sera from patients with early syphilis on Sephadex-G200 columns. Reactivity in the Kolmer WR was found in the IgG fractions, those from the IgM peak were anti-complementary. In the VDRL test, reactivity was found in the IgG fractions in 28 of 31 sera and in the IgM fractions in five of 14 primary and 10 of 17 secondary syphilitic sera. Immobilising antibody was found in the IgG fractions as also reported by Tringali et al (1968). Jobbágy (1970) fractionated primary syphilitic sera on Sephadex G200 and found that sera which originally gave negative TPI tests yielded fractions which would immobilise *T. pallidum*. He postulates the presence of an inhibitory factor in whole serum to account for this. Surjan et al (1971) studied the effect of 2-mercaptoethanol on the complement fixation titres of 79 syphilitic sera. Most sera contained both IgG and IgM activity but in a minority only one class was found. From a comparison of cold fixation with fixation at 37°C they conclude that IgG antibodies react more strongly in the former and IgM antibodies at the higher temperature. Tringali et al (1966) found that treatment with 2-mercaptoethanol did not affect the reactivity of syphilitic sera although it abolished the reactivity of sera giving BFP reactions due to the presence of IgM antibody. BFP sera from patients with connective tissue disorders lost activity in the Kolmer WR but not in the VDRL test after treatment with 2-mercapto-ethanol; in BFP sera found by chance or in association with liver disease or tumours, both tests became negative after exposure to this agent (Tringali and Valentino, 1971).

Julian and others (1970) used monospecific conjugates to study natural anti-treponemal antibodies in 36 presumed normal sera reacting with *T. pallidum* in the FTA test. The mean titres were IgG, 640; IgM, 5; and IgA 5. Inactivation of a 1 in 5 dilution of serum in buffered saline for 30 minutes at 56°C did not alter reactivity, but heating at 65°C for 1 hour reduced the IgG titre to 30 per cent and abolished reactivity with IgM and IgA. Jakubowski and Manikowska-Lesinska (1970) investigated group reactive antibody in 228 syphilitic sera in indirect fluorescence tests after absorption with Reiter ultrasonicate. In the primary stage group antibody was mainly IgG and IgA and the proportion of group IgG antibody fell in the later stages of the disease. The highest proportion of IgM group antibody was found in latent syphilis. A large proportion of the IgA antibody was group reactive at all stages.

Sartoris and others (1968) examined unabsorbed sera in the FTA test. In primary syphilis (16 sera) the IgG titre ranged from 150–2 500: IgM was present in all except one at titres of 150–450. Similar IgM titres were found in 40 secondary syphilitic sera but the IgG titres were higher, 450–8 000. IgA was inconstant, when present, the titre did not exceed 150. Julian et al (1969) studied early syphilitic sera and found that only IgG was detectable at dilutions in saline above 1 in 160, IgM and IgA were detectable at lower dilutions. When sorbent was used as the diluent, the IgG and IgM titres were lowered and IgA abolished. Hardy and Nell (1972) found that sorbent depressed the IgG titre more than that of IgM. Manikowska-Lesinska and Jakubowski (1970) tested unabsorbed sera from 305 patients with untreated syphilis. In primary syphilis most of the antibody was IgM but in the later stages the IgG rose; in late symptomatic syphilis IgM accounted for more than IgG. Atwood and Miller (1970) tested 147 syphilitic sera in FTA-ABS tests with monospecific conjugates; IgG was reactive at all stages, IgA was of little significance and IgM was found most often in early and late syphilis. They suggested that its presence in late syphilis may reflect persistence of treponemes. O'Neill and Nicol (1972) from a study of serial IgM titres after treatment of patients with early infections suggested that arrest of the disease may be associated with disappearance of IgM antibody. They found that although IgG persisted in almost all cases, IgM was only detectable for 3–6 months after treatment of secondary or early latent syphilis.

Thermostability of antibodies

Holst and Bentzon (1965) found that complement-fixing anti-lipoidal antibodies in early syphilis were more stable to heat than those in sera from patients with late syphilis; BFP antibody was heat-labile. Vaisman and Paris-Hamelin (1966, 1969) studied the effect of storage of sera at temperatures from $-180°C$ to $37°C$ on the reactivity of a range of serological tests. At $-20°C$ or below the titres of all tests remained unchanged for a year. They conclude that if sterile sera are stored at temperatures below $4°C$, valid results can be obtained for as long as a year. Blood dried on circles of absorbent paper (rondelles) can be eluted and used for FTA tests (Guthe, 1966). This has applications in field studies but transport and preservation of sera without deterioration is best achieved by storage in liquid nitrogen (Guthe, 1965).

The presence of other antibodies in syphilitic sera

In addition to anti-lipoidal and anti-treponemal antibodies syphilitic sera may contain rheumatoid factor and cryoglobulins. Mustakallio et al (1967) studied these in sera from 241 patients. Rheumatoid factor was found in 10·3 per cent; it was unrelated to previous treatment but was related to age, being found in only 2 per cent of patients under 24 but in 22 per cent of those over 51 years old. Cryoglobulins were found in 14·9 per cent of the patients and were more frequent in late infections and among older patients. Lassus (1969) detected rheumatoid factor in five of 101 primary and nine of 51 secondary syphilitic sera and cryoglobulins in 24 of the combined group. Only one patient had both antibodies. Their incidence increased with the length of the infection and they were commoner in sera with a high reagin titre. The significance of these antibodies is not known.

REFERENCES

AHO , K. (1967). *Brit. J. vener. Dis.*, **43**, 259.

AHO, K. (1968). *Brit. J. vener. Dis.*, **44**, 283.

ALFORD, C. A., POLT, S. S., CASSIDY, G. E., STRAUMFJORD, J. V. and RIMINGTON, J. S. (1969). *New Engl. J. Med.*, **280**, 1086.

ARMENIO, L. and CECIL, A. (1970). *Pediatria*, **78**, 246.

ATWOOD, W. G., MILLER, J. L., STOUT, G. W. and NORINS, L. C. (1968). *J. Amer. med. Ass.*, **203**, 549.

ATWOOD, W. G. and MILLER, J. L. (1970). *Int. J. Derm.*, **9**, 259.

BANFFER, J. R. J. (1972). *Lancet*, **1**, 996.

BEKKER, J. H., DEBRUIJN, J. H. and MILLER, J. N. (1966). *Brit. J. vener. Dis.*, **42**, 42.

BIRRY, A., CALONESCU, M. and KASATIYA, S. S. (1972). *Amer. J. clin. Path.*, **57**, 391.

BRADFORD, L. L., BODILY, H. L., KETTERER, W. A., PUFFER, J., THOMAS, J. E. and TUFFANELLI, D. L. (1965) *Publ. Hlth Rep.*, *Wash.*, **80**, 797.

BRADFORD, L. L., TUFFANELLI, D. L., PUFFER, J., BISSET, M. L., BODILY, H. L. and WOOD, R. M. (1967). *Amer. J. clin. Path.*, **47**, 525.

BROWN, W. J., DONAHUE, J. F. and PRICE, E. V. (1964). *Publ. Hlth Rep., Wash.*, **79**, 496.

BUCHANAN, C. S. and HASERICK, J. R. (1970). *Arch. Derm.*, **102**, 322.

BUCK, A. A. and MAYER, H. (1964). *Amer. J. Hyg.*, **80**, 85.

CANNEFAX, G. R. (1963). *Brit. J. vener. Dis.*, **39**, 121.

CANNEFAX, G. R., HANSON, A. W. and SKAGGS, R. (1968). *Publ. Hlth Rep., Wash.*, **83**, 411.

CARPENTER, C. M., KONYA, I. O. and LeCLAIR, R. A. (1966). *Calif. Med.*, **105**, 167.

CATE, T. R., TIEDMANN, G. G. and PRINCE, J. (1971). *Amer. J. clin. Path.*, **55**, 735.

CHANDLER, F. W. and CANNEFAX, G. R. (1969). *Brit. J. vener. Dis.*, **45**, 1.

CHANDLER, F. W. (1969). *Brit. J. vener. Dis.*, **45**, 305.

COFFEE, E. M., JUE, R. F., THOMAS, J. S., BRADFORD, L. L. and WOOD, R. M. (1970). *Brit. J. vener. Dis.*, **46**, 271.

COFFEE, E. M., NARITOMI, L. S., ULFELDT, M. V., BRADFORD, L. L. and WOOD, R. M. (1971). *Appl. Microbiol.*, **21**, 820.

COFFEE, E. M., BRADFORD, L. L., NARITOMI, L. S. and WOOD, R. M. (1972). *Appl. Microbiol.*, **24**, 26.

COLOMBANI, J. and RIPAULT, J. (1964). *Path. Biol.*, **12**, 56.

COX, P. M., LOGAN, L. C. and NORINS, L. C. (1969). *Appl. Microbiol.*, **18**, 485.

COX, P. M., LOGAN, L. C. and STOUT, G. W. (1971). *Publ. Hlth Lab.*, **29**, 43.

DANDOY, S. (1967). *Brit. J. vener. Dis.*, **43**, 105.

DAVIES, A. H. (1967). *Brit. J. vener. Dis.*, **43**, 197.

DEACON, W. E. and HUNTER, E. F. (1962). *Proc. Soc. exp. Biol. Med.*, **110**, 352.

DEACON, W. E., LUCAS, J. B. and PRICE, E. V. (1966). *J. Amer. med. Ass.*, **198**, 624.

DELHANTY, J. J. and CATTERALL, R. D. (1969). *Lancet*, **2**, 1099.

DIXON, J. M. S., GROCHOLSKI, J. J. and KADIS, E. M. (1972). *Canad. J. Publ. Hlth*, **63**, 257.

DUNCAN, W. P., JENKINS, T. W. and PARHAM, C. E. (1972). *Brit. J. vener. Dis.*, **48**, 97.

DUNCAN, W. P. and KUHN, U. S. G. (1972). *J. infect. Dis.*, **125**, 61.

ELSAS, F. J. (1971). *Brit. J. vener. Dis.*, **47**, 255.

ELSAS, F. J. (1972). *Brit. J. vener. Dis.*, **48**, 26.

ENGELBRECHT, E. and DENIS, C. (1970). *Path. microbiol.*, **36**, 44, 51.

ESCOBAR, M. R., DALTON, H. P. and ALLISON, M. J. (1970). *Amer. J. clin. Path.*, **53**, 886.

FALCONE, V. H., STOUT, G. W. and MOORE, M. B. (1964). *Publ. Hlth Rep., Wash.*, **79**, 491.

FISCHMAN, A. (1964). *Brit. J. vener. Dis.*, **40**, 225.

FISCHMAN, A. and MUNDT, H. (1971). *Brit. J. vener. Dis.*, **47**, 91.

FÖRSTRÖM, L. (1967). *Acta derm.-venereol., Stockh.*, **47**, Suppl. 59.

FÖRSTRÖM, L. and LASSUS, A. (1969). *Acta derm.-venereol., Stockh.*, **49**, 326.

FÖRSTRÖM, L., LASSUS, A. and JOKINEN, E. J. (1969). *Brit. J. vener. Dis.*, **45**, 126.

FRENK, E. (1972). *Schweitz. med. Wschr.*, **102**, 1898.

GAILLON, R., RIPAULT, J., STUDIEVIC, C. and DAUSSET, J. (1966). *Path. Biol.*, **14**, 953.

GARNER, M. F. (1967). *Med. J. Aust.*, **2**, 199.

GARNER, M. F. (1968). *Med. J. Aust.*, **1**, 672.

GARNER, M. F. and BACKHOUSE, J. L. (1971). *Brit. J. vener. Dis.*, **47**, 356.

GARNER, M. F. and BACKHOUSE, J. L. (1972). *J. clin. Path.*, **25**, 786.

GARNER, M. F., BACKHOUSE, J. L., DASKALOPOULOS, G. and WALSH, J. L. (1973). *J. clin. Path.*, **26**, 258.

GARNER, M. F., BACKHOUSE, J. L., DASKALOPOULOS, G. and WALSH, J. L. (1972a). *Brit. J. vener. Dis.*, **48**, 470; (1972b). *Ibid.*, 479.

GARNER, M. F., GRANTHAM, N. M., COLLINS, C. A. and ROEDER, P. J. (1968). *Med. J. Aust.*, **1**, 404.

GARNER, M. F. and GRANTHAM, N. M. (1968). *Brit. J. vener. Dis.*, **44**, 131.

GARNER, M. F. and ROBSON, J. H. (1968). *J. clin. Path.*, **21**, 576.

GLENN, J. H. and TURNBULL, A. R. (1971). *Brit. J. vener. Dis.*, **47**, 200.
GOLDMAN, J. N. and LANTZ, M. A. (1971). *J. Amer. med. Ass.*, **217**, 53.
GUDJONSSON, H. NEWMAN, B. and TURNER, T. B. (1970). *Brit. J. vener. Dis.*, **46**, 435.
GUDJONSSON, H., NEWMAN, B. and TURNER, T. B. (1972). *Brit. J. vener. Dis.*, **48**, 102.
GUDJONSSON, H. and SKOG, E. (1970). *Brit. J. vener. Dis.*, **46**, 318.
GUTHE, T. (1965). *Bull. Wld Hlth Org.*, **33**, 864.
GUTHE, T. (1966). *Acta derm.-venereol., Stockh.*, **46**, 72.
HARDY, P. H. and NELL, E. E. (1971). *Amer. J. clin. Path.*, **56**, 181.
HARDY, P. H. and NELL, E. E. (1972). *Amer. J. Epidemiol.*, **96**, 141.
HARNER, R. E., SMITH, J. L. and ISRAEL, C. W. (1968). *J. Amer. med. Ass.*, **203**, 545.
HEITMANN, H. J. (1972). *Z. Haut-u. Geschl.-Kr.* **47**, 433.
HOLST, E. and BENTZON, M. W. (1965). *Acta path. microbiol. scand.* **65**, 311.
HORNSTEIN, J. H., GATES, C. W. and BRANDON, S. M. (1971). *J. Lab. clin. Med.* **77**, 885.
HRNCIR, Z., KRAUS, Z. and TICHY, M. (1972). *Brit. J. vener. Dis.*, **48**, 108.
HUGHES, M. K., FUSILLO, M. H. and ROBERSON, B. S. (1970). *Appl. Microbiol.*, **19**, 425.
HUNTER, E. F., CREIGHTON, E. T. and LEWIS, J. S. (1971). *Hlth Lab. Sci.*, **8**, 35.
HUNTER, E. F., DEACON, W. E. and MAYER, P. E. (1964). *Publ. Hlth Rep., Wash.*, **79**, 410.
HUNTER, E. F., NORINS, L. C., FALCONE, V. H. and STOUT, G. W. (1968). *Bull. Wld Hlth Org.*, **39**, 873.
HUNTER, E. F., SMITH, J. F., LEWIS, J. S., McGREW, B. E. and SCHMALE, J. D. (1972). *Infect. Immunity*, **5**, 858.
JAKUBOWSKI, A. and MANIKOWSKA-LESINSKA, W. (1970). *Brit. J. vener. Dis.*, **46**, 383.
JENSEN, H. J. (1971). *Acta path. microbiol. scand.*, **79**, 124.
JOBBÁGY, A. (1970). *Brit. J. vener. Dis.*, **46**, 445.
JOHNSTON, N. A. (1972a). *Brit. J. vener. Dis.*, **48**, 464; (1972b). *Ibid.*, 474.
JOHNSTON, N. A. and WILKINSON, A. E. (1968). *Brit. J. vener. Dis.*, **44**, 287.
JOKINEN, E. J., LASSUS, A. and LINDER, E. (1969). *Ann. clin. Res.*, **1**, 77.
JUE, R., PUFFER, J., WOOD, R. M., SCHOCHLET, G., SMART, W. H. and KETTERER, W. A. (1967). *Amer. J. clin. Path.*, **47**, 809.
JULIAN, A. J., LOGAN, L. C. and NORINS, L. C. (1969). *J. Immunol.*, **102**, 1250.
JULIAN, A. J., LOGAN, L. C., NORINS, L. C. and COHEN, I. R. (1970). *Infect. Immunity*, **1**, 555.
JULIAN, A. J., PORTNOY, J. and BOSSAK, H. (1963). *Brit. J. vener. Dis.*, **39**, 30.
KASATIYA, S. S. and BIRRY, A. (1972). *Amer, J. clin. Path.*, **57**, 395.
KELLOGG, D. S. (1970). *Hlth Lab. Sci.*, **7**, 34.
KELLOGG, D. S. and MOTHERSHED, S. M. (1969). *J. Amer. med. Ass.*, **207**, 938.
KIPNIS, J., CAMARGO, M. E., NETTO, C. F., FERREIRA, A. W. and GUARNIERI, D. B. (1971). *Rev. Inst. Med. Trop. Sao Paulo*, **13**, 179.
KIRÁLY, K., JOBBÁGY, A. and KOVÁTS, L. (1967). *J. invest. Derm.*, **48**, 98.
KNOX, J. M., SHORT, D. H., WENDE, R. D. and GLICKSMAN, J. M. (1966) *Brit. J. vener. Dis.*, **42**, 16.
KRAUS, S. J., HASERICK, J. R. and LANTZ, M. A. (1970a). *J. Amer. med. Ass.*, **211**, 2140; (1970b). *New Engl., J. med.*, **282**, 1287.
KRAUS, S. J., HASERICK, J. R., LOGAN, L. C. and BULLARD, J. C. (1971). *J. Immunol.*, **106**, 1665.
LASSUS, A. (1969). *Int. Arch. Allergy*, **36**, 515.
LASSUS, A., JOHANSSON, E. and FÖRSTRÖM, L. (1970). *Acta derm.-venereol., Stockh.*, **50**, 148.
LAURELL, A.-B., OXELIUS, V.-A. and RORSMAN, H. (1968). *Acta derm.-venereol., Stockh.*, **48**, 268.
LECLAIR, R. A. (1971). *J. infect. Dis.*, **123**, 668.
LEWIS, J. S., DUNCAN, W. P. and STOUT, G. W. (1970). *Appl. Microbiol.*, **19**, 898.
LOCKYER, J. W. (1970). *Brit. J. vener. Dis.*, **46**, 290.

LOGAN, L. C. and COX, P. M. (1970). *Amer. J. clin. Path.*, **53**, 163.

MACKEY, D. M., PRICE, E. V., KNOX, J. M. and SCOTTI, A. (1969). *J. Amer. med. Ass.*, **207**, 1683.

MAHONY, J. D. H., HARRIS, J. R. W., McCANN, J. S., KENNEDY, J. and DOUGAN, H. J. (1972). *Acta derm.-venerol., Stockh.*, **52**, 71.

MAMUNES, P., CAVE, V. G., BUDELL, J. W., ANDERSON, J. A. and STEWARD, R. E. (1970). *Amer. J. Dis. Child.*, **120**, 17.

MANIKOWSKA-LESINSKA, W. and JAKUBOWSKI, A. (1970). *Brit. J. vener. Dis.*, **46**, 380.

MASSAWE, A. E. J., LOMHOLT, G., AHO, K. and LASSUS, A. (1972). *Brit. J. vener. Dis.*, **48**, 345.

MATTERN, P., SANDOR, G. and PILLOT, J. (1965). *Ann. Inst. Pasteur*, **109**, 120.

MATUHASI, T. and USUI, M. (1966). *Nature, Lond.*, **212**, 418.

McGREW, B. E., DUCROS, M. J. F., STOUT, G. W. and FALCONE, V. H. (1968). *Amer. J. clin. Path.*, **50**, 52.

METZGER, M. (1965). *Bull. Wld Hlth Org.*, **32**, 357.

METZGER, M. and PODWINSKA, J. (1965). *Arch. Immunol. Ther. exp.*, **13**, 516.

METZGER, M. and PODWINSKA, J. (1966). *Arch, Immunol. Ther. exp.*, **14**, 594.

MEYER, P. E. and HUNTER, E. F. (1967). *J. Bact.*, **93**, 784.

MILLER, J. N. (Ed.) (1971). 'Spirochaetes in Body Fluids and Tissues'. Charles C. Thomas, Springfield, Ill.

MORRIS, C. A. (1968). *J. clin. Path.*, **21**, 731.

MOTHERSHED, S. M. and BULLARD, J. C. (1968). *Brit. J. vener. Dis.*, **44**, 201.

MÜLLER, F. and SEGERLING, M. (1970). *Immunology*, **18**, 13.

MUSTAKALLIO, K. K., LASSUS, A. and WAGER, O. (1967). *Int. Arch. Allergy*, **31**, 417.

NEBLETT, T. R., BURNHAM, T. K. and FINE, G. (1966). *J. invest. Derm.*, **46**, 84.

NELL, E. E. and HARDY, P. H. (1972). *Cryobiology*, **9**, 404.

NIEL, G. and FRIBOURG-BLANC, A. (1965). *Bull. Wld Hlth Org.*, **33**, 89.

O'NEILL, P. JOHNSON, G. D. and NICOL, C. S. (1970). *Brit. J. vener. Dis.*, **46**, 278.

O'NEILL, P. and NICOL, C. S. (1972). *Brit. J. vener. Dis.*, **48**, 460.

ONISK, K. (1965). *Przegl. Derm.*, **52**, 373.

OVCINNIKOV, N. M. (1965). *Bull. Wld Hlth Org.*, **33**, 197.

OXELIUS, V.-A., RORSMAN, H. and LAURELL, A.-B. (1969). *Brit. J. vener. Dis.*, **45**, 121.

PARIS-HAMELIN, A., CATALAN, F. and VAISMAN, A. (1970). *Bull. Soc. franc. Derm. Syph.*, **77**, 474.

PARIS-HAMELIN, A., VAISMAN, A. and DUNOYER, F. (1968). *Bull. Wld Hlth Org.*, **38**, 808.

PILLOT, J., BETZ, A., COLOMBANI, J. and RIPAULT, J. (1965). *Brit. J. vener. Dis.*, **41**, 170.

PILLOT, J. and DUPOUEY, P. (1964). *Ann. Inst. Pasteur*, **106**, 456.

PODWINSKA, J. and METZGER, M. (1971). *Brit. J. vener. Dis.*, **47**, 81.

PORTNOY, J. (1963). *Amer. J. clin. Path.*, **40**, 473.

PORTNOY, J. (1965). *Publ. Hlth Lab.*, **23**, 43.

PORTNOY, J., BOSSAK, H. N., FALCONE, V. H. and HARRIS, A. (1961). *Publ. Hlth Rep., Wash.*, **76**, 933.

PORTNOY, J., BREWER, J. H. and HARRIS, A. (1962). *Publ. Hlth Rep., Wash.*, **77**, 645.

PORTNOY, J. and GARSON, W. (1960). *Publ. Hlth Rep., Wash.*, **75**, 985.

PUGH, V. H. and GAZE, R. W. T. (1965). *Brit. J. vener. Dis.*, **41**, 221.

PUTKONEN, T., JOKINEN, E. J. and FÖRSTRÖM, L. (1963). *Acta derm.-venereol., Stockh.*, **43**, 405.

RATHLEV, T. (1967). *Brit. J. vener. Dis.*, **43**, 181.

RATHLEV, T (1968). *Brit. J. vener. Dis.*, **44**, 295.

RATHLEV, T. and PFAU, C. J. (1965). *Scand. J. clin. Lab. Invest.*, **17**, 130.

RIPAULT, J. and COLOMBANI, J. (1964). *Path. et Biol.*, **12**, 276.

ROBERTS, M. E., MILLER, J. N., PRINGLE, T. C. and BINNINGS, G. E. (1968a). *J. Bact.*, **96**, 1507.

ROBERTS, M. E., MILLER, J. N. and BINNINGS, G. F. (1968b) *J. Bact.*, **96**, 1500.
RUCZKOWSKA, J. (1965). *Arch. Immunol. Ther. exp.*, **13**, 602.
RUCZKOWSKA, J. and KIERSNICKA, I. (1968). *Przegl. Derm.*, **55**, 287.
RYGAARD, J. and OLSEN, W. (1971). *Ann. N.Y. Acad. Sci.*, **177**, 430.
SALO, O. P., VALTONEN, V., JOKIPII, A. and AHO, K. (1967). *Brit. J. vener. Dis.*, **43**, 264.
SARTORIS, S., STRANI, G. F., PIPPIONE, M. and LEIGHEB, G. (1968). *Minerva Derm.*, **43**, 219.
SCOTTI, A. T. and LOGAN, L. (1968). *J. Pediat.*, **73**, 242.
SCOTTI, A., LOGAN, L. and CALDWELL, J. G. (1969). *J. Pediat.*, **75**, 1129.
SEE, I. M. (1972). *Hlth Lab. Sci.*, **9**, 197.
SEPETJIAN, M., GUERRAZ, F. T., MONIER, J. C., NIVELOU, J. L. and THIVOLET, J. (1970). *Brit. J. vener. Dis.*, **46**, 18.
SEQUEIRA, P. J. L. and ELDRIDGE, A. E. (1973). *Brit. J. vener. Dis.*, **49**, 242.
STEVENS, R. W. and STROEBEL, E. (1970). *Amer. J. clin. Path.* **53** 32.
STOUT, G. W., KELLOGG, D. S., FALCONE, V. H., McGREW, B. E. and LEWIS, J. S. (1967). *Hlth Lab. Sci.*, **4**, 5.
SURJAN, M., FUST, G. and BALOGH, I. (1971). *Brit. J. vener. Dis.*, **47**, 87.
TIO, B. S. 1970). *Brit. J. vener. Dis.*, **46**, 287.
TOMIZAWA, T. and KASAMATSU, S. (1966). *Jap. J. med. Sci. Biol.*, **19**, 305.
TOMIZAWA, T., KASAMATSU, S. and YAMAYA, S. (1969). *Jap. J. med. Sci. Biol.*, **22**, 341.
TRINGALI, G. (1970). *Ann. Sclavo*, **12**, 311.
TRINGALI, G. R. and COX, P. M. (1970). *Brit. J. vener. Dis.*, **46**, 313.
TRINGALI, G., DEL CARPIO, C. and GIAMMANCO, N. (1966). *Riv. Ist. Sieroter. Ital.*, **41**, 291.
TRINGALI, G., DEL CARPIO, C. and ZAFFIRO, P. (1968). *Riv. Ist. Sieroter. Ital.*, **43**, 161.
TRINGALI, G. and VALENTINO, L. (1971). *Ann. Sclavo*, **13**, 672.
TUFFANELLI, D. L., WUEPPER, K. D., BRADFORD, L. L. and WOOD, R. M. (1967). *New Engl. J. Med.*, **276**, 258.
UETE, T., FUKAZAWA, S., OGI, K. and TAKEUCHI, Y. (1971). *Brit. J. vener. Dis.*, **47**, 73.
VAISMAN, A. and PARIS-HAMELIN, A. (1966). *Bull. Wld Hlth Org.*, **34**, 461.
VAISMAN, A. and PARIS-HAMELIN, A. (1969). *Bull. Wld Hlth Org.*, **40**, 153.
WAGSTAFF, W., FIRTH, R., BOOTH, J. R. and BOWLEY, C. C. (1969). *J. clin. Path.*, **22**, 236.
WALKER, A. N. (1971). *Brit. J. vener. Dis.*, **47**, 259.
WEBERSCHINKA, J. and KITTNAR, E. (1966). *J. Hyg. Epidemiol.*, *Praha.*, **10**, 483.
WENDE, R. D., MUDD, R. L., KNOX, J. M. and HOLDER, W. R. (1971). *Sth. med. J.*, *Bgham. Ala.*, **64**, 633.
WEST, B. S., BRINKMAN, C. D. and HIBBERD, E. W. (1971). *Hlth Lab. Sci.*, **8**, 220.
WILKINSON, A. E. (1967). *Brit. J. vener. Dis.*, **43**, 186.
WILKINSON, A. E. (1973). *Brit. J. vener. Dis.*, **49**, 346.
WILKINSON, A. E. and COWELL, L. P. (1971). *Brit. J. vener. Dis.*, **47**, 252.
WILKINSON, A. E. and FERGUSON, H. G. (1968). *Brit. J. vener. Dis.*, **44**, 291.
WILKINSON, A. E. and RAYNER, C. F. A. (1966). *Brit. J. vener. Dis.*, **42**, 8.
WILKINSON, A. E., RODIN, P., McFADZEAN, J. A. and SQUIRES, S. (1967). *Brit. J. vener. Dis.*, **43**, 201.
WILKINSON, A. E., SCRIMGEOUR, G. and RODIN, P. (1972). *J. clin. Path.*, **25**, 437.
WILKINSON, A. E. and WISEMAN, C. C. (1971). *Proc. roy. Soc. Med.*, **64**, 422.
WOOD, R. M., INOUYE, Y., ARGONZA, W., BRADFORD, L., JUE, R., JEONG, Y., PUFFER, J. and BODILY, H. L. (1967). *Amer. J. clin. Path.*, **47**, 521.
WRIGHT, D. J. M., DONIACH, D., LESSOF, M. H., TURK, J. L., GRIMBLE, A. S. and CATTERALL, R. D. (1970). *Lancet*, **1**, 740.

11 Experimental Syphilis

J. R. W. Harris

Two excellent reviews on various aspects of experimental syphilis were published by Willcox and Guthe (1966) and Longhin and Podescu (1969). The most interesting and thought-provoking concept in syphilis during the last decade has been the discovery of the persistence of treponeme-like forms (Collart et al, 1962). This resulted in a critical reappraisal of methods for identifying the causative agent of syphilis as we know it today. Among the most definitive tests for the presence of syphilitic infection in man and laboratory animals is transfer of infection to laboratory animals (Turner et al, 1969). Hence there have been numerous technical advances in more specific methods of identifying *T. pallidum* in this situation. At the same time there has been much research into the diagnosis of infection in laboratory animals. Various workers have utilised electron microscopy and gas chromatography to define more clearly the nature of *T. pallidum* itself. Our inadequate knowledge of treponeme biology and the inability of research workers to make pathogenic organisms grow *in vitro* remain major obstacles in treponemal research.

The virulent treponeme, which is among the thinnest of the genus *Treponema*, has a cellular mass surrounded by two trilaminar membranous structures. These membranous structures are 7·5 to 15 μm in thickness and the organs of motility are situated between the two membranes. Ovčinnikov and Delektorskij (1969) believe that outside these membranous structures is a capsule which they have observed on electron microscopy and which they also found in their studies of *T. pertenue* (1970a). They postulate that this is a protective membrane. Christiansen (1963) suggested that this was a slimy layer that protected the organism from host defence mechanisms. Jones et al (1968) noted that material occluded on the outer surface of the treponeme and that this material prevented lysis under experimental conditions. However, other workers do not agree with their interpretation of these observations and feel that there is no capsule or protective layer (W.H.O. Tech. Ser. 455, 1970).

Pillot et al (1964) and Jepsen et al (1968) have demonstrated that the treponemes contain ribosomes, mesosomes and filamentous nuclear areas. Pillot (1965) also showed that the outer trilaminar membrane can be destroyed by glucosidases. He confirmed the impression of earlier workers that the inner membranous structure contains a mucopeptide layer.

Pillot et al (1964) demonstrated that the fibrils, which comprise the motility apparatus of the treponeme, arise from basal granules located subterminally in the cytoplasm at both ends of the cell. They penetrate the inner membranous structure and extend to the distal end of the cell. The fibrils arising from opposite ends of the cell overlap for most of the cell length. Ovčinnikov and Delektorskij (1969) believe that the fibrils are re-attached in the mid portion of the cell. *T. pallidum* and *T. pertenue* have both got three fibrils arising from each end (Ovčinnikov and Delektorskij, 1970a). The differences in appearance of the two ends of *T. pallidum* can be explained by stretching of the outer trilaminar structure during transverse fission.

Further electronmicroscopy studies of *T. pallidum* were made by Ovčinnikov and Delektorskij (1971) in which they described the development of L forms in cultivated strains under the influence of penicillin and antiserum. These forms reverted to normal when put in media lacking these agents. Abe (1969) and Azar et al (1970) had noticed that in chancre tissues *T. pallidum* was engulfed by polymorphonuclears and plasma cells. Ovčinnikov and Delektorskij (1969) observed that the *T. pallidum* were found in these cells and also demonstrated *T. pallidum* in macrophages, endothelial cells and monocytes. In 1970 they reported that the treponemes in plasma cells were in some instances surrounded by a multi-layered envelope (see Fig. 17). (Ovčinnikov and Delektorskij, 1970a). In 1972 the same workers described the results of their studies on the effect of crystalline penicillin or bicillin-I in experimental syphilis. They demonstrated that some of the treponemes, particularly those in the plasma and endothelial cells were remarkably well preserved despite 24-hour exposure to bicillin (see Fig. 18). Lauderdale and Goldman (1972) did not observe any treponemes in plasma cells but they did speculate that an intracellular habitat may provide another protective device for the treponemal invader against the action of drugs or the immunological reactions of the host. However, Izzat et al (1972) reported that rabbit macrophages actively phagocytose avirulent *T. pallidum*. From these reports it is evident that our knowledge of the cellular relationship of treponemes is limited.

The lipid composition of pathogenic and non-pathogenic treponemes has been studied by Vaczi et al (1966), using gas and thin-layer chromatography. The fatty acid spectra were simple and nearly identical. The phospholipid composition was quite complex and the authors felt that their findings indicated a ready permeability of the cell membrane. This

6

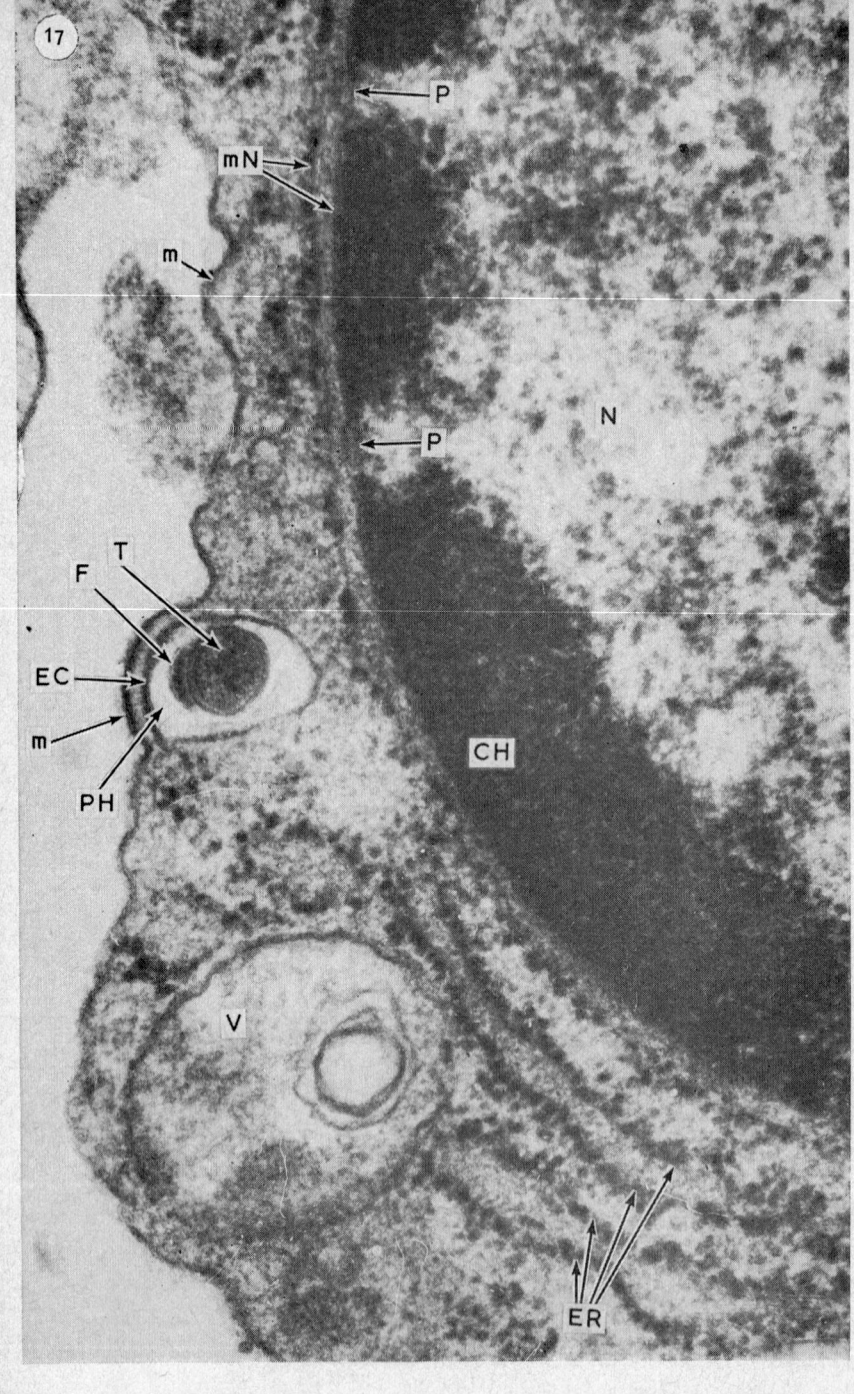

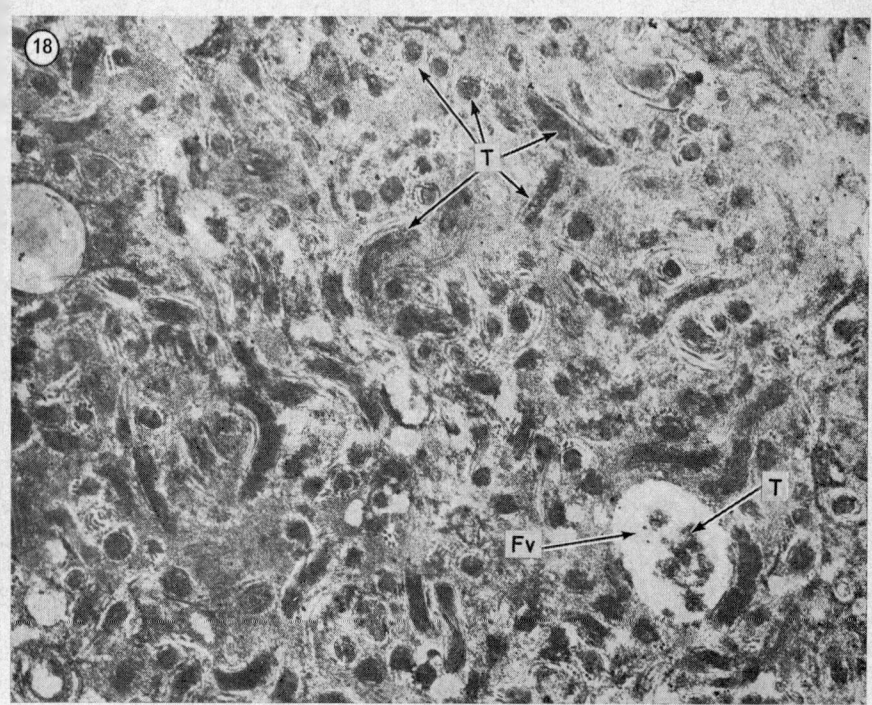

Fig. 18. Ultrathin section of tissue from a rabbit chancre 60 days after infection. Material taken 24 hours after administration of 84 000 units bicillin-1. Numberous treponemes (T) situated inside and outside the cells in various stages of preservation. Fv=food vacuoles. T=treponeme. × 14 000. (This illustration accompanies a paper by N. M Ovčinnikov and V. V. Delektorskij (1972). *Brit. J. vener. Dis.*, **48,** 327. Reproduced by kind permission of Professor Ovčinnikov and the Editor of the *Bnitish Journal of Venereal Diseases.*)

Fig. 17. Phagocytosis of *Treponema pallidum* by a plasma cell. Ultrathin section of rabbit hard-chancre tissue 47 days after infection. The phagocytosed treponeme (T) has a clear-cut structure. The fibrils (F) can be seen. There is a phagosome (PH) separated from the plasma membrane (m) by a narrow band of ectoplasm (EC). There is a large vacuole (V) with a residual body. The cell contents consist of marked endoplasmic reticulum (ER), a nucleus (N) with chromatin (CH), and outer and inner nuclear membranes (mN) and pores (P). × 70 000. (From an article by N. M. Ovčinnikov and V. V. Delektorskij (1972) *Brit. J. vener. Dis.*, **48,** 227. Reproduced by kind permission of the authors and the Editor of the *British Journal of Venereal Diseases.*)

could explain the high incidence of vulnerability to environmental influences. Cohen et al (1970) used gas chromatography to study the biochemical composition of a number of pathogenic and non-pathogenic treponemes and came to similar conclusions. Farshy et al (1970) carried out similar investigations.

Silver impregnation staining methods were reviewed by Blenden (1965) and Faine (1965) and modified by Walter et al (1969). Direct immunofluorescent techniques were used by Tringali and Mothershed (1969) to study T. pallidum. The reliability of a counting method for enumerating the organism was discussed by Artley and Clark (1969). Chandler and Cannefax (1969) evaluated dark-field and immunofluorescent techniques for demonstrating T. pallidum in fluids containing small numbers of organisms. Chandler and Clark (1970) showed that microscopically detectable T. pallidum would not pass a multipore membrane filter with a pore diameter of 0·22 μm. More motile organisms passed through larger filters than non-motile ones. Schmale et al (1970) used continuous particle electrophoresis to separate T. pallidum from rabbit testicular debris. Sternberger et al (1970) claimed that immuno-chemical staining of spirochaetes using a horseradish peroxidase and anti-horseradish peroxidase, as an antibody enzyme complex, in an unlabelled antibody enzyme method, is far superior in specificity and sensitivity to immunofluorescence. Obviously technical advances, such as those outlined above, which facilitate the recognition and specific identification of T. pallidum improve our research potential.

Alieva (1966) noted that 11·5 per cent of non-syphilitic rabbits gave positive reagin tests but that the TPI was negative. Pannu et al (1967) observed that up to half of sera from randomly selected rabbits may show reactive or weakly reactive VDRL reactions. It was suggested that this might be due to subclinical infection with T. cuniculi, (Smith and Pesetsky, 1967). Wells and Smith (1967) showed that it was possible for rabbits to be infected experimentally with syphilis and to develop lesions although the results of sensitive serological tests remained negative (Taylor et al, 1965). Clark (1970) in a study of 5 363 rabbits stated that 4·9 per cent of laboratory-raised rabbits, not apparently infected with T. cuniculi, reacted to the VDRL test in the U.S.A. In commercially produced rabbits 14·8 per cent reacted to the VDRL. Only 1·2 to 1·3 per cent reacted to the FTA-ABS test but 20 per cent reacted to the RPCFT test. Miller et al (1966) found that goats injected with normal rate testes developed low titre T. pallidum immobilising antibody, which could be absorbed by the Reiter treponeme. This suggested that rabbit testes shared non-specific immobilising antigen in common with the Nichols strain of T. pallidum.

Naumova (1969) made attempts to accelerate the development of syphilitic orchitis in rabbits. Smolin et al (1970) showed that anti-lymphocytic serum and steroids increased the infectivity of rabbit syphilis. Yano (1969) studied the mechanism of gumma formation in the animal. Izzat et al (1971) noted that in the rabbit an inoculum of 10 treponemes or more were required to infect all the animals. Also the incubation time was directly related to the total number of spirochaetes inoculated. Ragaishis (1964) described the renal changes in rabbits with experimental syphilis. Smith et al (1965) described the natural course of experimental ocular syphilis and neurosyphilis in the rabbit and Fribourg-Blanc et al (1966) followed the development of the fluorescent treponemal antibody in rabbit syphilis.

The work of Collart et al (1966), Collart and Dunoyer (1968) and Yobs et al (1968), must be viewed against the background of this research. Their views on persistent treponemes and the significance of these organisms have produced much controversy. The conclusion and the interpretation of animal infectivity tests were discussed at length in an excellent paper by Turner et al (1969).

Valuable work on experimental ocular syphilis in owl and marmoset monkeys has been carried out throughout the sixties in Miami, Florida. The unit of J. L. Smith have published several detailed papers on the subject (Smith et al, 1965; Wells and Smith, 1967; Elas et al, 1968; Clark and Yobs, 1968). It would appear that the owl monkey (*Aotus trivirgatus*) is preferable for studies of ocular and neurosyphilis (Levine et al 1970).

Gudjónsson and Skog (1970) in Stockholm reported that in rabbits infected with *T. pallidum* a fever developed 3 to 5 days after inoculation, and 50 per cent of the animals were dead within 2 weeks. This was thought to be a contaminating virus and when *T. pallidum* from Stockholm were used to inoculate nine rabbits in Baltimore, U.S.A., six of the rabbits died. This is an interesting observation as one wonders what less dramatic changes, due perhaps to other viruses, have been attributed to *T. pallidum* in the past.

REFERENCES

ABE, S. (1969). *Bull. Pharm. Res. Inst.* (*Takatsuki*), **79**, 6.
ALIEVA, S. G. (1966). *J. invest. Derm.*, **44**, 68.
ARTLEY, C. W. and CLARK, J. W. JR. (1969). *Appl. Microbiol.*, **17**, 665.
AZAR, H. A., PHAM, T. D. and KURBAN, A. K. (1970). *Arch. Path.*, **90**, 143.
BLENDEN, D. C. (1965). *J. invest. Derm.*, **45**, 68.
CHANDLER, F. W. and CANNEFAX, G. R. (1969). *Brit. J. vener. Dis.*, **45**, 1.
CHANDLER, F. W. and CLARK, J. W. JR. (1970). *Appl. Microbiol.*, **19**, 326.
CHRISTIANSEN, S. (1963). *Lancet*, i, 423.
CLARK, J. W. JR. and YOBS, A. R. (1968). *Brit. J. vener. Dis.*, **44**, 208.
CLARK, J. W. (1970). *Brit. J. vener. Dis.*, **46**, 191.
COHEN, P. G., MOSS, C. W. and FARSHTCHI, D. (1970). *Brit. J. vener. Dis.*, **46**, 10.
COLLART, P., BOREL, L. J. and DUREL, P. (1962). *Ann. Inst. Pasteur*, **102**, 596.
COLLART, P., POGGI, G. and DUNOYER, F. R. (1966). *Minerva Med.*, **57**, 4478.
COLLART, P. and DUNOYER, F. R. (1968). *Ann. Derm. Syph.*, (*Paris*), **95**, 285.

ELAS, F. J., SMITH, J. L., ISRAEL, C. W. and GAGER, W. E. (1968). *Brit. J. vener. Dis.*, **44**, 267.

FAINE, S. (1965). *J. clin. Path.*, **18**, 381.

FARSHY, D. C., THOMAS, M. L. and MOSS, C. W. (1970). *Brit. J. vener. Dis.*, **46**, 441.

FRIBOURG-BLANC, A., NIEL, G. and MOLLARET, H. H. (1966). *Bull. Soc. Path. exot.*, **59**, 54.

GUDJÖNSSON, H. and SKOG E. (1970). *Brit. J. vener. Dis.*, **46**, 318.

GUDJÖNSSON, H., NEWMAN, B. and TURNER, T. B. (1970). *Brit. J. vener. Dis.*, **46**, 435.

IZZAT, N. N., MUSHER, D. M. and MIN, K. W. (1972). *Brit. J. vener. Dis.*, **48**, 402.

IZZAT, N. N., KNOX, J. M., DACRES, W. G. and SMITH, E. B. (1971). *Acta derm.-vener.*, Stockh., **51**, 157.

JEPSEN, O. B., HOUGEN, H. H. and BIRCH-ANDERSON, A. (1968). *Acta path. microbiol. scand.*, **74**, 241.

LAUDERDALE, V. and GOLDMAN, J. N. (1972). *Brit. J. vener. Dis.*, **48**, 87.

LEVINE, B. M., SMITH, J. L. and ISRAEL, C. W. (1970). *Brit. J. vener. Dis.*, **46**, 307.

LONGHIN, S. and PODESCU, A. (1969). 'Biology of T. Pallidum', p. 224. Bucarest.

MILLER, J. N., BEKKER, J. H., DEBRUIJN, J. M. and ONVLEE, P. C. (1966). *J. immunol.*, **97**, 184.

NAUMOVA, D. (1969). *Vest. Derm. Vener.*, **43**, 40.

OVČINNIKOV, N. M. and DELEKTORSKIJ, V. V. (1969). *Bull. Wld Hlth Org.*, **35**, 322.

OVČINNOKOV, N. M. and DELEKTORSKIJ, V. V. (1970). *Brit., J. vener. Dis.*, **46**, 349.

OVČHINNIKOV, N. M. and DELEKTORSKIJ, V. V. (1970a). *Bull. Wld Hlth Org.*, **42**, 437.

OVČHINNIKOV, N. M. and DELEKTORSKIJ, V. V. (1971). *Brit. J. vener. Dis.*, **47**, 315.

OVČINNIKOV, N. M. and DELEKTORSKIJ, V. V. (1972). *Brit. J. vener. Dis.*, **48**, 327.

PANNU, J. S., ROSENBERG, M. A., ISRAEL, C. W. and SMITH, J. L. (1967). *Brit. J. vener. Dis.*, **43**, 114.

PILLOT, J., DUPOUEY, P. and RYTER, A. (1964). *Ann. Inst. Pasteur*, **107**, 663.

PILLOT, J. (1965). Contribution a l'étude du genre Treponema. Structures anatomique antigénique, Thesis No. 4571, University of Paris.

RAGAISHIS, S. L. (1964). *Vest. Derm. Vener.*, **38**, 58.

SCHMALE, J. D., KELLOGG, D. S. and MILLER, C. (1970). *Appl. Microbiol.*, **19**, 287.

SMITH, J. L. and PESETSKY, B. R. (1967). *Brit. J. vener. Dis.*, **43**, 117.

SMITH, J. L., SINGER, J. A., REYNOLDS, D. H., MOORE, M. B., YOBS, A. R. and CLARK, J. W. (1965). *Brit. J. vener. Dis.*, **41**, 15.

SMOLIN, G., NOZIK, R. A. and OKUMOTO, M. (1970). *Amer. J. Ophthal.*, **70**, 273.

STERNBERGER, L. A., HARDY, P. H. JR., CUCULIS, J. J. and MAYER, H. G. (1970). *J. Histochem. Cytochem.*, **18**, 315.

TAYLOR, W. H., SMITH, J. L. and SINGER, J. A. (1965). *Amer. J. Ophthal.*, **60**, 1093.

TRINGALI, G. R. and MOTHERSHED, S. M. (1969). *Riv. Ist. Sieroter Ital.*, **44**, 36.

TURNER, T. B., HARDY, P. H. and NEWMAN, B. (1969). *Brit. J. vener. Dis.*, **45**, 183.

VACZI, L., KIRALY, K. and RETHY, A. (1966). *Acta Microbiol. Acad. Sci. Hung.*, **13**, 79.

WALTER, E. K., SMITH, J. L., ISRAEL, C. W. and CAGER, W. E. (1969). *Brit. J. vener. Dis.* **45**, 6.

WELLS, J. A. and SMITH, J. L. (1967). *Brit. J. vener. Dis.*, **43**, 10.

WELLS, J. A. JR. and SMITH, J. L. (1967). 'Neuro-ophthalmology', Vol. 3, p. 262, Mosby, St. Louis.

WILLCOX, R. R. and GUTHE, R. (1966). *Bull. Wld Hlth Org.*, **35**, Suppl., 1–169.

W.H.O. TECH. REP. SERIES (1970). 455.

YANO, T. (1969). *Jap. J. Bact.*, **24**, 345.

YOBS, A. R. CLARK, J. W., MOTHCRSHED, S. E., BULLARD, J. C. and ARTLEY, C. W. (1968). *Brit. J. vener. Dis.*, **44**, 116.

12 Immunity in Syphilis

A. E. Wilkinson

It is well established that experimental infection with *T. pallidum*, if allowed to persist for 3 to 6 months before treatment, promotes the development of a substantial immunity to re-infection. This is confirmed by clinical experience in man. The mechanisms responsible for the development and maintenance of the immune state are still not clearly understood, despite much experimentation. For general reviews, the articles by Cannefax (1965), Wigfield (1965), Cannefax et al (1967) and Turner (1970) should be consulted.

Humoural immune mechanisms

Until recently, interest centred largely on humoural mechanisms of immunity in syphilis. The ability of sera containing immobilising antibody to immobilise and kill treponemes *in vitro* in the presence of complement naturally suggested that this antibody played a part in the maintenance of immunity *in vivo*. There is some correlation between the titre of immobilising antibody and immunity; the development of resistance to re-infection in the experimental animal roughly parallels the rise in titre of the TPI test (Turner and Hollander, 1957). However, Miller et al (1963b), Miller (1967), Metzger et al (1969) and Metzger and Smogor (1969) did not find such a correlation in experimentally immunised rabbits. Fribourg-Blanc (1956) has reported the presence of a heat-labile factor in both normal and syphilitic human sera which can immobilise and kill *T. pallidum in vitro*: this is distinct from complement and its possible role in immunity does not appear to have been studied. Anti-lipoidal antibodies are not related to the immunity of the host; their titre is often high early in the infection when resistance is poorly developed and low or even negative in late syphilis when there is a high level of immunity. These antibodies seem to be related to the amount of tissue response of the host to infection, and to reflect the activity of the disease process (Frederiksson et al 1968). Thivolet et al (1969) compared the development of serological reactivity of mice infected with *T. pallidum* with that in mice thymectomised shortly after birth. Positivity of the FTA-25 test developed rather more slowly in the thymectomised than in the control mice, but all of the animals which survived ultimately became FTA-positive. Hyperimmune sera have been shown to retard the course of experimental syphilis in rabbits (Sepetjian et al, 1973; Perine et al, 1973).

Cell mediated immunity

The part played by cell mediated immunity in syphilis has still to be determined, but this field is attracting increasing attention. In the non-immune animal, treponemes rapidly spread from the site of inoculation to the regional lymph nodes, but in an immune host they remain localised. Electron micrographic studies of testicular tissue from infected rabbits and from human primary and secondary lesions have shown *T. pallidum* within tissue cells, especially histiocytes and granulocytes (Sykes and Miller, 1971; Metz and Metz, 1972). *In vitro* studies have shown that rabbit peritoneal macrophages can take up *T. pallidum*; these were seen within vacuoles and sometimes showed evidence of degeneration (Musher et al, 1972). In this study treponemes were not seen within polymorphonuclear leucocytes or lymphocytes. These observations suggest that phagocytic cells play some part in the response of the host to infection; whether *T. pallidum* can persist within cells has yet to be determined.

The histological appearance of lesions following the intradermal injection of killed treponemes in patients with syphilis was studied by Temime et al (1966). The reaction was of the delayed hypersensitivity type; the epidermis was normal, the dermis showed perivascular infiltration with histiocytes and epithelioid cells with endothelial swelling. No local skin reactions were seen in 200 control patients but were produced in 124 of 391 patients thought to have syphilis on clinical or serological grounds. The test was positive in five of nine patients with late cutaneous syphilis, nine of 42 with tabes, 20 of 40 with aortitis, 10 of 15 with congenital syphilis and 59 of 203 with latent syphilis. A rise in titre of lipoidal antigen tests but not of the TPI test sometimes occurred after inoculation (Ranque et al, 1966). Laird and Thorburn (1966) carried out skin tests on 40 patients with late acquired or congenital syphilis but did not think the method was of value in the diagnosis or exclusion of syphilis. Cottini and Lazzaro (1965) injected Evans blue intravenously and 0·1 ml of a standardised suspension of *T. pallidum* intradermally. A positive reaction was shown by the development of a raised blue swelling 15 mm in diameter at the injection site within 20 minutes. They reported positive results in 30 of 32 patients with primary, all of 16 with secondary and 55 of 68 with latent syphilis. Cocuzza et al (1965) studied a passive cutaneous anaphylaxis test with syphilitic serum. Guinea-pigs were inoculated intradermally in the flank with the test serum and 4 hours later intravenously with Evans blue mixed with a suspension of *T. pallidum* or Reiter treponemes, Reiter protein antigen or cardiolipin antigen. Positive reactions were shown by the development of a blue coloration at the site of inoculation of serum; these were found with sera from patients with primary or secondary syphilis in animals challenged with *T. pallidum* or Reiter protein antigen. Negative results were found with sera from patients with latent syphilis, and in all animals challenged with intact Reiter treponemes or cardiolipin antigen.

The lymphocyte transformation reaction has been studied in syphilis by several workers. Sapuppo et al (1967) exposed lymphocytes from 17 patients with syphilis and 10 normal controls to a suspension of *T. pallidum*. No blast formation was found in the normal subjects or in patients with negative serological tests, but those patients whose TPI tests were positive showed increased blast formation. Chieregato and Faldarini (1968) used a cryolysate of *T. pallidum*, cardiolipin and preparations of Reiter treponemes as antigens. Transformation was found in two of 10 patients with primary syphilis, was maximal during the secondary stage but less marked in latency. Lymphocytes from some patients showed blast formation after exposure to *T. pallidum* but not to the other antigens. The intensity of transformation appeared to follow the behaviour of the TPI test. Similar results have been reported by Simon et al (1969), Badanoiu et al. (1969) and Badanoiu and Tardieu (1972). Janot et al (1971) considered a 4 per cent difference in blast formation in lymphocytes exposed to a saline suspension of *T. pallidum* from that in unexposed controls to be significant. With this criterion they found the test positive in four of six patients with primary syphilis, nine of 11 with secondary, five of six with congenital, all of 18 with cardiovascular or neurosyphilis, all of 30 with latent disease and in all of 12 patients with treated syphilis whose sera gave negative WR and TPI tests. The test was also found positive in three of 43 control patients with negative serological tests; these three patients were sensitive to penicillin and these results may have been due to cross-reactions to cephalothin incorporated in the culture medium. They consider that delayed hypersensitivity is established early in the course of syphilis, is maintained throughout the disease and persists in treated patients, even when conventional serological tests have become negative.

Levene et al (1969) compared blast formation of lymphocytes exposed to phytohaemagglutinin when cells from patients with syphilis were grown in their own plasma and in plasma from a single healthy donor. Cells from seven patients with primary syphilis, 12 with secondary, three with latent disease, one with a gumma and 12 healthy controls were studied. They found that transformation by phytohaemagglutinin was impaired in primary and secondary syphilis and that this was associated with a factor in the patients' sera which could also reduce the transformation ability of normal lymphocytes. Levene et al (1971) studied the histology of the spleen in 37 cases of congenital syphilis; moderate or gross depletion of lymphocytes in the area round the central arteriole was seen in 22 cases. Histological examination of inguinal lymph nodes from 20 patients with secondary syphilis showed depletion of lymphocytes in the paracortical areas; these appearances are thought to be associated with defective cell mediated immunity in man. A similar appearance has been seen in the spleens of rabbits infected after birth with *T. pallidum*; most of the animals died of a runting syndrome within 3 months (Festenstein et al, 1967). These findings are thought to reflect an impairment of cell mediated immunity in early acquired and congenital syphilis, possibly related to the widespread dissemination of the infective agent at these stages of the disease.

Studies of leucocyte migration after exposure to Reiter protein antigen have shown stimulation of migration of leucocytes from patients with primary syphilis and inhibition of migration in late active syphilis (Fulford and Brostoff, 1972). These results are interpreted as evidence of weak and strong delayed hypersensitivity at these two stages of the disease.

While both humoural and cell mediated mechanisms have been demonstrated which may contribute to immunity in syphilis, their relative importance is still uncertain. The demonstration of persisting treponeme-like forms in some patients with treated latent or late syphilis has also raised the question whether these may contribute to the immune state by presenting a continuing antigenic stimulus to the host. This implies a return to Neisser's concept of a 'chancre immunity' in syphilis.

IMMUNISATION AGAINST SYPHILIS

Attempts have been made to immunise rabbits against syphilis with commensal treponemes or material extracted from them. Reiter protein antigen (Miller et al, 1963a), cultivable Nichols strain treponemes with lysozyme or adjuvants (Izzat et al, 1970), a glycoprotein from the same strain with Freund's adjuvant (Izzat et al, 1971a), or ultrasonically disintegrated virulent Nichols strain treponemes with a lipopolysaccharide from *Esch. coli* as adjuvant (Izzat et al, 1971b); all failed to confer any immunity to challenge with virulent *T. pallidum*.

Metzger et al (1969) killed suspensions of the virulent Nichols strain of *T. pallidum* by leaving them exposed to the air for 10 days at 4°C. Animals given intravenous injections of such suspensions four times weekly for 7 weeks showed partial protection; none of 16 developed lesions after challenge but lymph node transfers showed that 10 of these animals had asymptomatic infections. No protection was conferred by suspensions stored at 4°C for 20–23 days or heated to 100°C. Protection was thought to be due to a labile surface component on the treponemes which was gradually lost on storage at 4°C or destroyed by heating. In further experiments rabbits were immunised by the intramuscular route four times weekly for 7 weeks with total doses varying from 3 to 12×10^9 treponemes treated to preserve this surface component. This conferred a degree of immunity as shown by the absence of lesions when challenged or a reduction in the number of lesions or prolongation of the incubation period. Solid immunity was produced in some animals as shown by the absence of lesions and negative lymph node transfers. The degree of protection increased with the larger immunising doses of treponemes. Immobilising antibody was not detected before challenge.

Miller (1965a, b) attenuated the virulent Nichols strain $T.\ pallidum$ by exposure to gamma radiation. Organisms so treated remained motile and were immobilised by syphilitic serum plus complement but failed to produce symptomatic or latent infections in rabbits inoculated with a single dose of 5×10^7 treponemes. Injections of these attenuated organisms once or twice weekly for 12 weeks failed to give immunity although immobilising antibody was present at titres of 208 to 7 680 in 13 of 15 rabbits. Extension of the immunising period to 24 weeks gave some degree of immunity by prolongation of the incubation period after challenge (Miller, 1967). Complete immunity to challenge could be achieved if the course of immunising injections were spread over 37 weeks. It is postulated that antibody to a weakly antigenic superficial mucopolysaccharide in the outer coat of the treponeme develops slowly during artificial immunisation in contrast to the more rapid development of treponemicidal antibody. Gamma radiation results in the inactivation of heat labile antigens and Miller thinks that heat stable antigens, presumably polysaccharides, play a dominant role in stimulating treponemicidal antibody or antibody associated with immunity, whether cellular or humoural. A polysaccharide isolated from Nichols strain $T.$ $pallidum$ has been shown to react with homologous rabbit antisera but not with human syphilitic sera; this suggests that there may be antigenic differences between the rabbit-adapted Nichols strain and 'street' strains of $T.\ pallidum$ (Miller, 1972).

Although these experiments have shown that active immunity can be produced in experimental animals, the prolonged course of immunisation is impracticable for use in man. Rabbits immunised with trepo-nemes extracted from rabbit testes have been shown to develop antibody against rabbit red cells and lymphocytes (Matej et al, 1973). If the suspensions are contaminated with testicular antigens, organ-specific antibody might also be produced during the immunisation of another species and cross-react with the host's testicular tissue. The use of a living, but attenuated treponeme which would multiply in the host offers an alternative approach, and Thatcher (1969) has suggested that $T.\ carateum$, the least pathogenic of the treponemes, might repay further study as a possible immunising agent. Jekel (1968) has reviewed the place of vaccine in the control of syphilis and pointed out the potential use of such a measure, if effective, in areas where mass campaigns against yaws have diminished the cross protection which this disease provides against syphilis.

The prospect of an effective vaccine against syphilis which could be used in man is still rather remote. Evaluation of its safety and efficacy will present formidable technical and ethical problems; such a vaccine might well have the positive disadvantage that the value of existing diagnostic serological tests would be compromised.

REFERENCES

BADANOIU, A. and TARDIEU, J. C. (1972). *Munch. med. Wschr.*, **25**, 1173.

BADANOIU, A., GAVRILESCO, M., NICOLAU, G. and CIRCIUMARESCO, T. (1969). *Arch. Roum. Path. exp. Microbiol.*, **28**, 419.

CANNEFAX, G. R. (1965). *Brit. J. vener. Dis.*, **41**, 260.

CANNEFAX, G. R., NORINS, L. C. and GILLESPIE, E. J. (1967). *Ann. Rev. Med.*, **18**, 471.

CHIEREGATO, G. and FALDARINI, G. (1968). *Minerva Derm.*, **43**, 264.

COCUZZA, G., NICOLETTI, G., LAZZARO, C. and GIARDINI, A. (1965). *Nuovi Ann. Ig.*, **16**, 187.

COTTINI, G. B. and LAZZARO, C. (1965). *G. ital. Derm.*, **106**, 77.

FESTENSTEIN, H., ABRAHAMS, C. and BOKKENHAUSER, V. (1967). *Clin. exp. Immunol.*, **2**, 311.

FREDERIKSSON, T., HEDERSTEDT, B. and ROSENGREN, S. (1968) *Acta path. microbiol. scand.*, **72**, 125.

FRIBOURG-BLANC, A. (1956). *Presse med.*, **64**, 1396.

FULFORD, K. W. M. and BROSTOFF, J. (1972). *Brit. J. vener. Dis.*, **48**, 483.

IZZAT, N. N., DACRES, W. G., KNOX, J. M. and WENDE, R. (1970). *Brit. J. vener. Dis.*, **46**, 451.

IZZAT, N. N., SMITH, E. B , JACKSON, S. W. and KNOX, J. M. (1971a). *Brit. J. vener. Dis.*, **47**, 335.

IZZAT, N. N., KNOX, J. M., DACRES, W. G. and SMITH, E. B. (1971b). *Acta derm.-venereol., Stockh.*, **51**, 157.

JANOT, C., GRANDIDIER, M., PUPIL, P., THOMAS, J.-L., BEUREY, J. and deLAVERGNE, J. (1971). *Presse med.*, **79**, 1901.

JEKEL, J. F. (1968). *Publ. Hlth Rep., Wash.*, **83**, 627.

LAIRD, S. M. and THORBURN, J. L. (1966). *Brit. J. vener. Dis.*, **42**, 119.

LEVENE, G. M., TURK, J. L., WRIGHT, D. J. M. and GRIMBLE, A. G. S. (1969). *Lancet*, **2**, 246.

LEVENE, G. M., WRIGHT, D. J. M. and TURK, J. L. (1971). *Proc. roy. Soc. Med.*, **64**, 426.

MATEJ, H., METZGER, M. and SMOGOR, W. (1973). *Arch. Immun. ther. Exp.*, **21**, 263.

METZ, J. and METZ, G. (1972). *Germ. Med.*, **2**, 56.

METZGER, M., MICHALSKA, E., PODWINSKA, J. and SMOGOR, W. (1969). *Brit. J. vener. Dis.*, **45**, 299.

METZGER, M. and SMOGOR, W. (1969). *Brit. J. vener. Dis.*, **45**, 308.

MILLER, J. N. (1965a). *Antonie van Leeuwenhoek*, **31**, 223.

MILLER, J. N. (1965b). *J. Bact.*, **90**, 297.

MILLER, J. N. (1967). *J. Immunol.*, **99**, 1012.

MILLER, J. N. (1972). *Med. Clin. N. Amer.*, **56**, 1217.

MILLER, J. N., WANG, S. J. and FAZZAN, F. P. (1963a). *Brit. J. vener. Dis.*, **39**, 195; (1963b). *Ibid.*, 199.
MUSHER, D. N., IZZAT, N. N., MIN, K.-W. and GYÖRKEY, F. (1972). *Acta derm.-venereol., Stockh.*, **52**, 349.
PERINE, P. L., WEISER, R. S. and KLEBANOFF, S. L. (1973). *Infect. Immunity*, **8**, 787.
RANQUE, J., TRAMIER, G., TEMIME, P. and LATOURELLE, P. (1966). *Proph. Sanit. morale*, **38**, 176.
SAPUPPO, A., CHIARENZA, A. and LAZZARO, C. (1967). *Minerva Derm.*, **42**, 12.
SEPETJIAN, M., SALASSOLA, D. and THIVOLET, J. (1973). *Brit. J. vener. Dis.*, **49**, 335.
SIMON, N., DOBOZY, A. and HUNYADI, J. (1969). *Arch. klin. exp. Derm.*, **236**, 1.
SYKES, J. A. and MILLER, J. N. (1971). *Infect. and Immunity*, **4**, 307.
TEMIME, P., TRAIMER, G. and PRIVAT, Y. (1966). *Proph. Sanit. morale*, **38**, 154.
THATCHER, R. W. (1969). *Brit. J. vener. Dis.*, **45**, 10.
THIVOLET, J., MONIER, J. C., SEPETJIAN, M. and SALUSSOLA, D. (1969). *Experientia*, **25**, 302.
TURNER, T. B. (1970). 'Infectious Agents and Host Resistance', ed. S. Mudd. W. B. Saunders Co.
TURNER, T. B. and HOLLANDER, D. H. (1957). Biology of the Treponematoses. *Wld Hlth Org. Monograph*, 35.
WIGFIELD, A. S. (1965). *Brit. J. vener. Dis.*, **41**, 275.

13 Therapy

J. R. W. Harris

PENICILLIN

Penicillin, after 30 years, still remains the drug of choice in the treatment of syphilis. Its mode of action has been particularly studied in recent years (Tipper and Strominger, 1965).

There is evidence that the antibiotic causes death of the micro-organisms by interfering with the synthesis of the glycopeptides that are essential constituents of the microbial cell wall. There appears to be strong affinity between the antibiotic and the transpeptidases produced by the growing micro-organisms. This lack of transpeptidase causes inhibition of the cell wall synthesis (*Lancet*, 1967). The defect on the cell wall results in death of the organism by osmotic lysis (Park, 1964). However, the bactericidal action only occurs during phases of growth. Hence if the bacteria are not exposed to a continuous concentration of penicillin the damage to the cell wall will not be complete. In these circumstances the sensitive micro-organisms may be transformed into insensitive spheroblasts or atypical forms (Park, 1964). In other circumstances they may be able to produce further transpeptidase and so recover. While there is no definite evidence that *T. pallidum* possesses such survival properties, there have been certain indications in the last decade that on occasions the treponeme-like forms found after treatment are *T. pallidum* (Dunlop, 1972).

Although a strain of *T. pallidum* resistant to penicillin has yet to be described, treponemes have been found after dosages of penicillin sufficient to maintain much higher concentrations than the 0·03 i.u./ml regarded as fully treponemecidal (Hardy et al, 1970). Various explanations have been advanced to explain both this and the fact that numerous workers have demonstrated treponeme-like forms in tissues from patients who have received apparently adequate treatment for early and late syphilis. These treponeme-like forms have been recovered from lymph nodes, arteries affected by temporal arteritis, aqueous humour, cerebrospinal fluid and bone, and have been extensively reviewed (Willcox,

1964; *Lancet*, 1968; Turner et al, 1969; Dunlop, 1970; W.H.O., 1970; Sparling, 1971).

McDermott (1958) in describing 'microbial persistence' noted that some organisms are able to survive attack by antibiotics to which they are sensitive. Thus occasional treatment failure may occur in a few patients after penicillin therapy for early syphilis. Ovčinnikov and Delektorskij (1971) and Lauderdale and Goldman (1971) observed that treponemes remain unchanged in fibroblasts; similar observations were made by Metz and Metz (1972) in leucocytes. Possibily organisms do survive within some cells and while treponemecidal levels of antibiotics are readily obtained in serum, relatively little is known about the levels obtained within cells. Because of the low levels of serum penicillin it seems that effective treponemecidal levels may not be attained in the C.S.F. and the eye. The intra-ocular level of penicillin and ampicillin may be increased by the administration of probenecid although even then adequate treponemecidal levels may only be maintained for 2 hours (Goldman et al, 1968).

While one may speculate that in late syphilis some organisms may survive because they are resting and so are insusceptible to treatment, the same hypothesis does not hold for early congenital syphilis. Yet Hardy et al (1970), obtained from a congenital syphilitic neonate an organism which had survived oxytetracycline, kanamycin and potassium penicillin G in a dosage of 800 000 i.u/kg. This strain of *T. pallidum* was pathogenic to rabbits and was sensitive to penicillin.

The inhibition of glycopeptides in the microbial cell wall is caused by free penicillin molecules only. Since part of the penicillin is reversibly bound to albumin in both serum and tissue, the total concentration of penicillin is the sum of the free and protein bound penicillin (Quinn, 1964; Knudsen, 1964). As there are variations in the binding capacity of the same penicillin, and the different penicillins have different binding capacities, the theoretical inhibiting concentration of penicillin is assumed to be 0·03 i.u./ml of serum. This safety margin is believed to cover other possible variations in serum concentration resulting from individual differences in rates and degrees of binding, absorption, excretion and tissue diffusion.

Only the free penicillin fraction is capable of diffusion into the tissues from the serum. The protein bound penicillin in serum and tissues thus represents a floating penicillin depot. Penicillin is liberated from this depot to maintain the equilibrium in the blood-tissue system (Rolinson, 1964). If this system is supplied from repository long-acting penicillin preparations the exposure of the organism is prolonged. The active free penicillin fraction in the serum can be assessed by determining the rate of treponemal immobilisation of the sera (Prieto and Jimon, 1965).

Since the multiplication time of *T. pallidum* was found to be 30–33 hours, at least during the first days of experimental infections (Collart, 1970), a minimal concentration of 0·03 i.u. of penicillin per ml of serum should be maintained for 7–10 days in early syphilis and the subtreponemecidal intervals during treatment should not exceed 24 hours. If this dose/time relationship is considered in any regime of therapy, any preparation of penicillin G will be effective in the treatment of early syphilis. This basic dose/tissue relationship is not adequately identified in many published reports on the results of penicillin therapy of syphilis. Thus the results of many of the series are open to discussion (Kern and Elste, 1966).

The long-acting repository penicillin preparations are the most commonly used methods of penicillin therapy for syphilis in the world today. Efforts to standardise these preparations have been fairly successful (W.H.O., 1964). The ideal dose/tissue relationship for penicillin therapy has not changed in the last decade. There has, perhaps, been an increasing appreciation of the value of benzathine penicillin G. Its effectiveness in symptomatic and asymptomatic human neurosyphilis has been demonstrated (U.S. Dept. of Health, Education and Welfare, 1965); also its ease of application in the treatment of neonatal and congenital syphilis has been appreciated (Harris and Cave, 1965).

In syphilis of more than 4 years duration (late latent and late symptomatic syphilis) the immunological pattern has been firmly established and can be influenced to a limited extent by treatment. The therapeutic aim here is to arrest the infection (Idsøe et al, 1972).

Capinski and his co-workers and Koh Kim Yam were reported by Idsøe et al (1972) as having found the following regimes completely successful in the treatment of seronegative and seropositive primary syphilis. Capinski and his colleagues found 6 mega i.u. of aqueous procaine penicillin given over 20 days satisfactory in the treatment of primary syphilis and 6 mega i.u. of aqueous procaine penicillin in association with 4·8 mega i.u. of procaine benzylpenicillin to be effective in the treatment of secondary syphilis. Koh Kim Yam found PAM 6 mega i.u. given over 10 days to be entirely satisfactory in the treatment of both primary and secondary syphilis. Idsøe et al (1972) reviewed 469 cases of late latent syphilis followed up for 12 years; C.S.F. findings were still normal and no evidence of cardiovascular syphilis was found. Progression from late latent to late symptomatic syphilis was prevented in all reported cases.

In the treatment of late symptomatic syphilis penicillin is the drug of choice in most countries. The U.S.A. (U.S. Dept of Health, Education and Welfare, 1968), the United Kingdom (King and Nicol, 1969), the Scandinavian countries (Perdrup, 1964), some clinics in the U.S.S.R. (Grobulev, 1966) and the Federal Republic of Germany (Braun-Falco and Petzoldt, 1970) all rely on penicillin. In France, while penicillin is the chief therapeutic agent (Pautrat and Wilhelm, 1966), there are still some workers who prefer to treat with penicillin and a heavy metal combination. The heavy metal used by Degos is an adjuvant (Degos, 1968), in order to reduce the intensity of a Jarish–Herxheimer reaction or to prevent therapeutic paradox (Bolgert and Poisson, 1965). However, it is the opinion of many that no advantages are gained by adding bismuth and/or arsenicals to penicillin. Treatment with penicillin alone is much safer and the actual curative effect of penicillin cannot be expected to improve by supplementation with bismuth. Pietro and Jimon (1965) showed that bismuth injections in healthy volunteers did not result in any treponemecidal effect on the serum.

Reference has been made above to the use of bismuth in an effort to reduce the intensity of the Jarish–Hexheimer reaction. Gudjónsson and Skog (1968) found that prednisone was of value in reducing or preventing the occurrence of a Jarish–Herxheimer. Viegas et al (1969), in a large series involving 187 patients with early syphilis and 257 patients with late syphilis, came to the conclusion that prednisone given with the antibiotic therapy was more effective in suppressing the JH reaction, than when the prednisone was given in advance of the antibiotic therapy. They felt that the hazards of steroid therapy outweighed the uncertain advantage of using it in allaying the JH reaction. They concluded that as corticosteroids stimulate the proliferation of treponemes, their administration before anti-syphilitic therapy was potentially dangerous. Arfouilloux (1969) believed that corticosteroids had some clinical use in reducing the intensity of the JH reaction and in preventing therapeutic paradox. Knudsen and Aastrup (1965) observed that several patients treated with bismuth as an adjuvant to penicillin had a 'double herxheimer', while none of the patients treated with penicillin had febrile reactions.

In the majority of cases of late symptomatic syphilis, penicillin treatment will arrest a pathological process which would frequently progress if not treated. Although duration of the infection is important, Vivas Salas (1966) described excellent results for penicillin therapy of non-complicated aortitis. Perdrup (1964) and Frishman (1967) found that asymptomatic neurosyphilis when treated with penicillin had similar good prognosis. Perdrup (1964) observed that penicillin treatment of gumma of internal organs was successful but the physician must be patient as the healing of the gumma is slow and may take up to one year, depending on the extent of infiltration and tissue destruction.

Patients with clinical neurosyphilis having irreversible brain damage can continue to deteriorate despite large doses of penicillin. This is particularly applicable to GPI (Wilner and Brody, 1968). This may well occur despite the fact that the active syphilitic process has been halted, As the level of penicillin in the C.S.F. after parenteral administration can be considerably lower than that in the serum (Collart, 1965), the physician will in these circumstances be concerned that he has not effectively halted the active process in the brain tissue. Oxelius et al (1969) feel that quantification of C.S.F. immunoglobulins at this stage may help to assess the activity of the neurosyphilis. O'Neill and Nicol (1972) indicate that assessment of the IgM class anti-treponemal antibody using fluorescent techniques may be of value in estimating continued activity of the syphilitic process. At the same time they feel that pre-antibiotic cortisone therapy will increase the susceptibility of the *T. pallidum* to penicillin, while Luger (1970) warns against the concomitant use of bacteriostatic preparations which inhibit growth and reduce the efficacy of the penicillin.

In the treatment of primary optic atrophy, Dowzenko and Owsianowski (1964) believe that the penicillin dosages should be higher and the treatment more prolonged than in neurosyphilis in general. Willcox (1964) and Huriez and Vanoverschelde (1965) feel that in an attempt to prevent oedema of the optic nerve following penicillin alone, corticosteroids should be administered in conjunction with penicillin.

Lightning pains continue to be a therapeutic dilemma. Ekbom (1966) found that carbamazepine (Tegretol) could be used with excellent effect. This has not been generally confirmed.

The present treatment practices with penicillin in syphilis as outlined by Idsøe et al (1972) are as follows. For primary, secondary and latent syphilis with non-reactive C.S.F. and adequate oppportunities for follow-up; a total of 2·4 mega i.u. benzathine penicillin stat. or a total of 4·8–6·0 mega i.u. procaine penicillin G in aluminium stearate solution (PAM) given as a stat. dose of 2·4 mega i.u. followed by 1·2 mega i.u. at 3-day intervals; a total of 6·0 mega i.u. procaine penicillin G given in dosages of 600 000 i.u. for 10 consecutive days.

For all other forms of syphilis, a total of 6–9 mega i.u. of benzathine penicillin given in doses of 2·4 mega i.u. at 7-day intervals; or a total of 6–9 mega i.u. PAM given in doses of 1·2 mega i.u. at 3-day intervals; or a total of 6–10 mega i.u. procaine penicillin G given in dosages of 600 000 i.u. daily.

For all cases of congenital syphilis up to 12 years of age, providing the patient weighs less than 32 kg (71 lb), a total of 50 000 i.u./kg benzathine penicillin given in one dose; or a total of 100 000 i.u./kg PAM given in three divided doses at 3-day intervals; or a total of 100 000 i.u./kg given as 10 000 i.u./kg for 10 consecutive days. All other cases can be treated with the same dosage/time regimes as adult latent syphilis.

It is important to remember that these treatment schedules are modified by the physician on consideration of his own experience and the clinical and social circumstances of the patient. Many would feel that in symptomatic neurosyphilis doses of 20–30 mega i.u. penicillin are required.

With the increasing antibiotic levels required to cure gonococcal infection, there was great concern among many workers in the sixties that concomitantly acquired syphilis might be masked as a result of the antibiotic therapy for gonorrhoea. Hallinger (1968) treated eight patients exhibiting dark field positive early syphilis with 5 mega i.u. sodium penicillin and 1 g probenicid. In all eight cases the syphilis regressed but relapsed in seven patients during the next 11 weeks. Degos et al (1968) reported an isolated case in which secondary syphilis occurred after a single injection of 2·4 mega i.u. benzathine penicillin for pre-serologic primary syphilis. Schroeter et al (1971) reviewed the situation and found PAM 2·4 mega i.u. or 3·0 mega i.u. completely success-ful in aborting incubating syphilis in 215 cases. Woodcock (1971) reviewed 281 patients treated for early syphilis and correlated this with a previous history of gonorrhoea. He was hesitant to draw firm con-clusions from the small numbers involved but inclined towards the interpretation that early syphilis may be accidentally cured by the treatment for gonorrhoea, rather than that it is being masked by the prolongation of the incubation period.

Adverse reactions to penicillin

At the outset it must be reiterated that among treponemecidal antibiotics penicillin is the least toxic (Stewart, 1964). Nevertheless, allergic reactions due to immunological responses to penicillin have become a major problem. Toxic reactions almost always occur when penicillin in high doses is given to patients with reduced renal function (Kurtzman et al, 1970). These are usually neurotoxic reactions especially if the brain tissue has been weakened by disease (Deisenhammer, 1969). The toxic effect is produced by the cations of the potassium or sodium salts (McGovern, 1970). Embolic toxic reactions following the accidental intravenous injection of procaine penicillin are rare (Freedman, 1965).

Penicillin is believed to be the commonest cause of drug allergy. Certain aspects of the various forms of allergic reaction have received attention. If the patient already has antibodies as a result of previous exposure to penicillin or related substances, then either immediate or accelerated reactions occur from seconds to 48 hours after adminis-tration (McGovern, 1970). The late allergic reactions tend to occur after 3 days in patients who may not have had penicillin before. They have been reviewed by McGovern (1970). Benzylpenicillin, having a low molecular weight combines with larger protein molecules to form hapten-protein conjugates (Levine, 1966). The major antigenic determinant has been indicted as being the penicilloyl protein conjugate (Parker, 1964). Other determinants appear to be macromolecules resulting from polymerisation of penicillin; these have been found in semisynthetic penicillins (Stewart, 1968).

Much evidence has been amassed that patients with past or present allergic diathesis, particularly bronchial asthma, are more disposed toward penicillin hypersensitivity than normal individuals (Idsøe et al, 1968). The indications for penicillin treatment in these patients should be severely restricted.

ANTIBIOTICS OTHER THAN PENICILLIN

Since penicillin should not be used in the treatment of syphilis in those known to be actual or potential reactors, there is a need for other drugs of proven treponemacidal ability in this context. While amino-benzylpenicillin (Ampicillin) has shown clinical and serological results compatible with those obtained with benzylpenicillin (Cannata, 1965), it is not suitable for the treatment of benzylpenicillin sensitised patients. Skin rashes occur more frequently after Ampicillin than with other penicillins (Krönig and Dennig, 1970). There has been some confusion between these skin rashes and Jarish–Herxheimer reactions in early secondary syphilis (Harris et al, 1972).

There is clinical and experimental evidence of cross sensitivity between conventional penicillins and the cephalosporins. This is on the basis of a shared lactam ring (Feinberg, 1970), which is thought to be the determinant factor in the occurrence of anaphylactic reactions following the initial injection of cephaloridine in patients previously documented as having penicillin allergy (Rothschild and Doty, 1966).

The other antibiotics of some proven value in the treatment of syphilis are chloramphenicol, erythromycin, spiramycin, spectinomycin, tetracyclines and cephalosporin derivatives. Pencillin and the cephalosporins are bacteriocidal while the broad spectrum antibiotics are usually bacteriostatic interfering with the synthesis of bacterial DNA and RNA and enabling the defence mechanism of the host to kill them (*Lancet*, 1967).

Chloramphenicol administered orally and parenterally is as effective as tetracyclines in all stages of syphilis. The high incidence of reported side effects including aplastic anaemia, have discouraged many workers from using it. Rangiah (1964) used it with effect in the treatment of pregnant women with syphilis. Twenty-three patients who had received 20 g chloramphenicol showed satisfactory clinical and serological response. The babies were well at 2-year follow-up.

Erythromycin stearate and erythromycin estolate are at present the erythromycin preparations of choice (Towpik, 1970). Satisfactory results have been obtained in early syphilis (Fernando, 1969). Lucas and Price (1967) presented a co-operative assessment of the results of treatment with erythromycin in the U.S.A. They proposed a dosage scheme of 30 g over 10 days. In prenatal syphilis and in neurosyphilis this dosage should be doubled to 60 g, as erythromycin diffuses less easily into the C.S.F. and the foetal circulation than chloramphenicol. Both the authors above and Dratwinski (1971) felt that doses of 20 g erythromycin were insufficient to adequately treat infectious syphilis.

Spiramycin has a bacteriocidal action and has been advocated by De Barros and Belda (1965) as being of some value in this situation. Its pharmacological properties have not yet been clearly outlined. It can be used orally, intramuscularly or intravenously. The total oral dosage used successfully is 16 g over 8 days and the total parenteral dose is 3 g over 6 days.

Spectinomycin sulphate is at present under investigation by the U.S. Public Health Service. Initial studies by Lucas and Price (1967) indicated that at levels of 32 g given over 8 days it was satisfactory. It requires parenteral administration (Walter and Heilmeyer, 1965) and high serum levels are achieved shortly after injection.

Tetracycline group antibiotics have been widely used in syphilis therapy. Recently parenteral oxytetracycline compounds have been used by Garnier et al (1965) and Luger (1968). While the clinical and serological results are acceptable the patients frequently experienced pain at the site of injection. Intravenous N-(pyrrolidinomethyl) tetracyline has been used to good effect in late and early syphilis by Kuhl (1965) and Luger (1968). The toxicity with this tetracycline derivative may exceed that of other tetracyclines. Lucas and Price (1967) found that tetracycline given orally to a dose of 30 g over a period of 10–15 days resulted in a 100 per cent cure rate in early syphilis; while Kimmig (1966) found that oral demethylchlortetracycline in a total dose of 10–15 g over 10 days was equally effective. The disadvantage with demethychlorotetracycline is that as it has a low renal excretion rate and there is thus a danger of blood and tissue accumulation. Doxycycline has an exceptionally good absorption and slow renal elimination. It has been used by Steppert (1968) and Wodniansky et al (1969) with effect in the treatment of early syphilis. The total dosage of 3 g is given orally over 10 days.

Since the isolation of cephalosporin nucleus (Abraham and Newton, 1961) various semi-synthetic derivatives have been defined, namely, cephaloglycin, cephalexin, cephalothin, cephalosporin C and cephaloridine. The immunochemical cross-reactivity between penicillin and these compounds has already been referred to in this section. In experimental syphilis cephaloridine has a lower treponemecidal activity than penicillin but the numerous clinical studies have shown that it is an effective agent in the treatment of early syphilis (Seftel, 1965; Flarer, 1967; Oller, 1967; Duncan and Knox, 1971). All the cephalosporins except cephaloglycin are given parenterally. Oller (1967) states that satisfactory blood levels can be maintained by intramuscular doses of 250–500 mg every 8–12 hours for 10 days, but Duncan and Knox (1971) advise that total doses greater than 15 g be given and advocate a total of 30 g. Apparently diffusion of cephaloridine from the blood to the spinal fluid is poor (Murdoch, 1965) and its value in the treatment of neurosyphilis awaits classification. Gonzalez-Ochou and Moreno (1967) have used cephaloridine in the treatment of five patients with a history of penicillin hypersensitivity. There were no ill effects. Glicksman et al (1968) have also treated five patients who had penicillin allergy without any evidence of cross sensitivity. Thus some patients with histories of penicillin hypersensitivity can be treated with cephaloridine but the reasons for this are obscure.

Apart from the cephaloridines, all other drugs used in the treatment of syphilis have much weaker treponemacidal effects. Thus patients undergoing treatment will remain dark field positive and potentially infectious for a longer period of time. This must be kept in mind if the patient is promiscuous and socially irresponsible. When these antibiotics are used instead of penicillin lesions heal more slowly. Erythromycin particularly has been indicted in protracted healing of indurated lesions of secondary syphilis (Isdøe et al, 1972).

The side effects of chloramphenicol have already been discussed. Tetracyclines should be avoided in pregnancy (*Lancet*, 1963). Acute fatty liver has been associated with high dose intravenous tetracycline therapy (Dowling and Leper, 1964). Superimposed candida infections are associated with tetracycline use and photosensitivity occurs particularly with demethylchlorotetracycline. Serious reactions following erythromycin treatment are rare. Children tolerate the drug well and even after prolonged therapy the only significant side effect is the sporadic occurrence of mild hepatitis (*Canad. med. Ass. J.*, 1963).

At present the drugs of choice in patients who do not tolerate penicillin are erythromycin and the tetracycline derivatives, with the proviso that tetracyclines should not be given during pregnancy or to young children.

Lest we feel complacent in our present-day management of syphilis, the report by Hardy et al (1970) of an isolated episode of complete failure to control early syphilitic infection must be remembered. In view of its significance the paper will be quoted in some detail.

A young woman was found to have secondary syphilis and treatment with tetracyclines was prescribed but not completed; 11 months later she was found to have gonorrhoea and as she was 7 months pregnant was treated with 2·4 mega i.u. benzathine penicillin G. She was admitted in labour to the Johns Hopkins Hospital 10 days later and a girl weighing 4 lb was born. The infant had hepatomegaly and splenomegaly, a distended abdomen and a small head; a petechial rash developed 12 hours after birth and there was increasing respiratory distress. As meconium peritonitis or generalised sepsis was suspected treatment was commenced with potassium penicillin G (50 000 i.u./kg/day to a total of over 800 000 i.u./kg) and kanamycin 15 mg/kg/day. Reports of VDRL, CWR, TPI and FTA-ABS tests on the cord blood were strongly positive at titres higher than maternal levels. Both clavicles and the long bones showed periostitis and irregular metaphyses. When the diagnosis of congenital syphilis was apparent treatment with kanamycin and cortiscosteroids were given from the second to the tenth day after birth as the infant had thrombocytopenia. On the second day after birth the spinal fluid showed 138 mononuclears per mm^3 and a protein level of 264 mg per cent. On the tenth day the cell count had fallen to 25 per mm^3 and a single non-motile treponeme was seen on dark ground microscopy.

The baby failed to thrive and bacterial sepsis was confirmed on the seventeenth day by isolation of *Klebsiella* from the blood, urine and spinal fluid. Penicillin was discontinued and kanamycin, colistin sulphate and prednisone were given. Death occurred on the twenty-second day after birth.

At post-mortem gross changes of congenital syphilis were seen in the long bones. The liver showed evidence of periportal fibrosis and interstitial scarring. The lungs showed the residue of pneumonia alba in the healing stage. Lesions in the brain were confined to the meninges and were typical of congenital syphilitic meningitis.

A non-motile treponeme was seen on dark ground in the aqueous humour removed immediately after death. Rabbits were inoculated intratesticularly with aqueous humour, ground ocular tissue and liver. After 75 days incubation the animals inoculated with aqueous humour and ocular tissue developed testicular lesions and a strain of *T. pallidum* highly virulent to the rabbit was isolated. Tests *in vitro* showed that this was not resistant to penicillin.

The demonstration of persistent virulent *T. pallidum* in this infant, who had been treated with penicillin, both *in utero* and after birth led the authors to question whether children born of syphilitic mothers should not be kept under observation for a number of years regardless of immediate clinical or serological evidence of disease.

REFERENCES

ABRAHAM, E. P. and NEWTON, G. G. F. (1961). *Biochem. J.*, **79**, 377.
ARFOUILLOUX, J. C. (1969). *Concours med.*, **91**, 437.
BOLGERT, M. and POISSON, R. (1965). *Bull. Soc. franç.*, *Derm. Syph.*, **72**, 392.
BRAUN-FALCO, O. and PETZOLDT, D. (1970). *Dtsch. Arztebl.*, **67**, 29.
BROWN, W. J. (1971). *J. Amer. med. Ass.*, **218**, 711.
CANAD. MED. ASS. J. (1963). **88**, 1173.
CANNATA, C. (1965). *Minerva derm.*, **40**, 50.
COLLART, P. (1970). *Rev. Med.*, *Paris*, **11**, 1265.
COLLART, P. (1965). *Proph. sanit. morale*, **37**, 49.

DE BARROS, J. M. and BELDA, W. (1965). *Rev. paul. Med.*, **66**, 214.

DEGOS, R., DELZANT, O. and GAIDMOUR, G. (1968). *Bull. Soc. franç. Derm. Syph.*, **75**, 289.

DEGOS, R. (1968). In: *XIII Congressus Internationalis Dermatologiae*, **1**, pp. 363–366. Springler, Munchen, Berlin.

DEISENHAMMER, E. (1969). In: *Hochmosierte Penicillin-Therapie Symposium*, Wien, Biochemie-Gesellschaft, p. 24.

DOWLING, H. F. and LEPER, M. M. (1964). *J. Amer. med. Ass.*, **188**, 307.

DOWZENKO, A. and OWSIANOWSKI, M. (1964). *Neurol. Neurochir. Psychiat. pol.*, **14**, 189.

DRATWINSKI, Z. (1971). *Przegl. Derm.*, **58**, 69.

DUNCAN, W. C. and KNOX, J. M. (1971). *Postgrad. med. J.*, **47**, 119.

DUNLOP, E. M. C. (1970). *Abst. Wld Med.*, **44**, 241.

DUNLOP, E. M. C. (1972). *Brit. med. J.*, **2**, 577.

EHRMANN, G. (1967). *Arch. klin. exp. Derm.*, **227**, 993.

EKBOM, K. (1969). *Acta med. scand.*, **179**, 251.

FEINBERG, J. G. (1970). In: 'Penicillin Allergy', Thomas, Springfield, Ill. p. 90.

FERNANDO, W. L. (1969). *Brit. J. vener. Dis.*, **45**, 200.

FLARER, F. (1967). *Postgrad. med. J.*, **43**, Suppl. 133.

FREEDMAN, M. A. (1965). *Rocky Mtn med. J.*, **62**, 34.

FRISHMAN, M. (1967). *Vestn. Derm. Vener.*, **41**, 76.

GARNIER, G., SISSMAN, R. and DASTAGUE, B. et al (1965). *Presse méd.*, **72**, 123.

GLICKSMAN, J. M., SHORT, D. H., and KNOX, J. M. (1968). *Arch. intern. Med.*, **121**, 342.

GOLDMAN, E. E., McLAIN, J. H. and SMITH, J. L. (1968). *Amer. J. Ophthal.*, **65**, 717.

GONZALEZ-OCHOU, A. and MORENO, J. B. (1967). *Postgrad. med. J.*, **43**, Suppl. 134.

GROBULEV, S. S. (1966). *Vestn. Derm. Vener.*, **39**, 75.

GUDJÓNSSON, H. and SKOG, E. (1968). *Acta derm.-venereol.*, Stockh., **48**, 15.

HALLINGER, L. (1968). *Acta derm.-venereol.*, Stockh., **48**, 260.

HARDY, J. B., HARDY, P. H., OPPENHEIMER, E. H., RYAN, S. J. and SHEFF, R. N. (1970). *J. Amer. med. Ass.*, **212**, 1345.

HARRIS, W. D. M. and CAVE, V. G. (1965). *J. Amer. med. Ass.*, **194**, 1312.

HARRIS, J. R. W., MAHONY, J. D. H. and McCANN, J. S. (1972). *Brit. med. J.* i, 687.

HURIEZ, C. and VANOVERSCHELDE, M. (1965). *Lille. méd.*, **10**, 348.

IDSØE, O., GUTHE, T. and WILLCOX, R. R. (1972). *Bull. Wld Hlth Org.*, **47**, Suppl. 12.

IDSØE, O., GUTHE, T., WILCOX, R. R. and WECK, A. L. DE (1968). *Bull. Wld Hlth Org.*, **38**, 159.

KERN, A. and SONNICHSEN, N. (1971). *Z. ärztl. Fortbild.*, Jena, **65**, 887.

KERN, A. and ELSTE, G. (1966). *Z. ärztl. Fortbild.*, Jena, **21/22**, 1201.

KIMMIG, J. (1966). *Therapiewoche*, **16**, 210.

KING, A. and NICOL, C. (1969). 'Venereal Diseases', 2nd ed., Canell, London.

KNUDSEN, E. L. T. (1964). *Postgrad. med. J.*, **40**, Suppl. 14.

KNUDSEN, K. A. and AASTRUP, B. (1965). *Brit. J. vener. Dis.*, **41**, 177.

KRÖNIG, B. and DENNIG, H. (1970). *Arzneimittel-Forsch.*, **20**, 1930–1938.

KUHL, M. (1965). *Hautatzt*, **16**, 78.

KURTZMAN, N. A., RODGERS, P. W. and HARTER, H. R. (1970). *J. Amer. med. Ass.*, **214**, 1320.

LANCET (1967), i, 321.

LANCET (1968), ii, 718.

LANCET (1963), ii, 283.

LAUDERDALE, V. and GOLDMAN, J. N. (1971). Quoted Dunlop, E. M. C. (1972). *Brit. med. J.*, ii, 577.

LEVINE, B. B. (1966). *New Engl. J. Med.*, **275**, 1175.

LUCAS, J. B. and PRICE, E. V. (1967). *Brit. J. vener. Dis.*, **43**, 244.

LUGER, A. (1968). In: 'Current Problems in Dermatology', Vol. 2, pp. 58–100. Karger, Basle and New York.

LUGER, A. (1970). *Hautarzt*, **21**, 531.

METZ, J. and METZ, G. (1972). *Germ. Med.*, **2**, 56.

MCDERMOTT, W. (1958). *Yale J. biol. Med.*, **30**, 257.

MCGOVERN, J. P. (1970). In: 'Penicillin Allergy', 1st ed. pp. 1–196. Thomas, Springfield, Illinois.

MURDOCH, J. McC. (1965). *Practitioner*, **195**, 109.

OLLER, L. Z. (1967). *Brit. J. vener. Dis.*, **43**, 39.

O'NEILL, P. and NICOL, C. S. (1972). *Brit. J. vener. Dis.*, **48**, 460.

OVČINNIKOV, N. M. and DELEKTORSKIJ, V. V. (1971). Quoted Dunlop, E. M. C. (1972). *Brit. med. J.*, ii, 577.

OXELIUS, V., RORSMAN, H. and LAURELL, A. B. (1969). *Brit. J. vener. Dis.*, **45**, 121.

PARK, J. T. (1964). *Postgrad. med. J.*, **40**, Suppl. 11.

PARKER, C.W. (1964). *Postgrad. med. J.*, **30**, Suppl. 141.

PAUTRAT, J. and WILHELM, V. (1966). *Presse méd.*, **74**, 269.

PERDRUP, A. (1964). *Arch. klin. exp. Derm.*, **219**, 160.

PRIETO, J. G. and JIMON, A. (1965). *Proceedings of the 24th General Assembly* and *Technical Meeting*, I.U.V.D.T., Lisbon, p. 289.

QUINN, E. L. (1964). *Postgrad. med. J.*, **40**, 23.

RANGIAH, P. N. (1964). In: *Proceedings of the World Forum on Syphilis and other Treponematoses*, Washington, D.C., U.S. Government Printing Office (Public Health Service Publication No. 997), p. 302.

ROLINSON, G. N. (1964). *Postgrad. med. J.* **40**, Suppl. 20.

ROTHSCHILD, P. D. and DOTY, D. B. (1966). *J. Amer. med. Ass.*, **196**, 372.

SCHROETER, A. L., TURNER, R. H., LUCAS, J. B. and BROWN, W. J. (1971). *J. Amer. med. Ass.*, **218**, 711.

SEFTEL, H. C. (1965). *Med. Proc.*, **11**, 44.

SPARLING, P. F. (1971). *New Engl. J. Med.*, **284**, 642.

STEPPERT, A. (1968). *Wien. med. Wschr.*, **118**, 599.

STEWART, G. T. (1964). *Postgrad. med. J.*, **40**, Suppl. 160.

STEWART, G. T. (1968). *Pediat. Clin. N. Amer.*, **15**, 13.

TIPPER, D. J. and STROMINGER, J. L. (1965). *Proc. nat. Acad. Sci., Wash.*, **54**, 1133.

TIPPER, D. J. and STROMINGER, J. L. (1968). *J. biol. Chem.*, **243**, 3169.

TOWPIK, J. (1970). *Pol. Tyg. lek.*, **25**, 1033.

TURNER, T. B., HARDY, P. H. and NEWMAN, B. (1969). *Brit. J. vener. Dis.*, **45**, 183.

U.S. DEPARTMENT OF HEALTH, EDUCATION AND WELFARE (1965). *V.D. Fact Sheet*, Public Health Service Publication **341**, 22nd rev. Washington, D.C.

U.S. DEPARTMENT OF HEALTH, EDUCATION AND WELFARE (1968). *Syphilis: A Synopsis*, Public Health Service Publication No. 1660. Washington, D.C.

VIEGAS, L. C., LISBOA, M. S. S. and AGUIARIS, S. (1969). *J. med., Porto*, **68**, 349.

VIVAS, SALAS E. (1966). *Arch. Inst. Cardiol. Mex.*, **36**, 316.

WALTER, A. M. and HEILMEYER, L. (1965). 'Antibiotika-Fibel', p. 268. Georg Thieme, Stuttgart.

W.H.O. EXPERT COMMITTEE ON BIOLOGICAL STANDARDISATION (1964). *Wld Hlth techn. rep. Ser.*, **274**, Annex 2.

W.H.O. SCIENTIFIC GROUP, TREPONEMATOSES RESEARCH (1970). *Wld Hlth Org. techn. rep. Ser.*, 455.

WILLCOX, R. R. (1964). *Brit. J. vener. Dis.*, **40**, 90.

WILLCOX, R. R. (1964). 'A Textbook of Venereal Diseases and Treponematoses', 2nd ed. Heinemann Medical Books Ltd., London.

WILNER, E. and BRODY, J. A. (1968). *Lancet*, ii, 1370.

WOODCOCK, K. R. (1971). *Brit. J. vener. Dis.*, **47**, 95.

WODNIANSKY, P., HOLUBAR, K. and PHILIPPU, G. (1969). *Z. Haut-u. Geschl.-Kr.*, **44**, 571.

14 The Chronic Biological False Positive Reaction

R. D. Catterall

Introduction

Some of the most important developments in medicine during the past decade have occurred in immunology and progress has been particularly rapid in the demonstration and characterisation of both antigens and antibodies. This has resulted in a better understanding of those immune reactions, which are harmless to the individual, and of the reactions, which may cause tissue damage and destruction, leading eventually to serious illness. It is now quite clear that both humoral antibodies and cell-mediated immune mechanisms are involved in the pathogenesis of diseases related to immune injury, and, if the immune system is defective, the body mechanisms which prevent immunocytes and antibodies from reacting with normal components of the body may break down, leading to the development of autoimmune disease. The exact aetiology of most immunopathological lesions is still unknown and external or genetically determined responses frequently complicate the situation.

Shortly after the introduction of the Wassermann reaction in 1906 it was suspected that false positive reactions to the test occurred with the sera of some patients. This observation was confirmed during the next 40 years when the principal tests employed in the diagnosis of syphilis and other treponemal diseases were tests measuring reagin and employing lipoidal antigens. False positive results were obtained with both the complement fixation tests and the flocculation tests, but the patients in whom these reactions occurred were not studied because of the lack of a suitable confirmatory test. Physicians were only able to guess, on the basis of the patient's history, the results of physical examination and the pattern of the serological tests, whether a particular patient had a true treponemal reaction or a false positive reaction.

The description of the treponemal immobilisation test (TPI) by Nelson and Mayer in 1949, provided for the first time a reliable method of distinguishing between these two reactions and from that moment onwards patients with biological false positive (BFP) reactions have been investigated and studied in many centres throughout the world. The development of the fluorescent treponemal antibody absorbed test (FTA-ABS) by Hunter et al in 1964 and the more recent *Treponema pallidum* haemagglutination test (TPHA) by workers in Copenhagen and later by Tomizawa and his colleagues in 1969 have made it possible to distinguish between false positive and treponemal reactions with a considerable measure of accuracy.

FALSE POSITIVE REACTIONS

It soon became apparent that a considerable proportion of the population could develop a biological false positive reaction under appropriate circumstances and Moore and Mohr (1952) estimated that 20 per cent of people are potential false positive reactors. The same authors distinguished between acute and chronic BFP reactors and showed that the acute reaction, which usually persists for only a few weeks, and never longer than 6 months, was harmless to the patient and was not associated with the development of subsequent disease. The acute reaction occurs during or shortly after any of a variety of immunological procedures or acute, infectious illnesses. These include recent vaccination against smallpox, inoculation with TAB vaccine, infective hepatitis, infectious mononucleosis, virus pneumonia, chicken-pox, measles, malaria, enterovirus infections and variety of other conditions. It is frequently found in pregnant women but in many cases no cause can be found.

There is general agreement that the acute BFP reaction is without serious significance to the patient and, provided the diagnosis is clearly established, the patient can be safely reassured that the reaction is benign and harmless.

Significance of Chronic BFP reaction

Moore and Mohr (1952) and Moore and Lutz (1955) showed that the chronic BFP reaction was commoner in women than in men and was frequently detected for the first time between the ages of 20 and 35 years. Patients with the chronic reaction had a high incidence of autoimmune disease, especially systemic lupus erythematosus, Sjögren's disease, autoimmune haemolytic anaemia, Hashimoto's thyroiditis, purpura and rheumatoid arthritis. Other less clear-cut connective tissue diseases were found to develop in a proportion of the patients with the chronic reaction. Haserick and Long (1952) showed that the chronic BFP reaction may occur many years before the onset of a collagen disease.

Schulman and Harvey (1964) confirmed these findings and later Harvey and Schulman (1966) produced evidence that a genetic factor may be involved in the development of the chronic reaction, describing 11 patients with one or more close relatives with the BFP reaction. Later Tuffanelli (1968) found a higher incidence of raised serum gamma globulin levels, antinuclear factors and rheumatoid factors in 199 relatives of 103 chronic BFP reactors than in a series of control patients.

In 1972, Catterall described the findings in 130 patients with chronic BFP reactions, who had been kept under observation for a period of from 1 to 12 years. Ten women developed or already had systemic lupus erythematosus, and other connective tissue disorders such as rheumatoid arthritis, rheumatic heart disease, discoid lupus erythematosus, hepatic cirrhosis, haemolytic anaemia, polyarteritis nodosa, Hashimoto's thyroiditis, Sjögren's disease, chronic nephritis and a variety of other conditions were diagnosed. Seventy-four patients could not have an accurate diagnosis made but 14 of them had developed symptoms whilst under observation.

Hypersensitivity to a variety of drugs had occurred in 26 of the patients and a history of sensitivity to penicillin was obtained in 20 patients. Six of these had suffered immediate reactions and 14 delayed reactions. The onset of symptoms of autoimmune disease was related to the administration of penicillin in five patients.

Fulford et al (1972) described six youngish women, who presented with signs and symptoms of a neurological disorder resembling multiple sclerosis associated with laboratory findings suggestive of systemic lupus erythematosus. Five had developed a progressive spastic paraplegia 8 months to 3 years before they were found to have the chronic BFP reaction and other evidence of a connective tissue disease. The cerebrospinal fluid showed a slight excess of protein together with a paretic Lange curve. They all had antinuclear antibodies, mitochondrial antibodies, raised serum IgM levels, thyroid and gastric organ-specific antibodies and, in the majority, LE-cells in the peripheral blood. The authors suggested that these patients represent a distinct variant of systemic lupus erythematosus for which they proposed the name 'lupoid sclerosis', the principal characteristics of which are as follows. The patients are young women, who develop symptoms and signs resembling multiple sclerosis with minimal evidence of involvement of the other systems of the body, associated with the BFP reaction, moderate elevation of the E.S.R., weakly positive tests for antinuclear factor and other autoantibodies, raised serum IgM levels, moderate elevation of C.S.F. protein levels, a paretic Lange curve and, in the majority, LE-cells in the peripheral blood.

Laboratory abnormalities frequently found in the sera of patients with chronic BFP reactions include a raised serum globulin level, anaemia, a raised erythrocyte sedimentation rate (E.S.R.), abnormal liver function tests, abnormal immunoglobulins, antinuclear, rheumatoid and LE-cell factors. Thyroid antibodies are often present in appreciable amounts and Harvey and Schulman (1966) showed that there might be a high level of a circulating anticoagulant in the serum of some patients.

The antibodies are usually IgM in type, but may also be of IgG type or a combination of the two (Tringali et al, 1969; Delhanty and Catterall, 1969). Anticomplementary activity in complement fixation tests occurs in the presence of raised gamma globulins and when the serum contains antigen–antibody complexes such as cryoglobulins and rheumatoid factors (Lassus, 1969).

False positive reactions with lipoidal antigens are usually of low titre, although rarely they may occur at high titre. Tringali et al (1966) found that the titres were abolished with mercaptoethanol, whereas they were not affected in syphilis. Unfortunately, Delhanty and Catterall (1969) found that there were too many exceptions in both groups to make this a reliable diagnostic test.

The antibodies responsible for the BFP reaction cross the placenta into the foetal circulation during pregnancy. There is some evidence that the antibodies detected by complement fixation tests cross the placenta more readily than those responsible for flocculation reactions. These passively transferred antibodies disappear from the infants serum within a few weeks of birth. IgM antibodies are believed not to cross the placental barrier and the presence of IgM anti-treponemal antibody in the serum of an infant is believed to indicate that the infant is responding to an infection. In cases where the diagnosis is in doubt in the mother, the use of the FTA-ABS test, employing a specific anti-IgM conjugate may be helpful, because if this test is positive on the infant's serum, it is reasonable to assume that the infant is infected with syphilis and that the antibody is not due to passive transfer of antibody from the mother (Scotti and Logan, 1968; Alford et al, 1969).

Although little data is available, biological false positive reactions are believed to be uncommon in tests on the cerebrospinal fluid.

Mechanism of chronic BFP reaction

Standard serological tests for syphilis detect antibodies to cardiolipin, which is a complex of diphospholipids found mainly on the mitochondrial inner membrane. It is probable that Wassermann reagins are a type of auto-antibodies produced as a result of the adjuvant effect of treponemes in the body. Auto-antibodies found consistently in patients with primary biliary cirrhosis, which react with a lipoprotein component of the mitochondrial inner membrane, but not with cardiolipin, have been described by Doniach and Walker (1969) and produce 'M' fluorescence with Coon's technique. Recently Doniach et al (1970) and

Catterall (1973) studied 60 patients with chronic BFP reactions and found 'M' fluorescence, similar to that seen in primary bilary cirrhosis in 34 (56 per cent) at titres varying from 1 in 5 to 1 in 50. Of all the 60 patients 58 (96 per cent) had one or more positive tests for auto-antibodies, which were mainly of the IgM class in 10 cases, of both IgM and IgG classes in eight and mainly of the IgG class in three. Non-organ specific complement fixation reactions were obtained with rat kidney homogenates in 27 cases. Antinuclear antibodies were found in 28 patients (46 per cent), 16 of whom had high titres. The antinuclear antibodies were predominately of the IgG class and of the so-called 'homogenous' type, similar to that seen in systemic lupus erythematosus, 'lupoid' hepatitis and other connective tissue disorders. Smooth muscle fluorescence, which is another antibody marker, was present in 16 cases (28 per cent). This antibody is uncommon in patients who do not have liver disease. Rheumatoid antiglobulins and thyroid-specific antibodies had an incidence only slightly above that found in normal controls and organ-specific gastric parietal cell fluorescence was present in only six of the 30 patients tested.

The high incidence of tissue antibodies in the series was thought to be related to the high incidence of systemic disease. The mitochondrial fluorescence was most frequently of low titre and the antibodies were present mostly in the IgM immunoglobulins. Both the cardiolipin antigen and the lipoprotein reactive in 'M' fluorescence are situated on the inner mitochondrial membranes in close proximity to each other. They are uncommon in the normal population and, although their true pathological significance is not understood, they are considered to be useful markers of a special immunological abnormality related to connective tissue disease. The presence of 'M' fluorescence in this series of patients usually indicated the development or actual presence of systemic disease and the authors considered that tests for tissue anti-bodies and 'M' fluorescence may be helpful in detecting those patients likely to develop connective tissue disease and should form part of the follow-up assessment of all patients with the chronic BFP reaction.

Johansson et al (1972) tested 68 patients with chronic BFP reactions for immunoglobulins bound to the dermo-epidermal junction and for serum antinuclear factors. Nine of the patients had definite systemic lupus erythematosus and 11 probably had the disease. Twenty-three patients were found to have skin-bound immunoglobulins and 35 antinuclear factors in the serum. Both of these abnormalities were more common in cases of systemic lupus erythematosus. The immunoglo-bulins found both in the dermo-epidermal junction and in the tests for antinuclear factors were usually of IgM class. Circulating auto-anti-bodies occurred more frequently in patients with bound immuno-globulins than in those without this phenomen. Immunoglobulins bound to the basal membrane area were not found in any of the patients who only showed false positive reactions to complement fixation tests but otherwise had no other abnormality.

Chronic BFP reactions are known to occur among patients with leprosy, particularly those with the lepromatous form of the disease. Scotti et al (1970) reported on the results of testing sera from 206 patients with leprosy. Their results suggested that of the 82 sera which gave positive results with tests for reagin, 16 per cent had treponemal disease while 24 per cent had given BFP reactions with the standard tests.

DISCUSSION

It is important to remember that the commonest cause of positive serological tests for syphilis is still syphilis, although the incidence of BFP reactions is sufficiently high to warrant the careful investigation of all patients with positive serological tests before a diagnosis of latent syphilis is made and anti-syphilitic treatment is given. This is particularly the case if the patient is a youngish woman and the titre of the positive tests is low. No satisfactory studies are available to indicate the true incidence of chronic BFP reactions among the general population.

The chronic BFP reaction should only be diagnosed if the standard serological tests for reagin are positive on repeated testing for more than 1 year, if there is no history of congenital or acquired syphilis or other treponemal disease, if detailed and careful physical examination does not reveal any evidence of treponemal disease, if tests of the cerebrospinal fluid and radiological examination of the heart and aorta are normal and if the specific serological tests, the treponema immobilisation test (TPI) and the absorbed fluorescent treponemal antibody test (FTA-ABS) are negative, preferably on more than one specimen of serum. Preliminary evidence indicates that the *Treponema pallidum* haemagglutination test (TPHA) will also be negative in the majority of cases. Positive findings which will help to confirm the diagnosis will be found in some of the patients. These include a history suggestive of a collagen disease, abnormal physical signs on examination, abnormal haematological and immunological tests, and in those who already have or may develop serious disease, the presence of mitochondrial fluorescence. If these principles are carefully followed in all cases, the margin of error in diagnosis can be reduced to about 5 per cent, especially if the patients are carefully followed up.

It is very difficult to predict the course of the condition in any individual patient after the discovery of the chronic BFP reaction. Harvey and Schulman (1966) and Catterall (1972) have shown that, in addition to the clinical progress of the disease, a consistent sequence of laboratory investigations tend to become abnormal. The chronic BFP reaction usually, but not invariably, appears first and is followed by an increase in the E.S.R. Frequently the situation does not change for months or years, but in some patients a microcytic hypochromic anaemia develops, followed by abnormalities of the plasma proteins, especially of the gamma and to a lesser extent of the beta fractions. In some cases a variety of auto-antibodies and antinuclear factors appear at this stage, but the exact time at which they most frequently develop is not yet known. Later LE-cells may be found. There is still uncertainty as to when mitochondrial antibodies of the IgM class first make their appearance, but their association with systemic disease suggests that tests for their presence may be of value in distinguishing between those who are likely to develop systemic illnesses and connective tissue disorders in the future and those in whom the condition is likely to remain benign and symptomless.

The concept of the chronic biological false positive reaction depends upon the use of screening tests employing lipoidal antigens and measuring syphilitic reagin. With the rapid growth of automated laboratory techniques and the consequent reluctance to carry out manual tests, it is probable that complement fixation tests for syphilis will be employed much less frequently and may eventually disappear altogether. Flocculation tests, which can be satisfactorily automated, will be the only reagin tests used and the other screening tests will probably be one or more of the specific, treponemal tests, such as the FTA-ABS test or the TPHA test. It is important to remember that both these tests can give false positive and false negative reactions (Mackey et al, 1969). Atypical fluorescence of either a homogenous or beaded type may occur when the FTA-ABS is performed on the sera of patients with certain non-treponemal abnormalities (Kraus et al, 1971) and can result in errors of diagnosis. More recently false positive results in the TPHA test have been increasingly observed and it is becoming clear that the TPI test remains the most specific test available although it is insensitive in early syphilis and in some cases of treated and untreated late acquired and congenital syphilis (Förström and Lassus, 1969).

The diagnosis of the chronic BFP reaction depends upon a careful medical history, a detailed physical examination, repeated serological testing, using non-treponemal reagin tests and specific treponemal tests, tests of the cerebrospinal fluid, radiological examination of the heart and aorta and a variety of immunological investigations. In many instances the differential diagnosis from latent treponemal disease may be extremely difficult and prolonged follow-up with repeated examination and testing will be necessary before an accurate diagnosis can be made.

When evidence of systemic disease is present, the question of prophylactic or symptomatic treatment should be considered. In practice effective forms of treatment are restricted to corticosteroids and immunosuppressive drugs. Their use is usually limited because of the chronic and slowly progressive nature of most of the diseases associated with the chronic BFP reaction. With the corticosteroids the risks involved with prolonged treatment may be greater than the advantages to the patient. The side effects of immunosuppressive drugs are such that they are probably indicated in only a few cases with severe and rapidly progressive symptoms.

The chronic BFP reaction is an immunological phenomenon of considerable importance. It presents a unique situation in medicine, in that it is possible to predict years in advance that a number of patients with the reaction will develop serious and sometimes fatal disease in the future. This offers a special opportunity for the study of the presymptomatic stages, evolution and natural history of the autoimmune diseases and the responsibility for developing safe and effective methods of preventive treatment.

REFERENCES

ALFORD, C. A. JR., POLT, S. S., CASSADY, G. E., STRAUMFJORD, J. V. and REMINGTON, J. S. (1969). *New Engl. J. Med.*, **280**, 1086.
CATTERALL, R. D. (1972). *Brit. J. vener. Dis.*, **48**, 1.
CATTERALL, R. D. (1973). *9th Symposium on Advanced Medicine.* Royal College of Physicians, London.
DELHANTY, J. J. and CATTERALL, R. D. (1969). *Lancet*, **2**, 1099.
DONIACH, D. and WALKER, J. G. (1969). *Lancet*, **1**, 813.
DONIACH, D., DELHANTY, J., LINDQUIST, H. J. and CATTERALL, R. D. (1970). *Clin. exp. Immunol.*, **6**, 871.
FÖRSTRÖM, L. and LASSUS, A. (1969). *Acta derm.-venereol., Stockh.*, **49**, 326.
FULFORD, K. W. M., CATTERALL, R. D., DELHANTY, J. J., DONIACH, D. and KREMER, M. (1972). *Brain*, **95**, 373.
HARVEY, A. M. and SCHULMAN, L. E. (1966). *Med. Clin. N. Amer.*, **50**, 1271.
HASERICK, J. R. and LONG, R. (1952). *Ann. intern. Med.*, **37**, 559.
HUNTER, E. F., DEACON, W. E. and MAYER, P. E. (1964). *Publ. Hlth Rep., Wash.*, **69**, 410.
JOHANSSON, E. A., LASSUS, A. and SALO, O. P. (1972). *Acta derm.-venereol., Stockh.*, **52**, 196.
KRAUS, S. J., HASERICK, J. R., LOGAN, L. C. and BULLARD, J. C. (1971). *J. immunol.*, **106**, 1665.
LASSUS, A. (1969). *Int. Arch. Allerg.*, **36**, 515.
MACKEY, D. M., PRICE, E. V., KNOX, J. M. and SCOTTI, A. (1969). *J. Amer. med. Ass.*, **207**, 1683.
MOORE, J. E. and LUTZ, W. B. (1955). *J. chron. Dis.*, **1**, 297.
MOORE, J. E. and MOHR, C. F. (1952). *J. Amer. med. Ass.*, **150**, 467.
NELSON, R. A. JR. and MAYER, M. M. (1949). *J. exp. Med.*, **89**, 369.
SCOTTI, A. T. and LOGAN, L. (1968). *J. Pediat.*, **73**, 242.
SCOTTI, A. T., MACKEY, D. M. and TRAUTMAN, J. R. (1970). *Arch. Derm., Chicago*, **101**, 328.
SCHULMAN, L. E. and HARVEY, A. N. (1964). *Amer. J. Med.*, **36**, 174.
TOMIZAWA, T. S., KASAMATSU, S. and YAMAYA, S. (1969). *Jap. J. Med. Sci. Biol.* **22**, 341.
TRINGALI, G. R., DEL CARPIO, C. and GIMMANCO, N. (1966). *Riv. Ist. sieroter. Ital.*, **41**, 291.
TRINGALI, G. R., JULIAN, A. J. and HALBERT, W. M. (1969). *Brit. J vener. Dis.*, **45**, 202.
TUFFANELLI, D. L. (1968). *Arch. Derm., Chicago*, **98**, 606.
WASSERMANN, A., NEISSER, A. and BRUCK, C. (1906). *Dtsch. med. Waschr.*, **32**, 745.

Part 3
Chancroid, Lymphogranuloma Venereum and Granuloma Inguinale (Donovanosis)

15 Chancroid (Soft Sore)

R. R. Willcox

Introduction

Chancroid is an auto-inoculable sexually transmitted disease characterised by necrotising genital ulceration with inflammatory enlargement and suppuration of the regional lymph nodes.

The infective agent is *Haemophilus ducreyi*, a Gram-negative coccoid bacillary rod with rounded ends and a tendency to group in short chains.

At one time a very prevalent disease with worldwide distribution chancroid remains common in some tropical and sub-tropical countries, *eg* in Vietnam (Kerber et al, 1969) and parts of the Far East, but elsewhere has become or is becoming rare. In the United States (U.S.P.H.S., 1972) in 1971 some 1 507 cases were reported (case rate 0·7 per 100 000), there were 55 cases (50 in males) reported from the clinics of England and Wales, and 93 (83 in males) in France (Martin-Bouyer et al, 1972).

Epidemiological and social aspects

It has been described as 'a disease of the unenlightened and the common poor' (Greenblatt et al, 1953), of the unclean and unwashed. At one time the prostitute was the main source of infection. The disproportionate numbers of reported male and female cases may indicate that the female can remain an infective carrier after the lesions have healed.

Clinical aspects

After an incubation period of 3–7 days a vesico-pustule develops on the genitals which soon breaks down to leave a sharply circumscribed ulcer often surrounded by an erythematous halo. The sores then multiply rapidly by auto-inoculation. Preputial lesions which are common (Willcox, 1951) may present as a rosette and be complicated by phimosis or paraphimosis and rapid destructive ulcerations may occur.

185

Inguinal adenitis is present in approximately one-half of cases (Kerber et al, 1969) the glands rapidly becoming tender and developing into unilocular buboes which, if the condition is untreated, rupture and the ulceration continues in the groin.

Anal (Rivoire, 1971) and extra-genital infections (Greenblatt et al, 1953) are occasionally encountered.

Leading laboratory aspects

Diagnosis is by means of Gram-stained smear of material taken from the lesions, by culture and skin test together with the exclusion of other genital conditions particularly syphilis, granuloma inguinale and herpes genitalis.

Smear diagnosis offers difficulty because of other confusing organisms (Willcox, 1951). According to Borchardt and Hoke (1970) the lesion should be first cleaned with normal saline and the serous exudate from the undermined border of the ulcer collected on sterile cotton-tipped applicator sticks which should be rolled on the slides through 180° in one direction in order to maintain the morphological integrity of the chained organisms.

In culture *H. ducreyi* is a fastidious organism requiring a constituent of blood for growth (Barile et al, 1962; Kerber et al, 1969). A medium using inactivated serum from the patient was successfully used by Borchardt and Hoke (1970).

The skin test, using an intradermal injection of vaccine of Ducrey's bacillus (Dmelcos), and read after 48 hours does not become positive until an average of 12–14 days after the appearance of the lesion and once positive may remain so for life. It is thus of limited value in the individual case but is a very useful guide to the prevalence of the disease on a group basis (Willcox, 1951a). Unfortunately the skin test antigen is no longer commercially available.

Treatment

Treatment (see Rama Ayyangar, 1964; McDaniel, 1964; Willcox, 1963; Boutet and Reboul, 1965) is by means of sulphonamides, tetra-cyclines or streptomycin which contrasts with the white hot cautery, pure bromine or other locally applied caustics of former days (Hammond 1864). Penicillin in high doses has been found to have some effect in the experimental condition (Willcox, 1952) and has been used for the treatment of genital sores in endemic areas of Africa under condition when dark-field tests to exclude syphilis were unavailable.

Streptomycin (1·0 g daily for 5 days) has been shown to be very effective in the Far East (Asin, 1952). Sulphonamides, including long-acting preparations (Narang et al, 1964) and tetracyclines are usually given for 7–14 days. The sulphonamides are preferred as they do not mask undiagnosed syphilis and indeed, in Vietnam, contrary to experience elsewhere, Kerber et al (1969) have recently reported indifferent results with tetracycline.

REFERENCES

ASIN, J. (1952). *Amer. J. Syph.*, **36**, 483–487.
BARILE, M. F., BLUMBERG, J. M., KRAUL, C. W. and YAGUCHI, R. (1962). *Arch. Derm., Chicago*, **86**, 273–281.
BORCHARDT, K. A. and HOKE, A. W. (1970). *Arch. Derm., Chicago.*, **102**, 188–192.
BOUTET, R. and REBOUL, E. (1965). *Bull. Soc. Med. Milit. Franç.*, **59**, 232–234.
GREENBLATT, R. B., POND, E. R., SANDERSON, E. S., TORPIN, R. and DIENST, R. D. (1953). Management of chancroid, granuloma inguinale, lymphogranuloma venereum in general practice. *Pub. Hth Service Publication* No. 255, Washington.
HAMMOND, W. A. (1864). 'Lectures on the Venereal Diseases'. J. G. Lippincott, Philadelphia.
KERBER, R. E., ROWE, C. E. and GILBERT, K. R. (1969). *Arch. Derm., Chicago*, **100**, 604–607.
MCDANIEL, W. E. (1964). *S. Kentucky med. Ass.*, **62**, 281–284.
MARTIN-BOUYER, GAIGNOUS, Y. and VEIGA-PIRES, H. (1972). *La Prophyl. Sanit. Morale*, **44**, 136–146.
NARANG, S. S., BHARGUA, N. C. and SESHAGIRI, M. (1964). *Indian J. Derm.*, **30** 246–250.
RAMA AYYANGAR, M. C. (1964). *Med. Digest, Bombay*, **32**, 61–66.
RIVOIRE, M. J. (1971). *Bull. Soc. Franc. Derm. Syph.*, **78**, 203.
UNITED STATES PUBLIC HEALTH SERVICE (1972). VD Fact Sheet, 1971. Atlanta.
WILLCOX, R. R. (1951). *East Afr. med. J.*, **28**, 483–491.
WILLCOX, R. R. (1951a). *Bull. Wld Hlth Org.*, **4**, 283–290.
WILLCOX, R. R. (1952). *Postgrad. med. J.*, **28**, 107–116.
WILLCOX, R. R. (1963). *Brit. J. clin. Pract.*, **17**, 455–460.

16   Lymphogranuloma Venereum

R. R. Willcox

Introduction

Lymphogranuloma venereum is a venereal disease of the lymph channels characterised by a small fleeting primary lesion followed by the development of a usually suppurative regional adenitis in the male and distressing late complications in the female. Monographs on the subject include those of Stannus (1933), Greenblatt and colleagues (1953), Favre and Hellerstrom (1954) and Sigel (1962).

The causative agent belongs to the genus Chlamydia, members of which are responsible for a wide range of infections in the animal kingdom. In man these include lymphogranuloma venereum, psittacosis and trachoma while one member (TRIC agent) is found in cases of inclusion conjunctivitis, cervicitis and proctitis and a substantial proportion of cases of non-gonococcal urethritis (*qv*).

The condition has worldwide distribution, being endemic in the South American ports, the West Indies, the West African coast and Madagascar, but generally it seems to be a dying disease (Duhamel and Cohen, 1970).

In the U.S.A. in 1971 there were 615 reported cases (0·3 per 100 000) compared with 2 858 in 1944 (U.S.P.H.S., 1972) while in the clinics of England and Wales in 1971 there were only 47 cases seen, all but two being in males.

Epidemiological and social aspects

Clinical cases are encountered more often in males than in females. There is an association with other venereal disorders and a high proportion of female prostitutes have been shown to have antibodies to the disease (Placido de Sousa and Norton Brandâo, 1961; Saad et al, 1962).

Rectal involvement, usually found in the female, is insidious in onset, infectious and may progress towards severe disability thereby representing both a social and public health problem (Miller, 1965). Sodomy has been suspected as being important in the aetiology of this complication (Duhamel and Cohen, 1970) but others (*eg* Annamunthodo, 1962) have considered otherwise.

Clinical aspects

After an incubation period of usually 2–5 days, although longer intervals up to 5 weeks have been described, the primary lesion, a small evanescent vesicle sore, is observed in about one-quarter of males (Willcox, 1952; Alergant, 1957) but is less frequently encountered in females.

In the male, following a further interval of from 4 days to 4 months, the inguinal glands enlarge, become matted together and tender forming a multilocular bubo characteristically grooved by the inguinal ligament.

The inflammation may regress and on occasion flare again after even a lapse of years (Oller, 1968) but commonly individual glands burst to discharge a purulent thin milky fluid through a number of sinuses in one or both groins. Damage to the lymphatics may later result in lymphatic obstruction and oedema of the penis. Distortion of the penis ('Saxophone penis') and scrotum may ensue.

Urethral infections may occur (Riggs and Sanford, 1962) resembling non-gonococcal urethritis (Harkness, 1950) and urethral stricture and fistula may follow. The course of stricture resembles that of post-gonorrhoeal stricture (Pierre-Louis, 1960).

Proctitis with peri-rectal abscess or fistula-in-ano may be encountered in the male homosexual and lymphogranuloma venereum should be considered in homosexuals with these conditions (Greaves, 1963). Rectal strictures are rare in the male.

In women, in whom the lymphatics involved differ from those of the male, inguinal buboes are less commonly seen and the disease is usually manifest at a later stage by ulceration and tissue destruction, polypoid growths or by elephantiasis (esthiomène) of the vulvar tissues. Following involvement of the ano-rectal glands, proctitis and perio-proctitis occur which lead to rectal stricture, abscesses and perineal and recto-vaginal fistulae. Extensive damage and tissue loss of the urethal and rectal areas with incontinence may ensue if the disease is not adequately controlled (Lawson, 1963; Weinstein et al, 1966).

The lowest point of the rectal stricture, which is usually tubular, is 3–5 cm from the anal verge (Miles, 1959; Annamunthodo, 1962). There is controversy as to whether this condition predisposes to malignancy (Stewart, 1959) although cases of malignancy superimposed on chronic stricture have been reported (Morson, 1964).

In both sexes constitutional symptoms (including fever, rigors, anorexia, nausea, loss of weight, backache, joint pains, lassitude, epistaxis, erythema nodosum) may be noted or may be absent. A raised erythrocyte sedimentation rate is common being very high in late cases.

Laboratory aspects

A definitive diagnosis is by culture of the infective agent from bubo fluid or other material, by skin and serological tests and by histology. In routine practice in most clinics the diagnosis usually rests on skin and serological tests confirming the clinical findings.

The *Chlamydia* of lymphogranuloma venereum can be cultured in the yolk sacs of embryonated chicks (Philip et al, 1971) but more satisfactorily in tissue culture using irradiated McCoy cells (Gordon et al, 1969). The cultures are examined under the low-power microscope for glycogen-containing inclusions (by periodic acid–Schiff (PAS) stains).

Inclusions of sub-group A Chlamydia (including strains of lymphogranuloma venereum, trachoma and TRIC agents) contain glycogen while those of sub-group B which includes the agent of psittacosis do not (Gordon and Quan, 1965). The two sub-groups have also been shown to have differences in ribonucleic acid homogenicity (Kingsbury and Weiss, 1968) and in drug sensitivity (Lin Hsiu-San and Moulder, 1966). Lymphogranuloma venereum strains have been shown capable of differentiation from those obtained from cases of non-gonococcal urethritis by their greater pathogenicity for chick embryos and mice (Philip et al, 1971). However strains have been isolated from patients with lymphogranuloma venereum which show atypical properties (Schachter, 1967).

In the Frei skin test, 0·1 ml of antigen ('Lygranum') containing killed 'virus' is injected intradermally into one forearm with a like amount of control without 'virus' into the other. A papule 0·5 cm or greater at 48–72 hours resulting from the test material only indicates a positive result.

The reaction usually takes 1 week to 6 months to become positive after which it may remain so for life. There may be no correlation with clinical severity (Abrams, 1968) and positivity may be abolished during a course of corticosteroids (Grace et al, 1952). A negative result does not necessarily exclude the disease (Willcox, 1952; Schachter et al, 1969) and neither does the result of the skin test always agree with that of the complement-fixation test (King et al, 1956; Placido de Sousa and Norton Brandào, 1961; Hill, 1965; Abrams, 1968).

The skin test may show cross-reactions in infections with other members of the genus *Chlamydia* and positivity rates of 17–26 per cent have been reported in patients with present or past non-gonococcal urethritis (Willcox, 1954; King et al, 1956).

Antigens for the complement-fixation test are group-specific. An antigen obtained from the agent of enzootic abortion in ewes (EAE) gives a similar pattern (Willcox and Stamp, 1954) and has been found to be more sensitive (Grist and McLean, 1964; Philip et al, 1971). Titres of 1 : 16 or more are now regarded as positive.

The complement-fixation test is considered more sensitive than the skin test in active cases. In the acute form of the disease the titres can be expected to be high but unlike the skin test, positivity falls off rapidly with effective treatment or more slowly with time lapse (Sigel, 1962). Titres remain high in chronic cases.

As with complement-fixation tests for syphilis, false positive reactions are encountered and low titre positivity has been reported in narcotic addicts (Cherubin and Millian, 1968).

Cross-reactions may occur in chlamydial infections of the ornithosis group (Eddie et al, 1966) although these may occur at low titre (Stallman and Dwyer, 1963): indeed the ornithosis antibodies may be present in the guinea-pig complement (Terzin, 1964). Low titre (up to 1 : 8) sub-positivity and sometimes higher titres have been reported from venereal disease patients (King et al, 1956) especially those with non-gonococcal urethris (Macrae and Willcox, 1953; Stallman and Dwyer, 1963; Philip et al, 1971).

Newer serological tests include the radioisotope precipitation test (Gerloff and Watson, 1967) which evokes very high titres (up to 1 : 1 024 or above) in sera from patients with lymphogranuloma venereum (Philip et al, 1971) but this test also only detects group and not specific antibody.

More recently the micro-immunofluorescence typing test (Wang and Grayston, 1970) which also gives high titres, has shown promise and three sub-types of lymphogranuloma agent and at least six of TRIC agent have been described (Dwyer et al, 1972) although some overlap was still noted.

Histopathological studies may be useful in doubtful cases (Greenblatt et al, 1953) but the findings are not specific and 'positive' reports may be obtained in other diseases.

Treatment

The most widely used drugs are the sulphonamides and the tetracyclines. Although the sulphonamides have the advantage that they will not mask co-existing syphilis the tetracyclines are often preferred as they can be given for longer periods with the minimum of side effects.

Sulphonamides over periods of 5–10 days have proved effective in the early stages with bubo (Willcox, 1952; Greenblatt et al, 1953; Krishnamurthi et al, 1959) although repeated courses may be required (Erskine, 1958). The conventional tetracyclines in a dosage of 500 mg orally four times a day for 10–14 days also give good results (Greenblatt et al 1953; McDaniel, 1964).

Longer treatments are required for 30 days or more in chronic cases (Greenblatt et al 1953; Boutet and Reboul, 1965; Pierre-Louis, 1960).

Chloramphenicol (Miles, 1956)—which is seldom used because of side effects—erythromycin (Alexander and Schoch, 1954) and triacetylo-leandomycin (Fluker, 1963) are also active. Penicillin has some but only slight action (Willcox, 1946; Oller, 1968; Matsumoto and Manire, 1970) while streptomycin is generally considered to be ineffective (King, 1964).

Buboes should be aspirated before they burst. Surgical removal or vulvectomy may be required for polypoid growths and vulvar ele-phantiasis but is frequently unsuccessful in the chronic disabling lesions in the female on account of fibrosis and impaired blood supply.

The options for the treatment of rectal stricture, as indicated by Annamunthodo (1962), are periodic dilatation, colostomy and various forms of excision, including abdomino-perineal but preserving the sphincter where possible.

Colostomy is required for intestinal obstruction (Miles, 1957) and prior to attempted repair of recto-vaginal fistula. Abdomino-perineal resection is indicated should malignancy supervene but for the detection of early cancer proctosigmoidoscopy with biopsy and X-ray examination are necessary (Levin and colleagues, 1964).

REFERENCES

ABRAMS, A. J. (1968). *J. Amer. med. Ass.*, **205**, 199–202.
ALERGANT, C. D. (1957). *Brit. J. vener. Dis.*, **33**, 47.
ALEXANDER, L. J. and SCHOCH, A. G. (1954). *Amer. J. Syph.*, **38**, 107.
ANNAMUNTHODO, H. (1962). *West Indian med. J.*, **11**, 73–85.
BOUTET, B. and REBOUL, E. (1965). *Bull. Soc. Med. Mil. Franç.*, **59**, 232–234.
CHERUBIN, C. E. and MILLIAN, S. J. (1968). *Ann. intern. Med., Philadelphia*, **69**, 739–742.
DUHAMEL, J. and COHEN, M. (1970). *Arch. Franç. Mal. Appar. Dig., Paris*, **59**, Suppl. 7–8, 55.
DWYER, R. ST. C., TREHARNE, J. D., JONES, B. R. and HERRING, J. (1972). *Brit. J. vener. Dis.*, **48**, 452–459.
EDDIE, B., SLADEN, W. J. L., SLADEN, B. K. and MEYER, K. F. (1966). *Amer. J., Epid.*, 405–410.
ERSKINE, D. (1958). *Brit. J. vener. Dis.*, **34**, 163.
FAVRE, M. and HELLERSTROM, S. (1954). The epidemiology, aetilogy and prophylaxis of lymphogranuloma inguinale. *Acta derm.-venereol., Stockh.*, **34**, Suppl. 30.
FLUKER, J. L. (1963). *Brit. J. vener. Dis.*, **39**, 24–27.
GERLOFF, R. K. and WATSON, R. V. (1967). *Amer. J. Ophthal.*, **63**, 1492.
GORDON, F. B. and QUAN, A. L. (1965). *J. Infect. Dis.*, **115**, 186–196.
GORDON, F. B., HARPER, I. A., QUAN, A. L., TREHARNE, J. D., DWYER, R. ST. C. and GARLAND, J. A. (1969). *J. infect. Dis.*, **120**, 451.
GRACE, A. W., FRANK, L. and WYSE, R. J. (1952). *Arch. Derm. Syph., Chicago*, **65**, 248.
GREAVES, A. B. (1963). *Bull Wld Hlth Org.*, **29**, 797–801.
GREENBLATT, R. B., PUND, E. R., SANDERSON, E. S, TORPIN, R. and DIENST, R. B. (1953). Management of chancroid, granuloma inguinale, lymphogranuloma

venereum. U.S. Depth Hlth Education Welfare, *Public Health Service Publication*, 255, Washington.
GRIST, N. R. and McLEAN, C. (1964). *Brit. med. J.*, 4 July, 21–5.
HARKNESS, A. H. (1950). 'Non-Gonococcal Urethritis'. E. & S. Livingstone, Edinburgh.
HILL, D. (1965). *Nurs. Times, London*, **61**, 1000–1003.
KING, A. J. (1964). In: 'Recent Advances in Venereology, pp. 304–333. Churchill, London.
KING, A. J., BARWELL, C. F. and CATTERALL, R. D. (1956). *Brit. J. vener. Dis.*, **32**, 209–216.
KINGSBURY, D. Y. and WEISS, E. (1968). *J. Bact.*, **96**, 1421–1423.
KRISHNAMURTHI, M. V., SOBHANADRI, C. and SOWMINI, C. N. (1959). *J. Indian med. Ass.*, **22**, 402.
LAWSON, J. B. (1963). *West African med. J.*, **3**, 89–98.
LEVIN, I., ROMANO, S., STEINBERG, M. and WELSH, R. A. (1964). *Dis. Colon Rect.*, 7, 129.
LIN HSIU-SAN and MOULDER, J. W. (1966). *J. Infect. Dis.*, **116**, 372–376.
MACRAE, A. D. and WILLCOX, R. R. (1953). *Brit. J. vener. Dis.*, **29**, 231–235.
McDANIEL, W. E. (1964). *J. Kentucky med. Ass., Louisville*, **62**, 281–283.
MATSUMOTO, A. and MANIRE, G. P. (1970). *J. Bact.*, **101**, 278–285.
MILES, R. P. M. (1956). *West Indian med. J.*, **5**, 183.
MILES, R. P. M. (1957). *Brit. J. Surg.*, **45**, 180.
MILES, R. P. M. (1959). *Postgrad. med. J.*, **35**, 92.
MILLER, H. (1965). *Amer. J. Proct., N.Y.*, **16**, 291–296.
MORSON, B. C. (1964). *Proc. roy. Soc. Med., London*, **57**, 179–180.
OLLER, L. Z. (1968). *Brit. J. vener. Dis.*, **44**, 154–156.
PHILIP, R. N., HILL, D. A., GREAVES, A. B., GORDON, F. B., QUAN, A. L., GERLOFF, R. K. and THOMAS, L. A. (1971). *Brit. J. vener. Dis.*, **47**, 114–121.
PIERRE-LOUIS, C. (1960). *Rev. Confed. Med. Panamer., Havana*, **7**, 196–197.
PLACIDO DE SOUSA, C. and NORTON BRANDÃO, F. (1961). *Brit. J. vener. Dis.*, **37**, 179–182.
RIGGS, S. and SANFORD, J. P. (1962). *New Engl. J. Med.*, 10 May, 992.
SAAD, E. A., DE GOUVEIA, O. F., FILHO, P. D., TEIXEIRA, D. and ERTHAL, A. (1962). *Gastro-enterologica, Basel*, **97**, 89–102.
SCHACHTER, J. (1967). *Amer. J. Ophthal., Chicago*, **63**, 1049–1053.
SCHACHTER, J., SMITH, D. E., DAWSON, C. R., ANDERSON, W. R., DELLER, J. J., HOKE, A. W., SMARTT, W. H. and MEYER, K. F. (1969). *J. Infect. Dis., Chicago*, **120**, 372–375.
SIGEL, M. M. (1962). 'Lymphogranuloma Venereum. Epidemiological, Clinical, Surgical and Therapeutic Aspects Based on a Study in the Caribbean'. University of Miami Press, Florida, U.S.A., 197 pp.
STALLMAN, N. D. and DWYER, R. St. C. (1963). *Med. J. Aust.* **2**, 1043–1046.
STANNUS, H. S. (1933). 'A Sixth Venereal Disease'. Ballière Tindall and Cox, London, 270 pp.
STEWART, D. B. (1959). *West Indian med. J., Jamaica*, **8**, 55–62.
TERZIN, A. L. (1964). *J. Hygiene*, **62**, 179–184.
UNITED STATES PUBLIC HEALTH SERVICE (1972). V.D. Fact Sheet, 1971, U.S. Dept of Health, Education and Welfare, Public Health Service, Center for V.D. Control, Atlanta, Georgia.
WANG, S. P. and GRAYSTON, J. T. (1970). *Amer. J. Ophthal.*, **70**, 367.
WEINSTEIN, E. L., NAYASHIDA, T. and LeMON CLARK, P. (1966). *J. Amer. Geront. Soc., Baltimore*, **14**, 80–84.
WILLCOX, R. R. (1946). *Postgrad. med. J.*, **22**, 96–98.
WILLCOX, R. R. (1952). *Trans. roy. Soc. Trop. Med. Hyg.*, **46**, 658–651.
WILLCOX, R. R. (1954). *Acta derm. venereol., Stockh.*, **34**, 430–438.
WILLCOX, R. R. and STAMP, J. T. (1954). *Amer. J. Syph.*, **38**, 459–468.

17 Granuloma Inguinale (Donovanosis)

R. R. Willcox

Introduction

A chronic slowly progressive, auto-inoculable, mildly contagious disease characterised by velvety, beefy granulations affecting the genitalia and surrounding skin, occasionally elsewhere.

The causative agent is *Donovania granulomatis* a non-spore forming ovoid encapsulated body 1–1·5 μ long and 0·5–0·7 μ wide, which has a number of properties, including ultrastructure, of Gram-negative bacteria (Davis and Collins, 1969).

The disease is endemic in Southern India particularly along the eastern seaboard (Rajam and Rangiah, 1954; Serma, 1957; Rama Ayyangar, 1961; Rangiah, 1962; Lal and Nicholas, 1970) and in New Guinea (Maddocks, 1967) where epidemics have been earlier described (Vogel, 1965). Elsewhere it is widespread but relatively few cases are reported. For example, Willcox (1950, 1951) found 17 cases during a 6-month survey involving the examination of some 1 500 venereal disease patients in Rhodesia.

In the U.S.A. 103 cases were reported in 1971 giving an incidence of 0·1 per 100 000 compared with 2 403 cases in 1947 (U.S.P.H.S., 1972) but in Europe it is rare, only five (all male) cases being encountered in the clinics of England and Wales in 1971.

Epidemiological and social aspects

There is a marked sex bias, approximately two-thirds of cases being found in males (Rajam and Rangiah, 1954; Lal and Nicholas, 1970). There are no limitations as to race but whether there is a racial susceptibility, as might be inferred from its markedly higher incidence in certain world areas, is unclear. The disease is usually one of unhygienic promiscuous persons of low socio-economic status and behavioural factors (*eg* pederasty) are likely to be more important.

As was pointed out by Stewart (1964) Koch's postulates have not been completely met as it has not so far been found possible to produce the clinical disease by means of the cultured organism either in experimental animals or in human volunteers in spite of many attempts (Greenblatt et al, 1953) although the disease has been produced in humans by the transfer of aspirated pus from pseudobuboes (Dienst et al, 1950).

There is controversy as to how the disease is spread although the conflicting theories both involve the sexual act. In many series there is an apparent rarity of its direct transmission between established sexual partners (Rajam and Rangiah 1952; Goldberg, 1964) but this finding was not supported by Lal and Nicholas (1970) who found co-existing conjugal disease in more than half of their cases.

Goldberg (1964) believed that *D. granulomatis* is an intestinal inhabitant causing no local lesions but by auto-inoculation of faecal material will establish itself on skin injured by trauma or bacterial inflammation. Certainly a high proportion of reported cases are in male pederasts (Marmell, 1958; Goldberg and Bernstein, 1964; Peck, 1968; Davis, 1970). Moreover Goldberg (1964) showed that a quarter to one-third of female patients attending venereal disease clinics had had heterosexual anal coitus at least once and approximately one-half of those investigated carried faecal organisms in the vaginal tract.

Clinical aspects

The incubation period has been reported to vary from a few days to several months. The lesion commences in the genitalia as a vesicle or papule, the surface of which becomes eroded to form a sharply defined ulcer which fills with beefy, smooth, red granulation tissue, later becoming raised with rolled edges. Subsequent spread occurs by extension along the skin, by autoinoculation of opposing surfaces or by mediate transmission through infected clothes or finger nails. It sometimes commences as a subcutaneous nodule which slowly becomes an abscess ('pseudobubo') which bursts to form an ulcer.

In the female the lesion may occur internally on the cervix or in the vagina (Stewart, 1964) or in either sex the mouth may be involved (Lal and Nicholas, 1970).

The absence of lymph gland enlargement has been regarded as 'one of the diagnostic hallmarks of the disease' (Rajam and Rangiah, 1954) although that such may be produced by secondary infection was noted by Maddocks (1967). Secondary infection with fuso-spirochaetal organisms can result in much tissue destruction, even including loss of the phallus (Serma, 1962).

The ulcerative process normally extends slowly, with exacerbations, or it may remain stationary for many years. Scars may form, pseudo-elephantoid enlargement of penis and scrotum may occur (which may be falsely attributed to esthiomène of lymphogranuloma venereum—

Stewart, 1964) and carcinomatous change may supervene. Ultimately the general health may be impaired with anorexia and anaemia and even death can result (see Moore et al, 1963; Brauer et al, 1966).

The development of malignancy is not uncommon (Stewart, 1964; Rangiah et al, 1966; Davis, 1970). Goldberg and Annamuthodo (1966) found antibodies to *D. granulomatis* in nine of 62 cases of cancer of the penis but in none of controls.

Metastatic haematogenous spread to the bones has been reported in about 6 per cent of cases (Sieber, 1965). Such a diagnosis should be considered in any female patient presenting with genital lesions and radiographic bone defects otherwise the genital lesions might be mistaken for carcinoma with unhappy consequences (Kirkpatrick, 1970).

Laboratory aspects

A definitive diagnosis is best made by finding Donovan bodies of tissue spreads made from small pieces of granulation tissue obtained by biopsy punch from deep in the ulcer, stained by Leishman, Giemsa or Wright's stain. Typically they have intense polar staining and resemble closed safety pins.

The organism is difficult to culture and will not grow on a solid medium. Following the achievement of growth in the yolk sac of the developing chick embryo (Anderson, 1943) its dependence in egg-yolk material was appreciated and it subsequently has been cultured in liquid media. The growth factor in egg yolk can be replaced by lactalbumen hydrolysate or an enzymatic digest of soya meal suggesting it is a peptide (Goldberg, 1962).

Skin tests have been used although a significant number of false positive reactions are encountered (Greenblatt et al, 1953) as have complement-fixation serological tests (Greenblatt et al, 1953; Goldberg and Annamunthodo, 1966). A practical difficulty for both procedures is the non-availability of antigen except in the few centres where the disease is being studied.

Biopsy may be helpful, particularly in distinguishing from lymphogranuloma venereum (Serma, 1962; Stewart, 1964).

Treatment

Streptomycin or the tetracyclines are the drugs of choice.

Streptomycin in doses of 1·0 g is usually given daily for 20 days or twice daily for 10 days (Serma, 1962) and although some resistance may be expected in 9–17 per cent of cases (Lal et al, 1967; Rama-Rao and Patnaik, 1966) it has been considered that in India this problem has not worsened through the years (Lal, 1971).

The conventional tetracyclines have usually been given in a dose of

2 g daily for 12–21 days (McDaniel, 1964; Davis, 1970). The newer tetracyclines have also been successful in small numbers of cases, *eg* methacycline (Marmell and Prigot, 1964), as have chloramphenicol, erythromycin, carbomycin, gentamicin and also ampicillin (Thew et al, 1969).

REFERENCES

ANDERSON, K. (1943). *Science*, **97**, 500.

BRAUER, U., KLEINE-NATROP, E. and RODER, H. (1966). *Derm. Wschr., Leipzig*, **152**, 780–784.

DAVIS, C. M. (1970). *J. Amer. med. Ass.*, v. **211**, 632–636.

DAVIS, C. M. and COLLINS, C. (1969). *J. Invest. Derm., Baltimore*, **53**, 315–321.

DIENST, R. B., GREENBLATT, R. B. and CHEN, C. H. (1950). *Amer. J. Syph*, **34**, 189.

GOLDBERG, J. (1962). *Brit. J. vener. Dis.*, **38**, 99–102.

GOLDBERG, J. (1964). *Brit. J. vener. Dis.*, **40**, 140–146.

GOLDBERG, J. and ANNAMUNTHODO, H. (1966). *Brit. J. vener. Dis.*, **42**, 205–209.

GOLDBERG, J. and BERNSTEIN, R. (1964). *Brit. J. vener. Dis.*, **40**, 137–139.

GREENBLATT, R. B., PUND, E. R., SANDERSON, E. S., TORBIN, R. and DIENST, R. B. (1953). Management of chancroid, granuloma inguinale, lymphogranuloma venereum in general practice. *U.S. Public Health Service Publication*, No. 255, Washington, D.C.

KIRKPATRICK, D. J. (1970). *Clin. Radiol., London*, **21**, 101–105.

LAL, S. (1971). *Brit. J. vener. Dis.*, **47**, 454–455.

LAL, S. and NICHOLAS, C. 1970). *Brit. J. vener. Dis.*, **46**, 461–463.

LAL, S., PADMA, N. S. and VELOV, A. (1967). *Indian J. Derm. Vener.*, **33**, 65.

MCDANIEL, W. E. (1964). *J. Kentucky Med. Ass., Louisville*, **62**, 281–283.

MADDOCKS, I. (1967). *Papua New Guinea med. J.*, **10**, 49–54.

MARMELL, M. (1958). *Brit. J. vener. Dis.*, **34**, 213.

MARMELL, M. and PRIGOT, A. (1964). *N.Y. J. Med., N.Y.*, **64**, 304–305.

MOORE, M. B., FERGUSON, J. P., FREEMAN, R. G. and KNOX, J. M. (1963). *Sth. med. J., Birmingham, Alabama*, **56**, 860–863.

PECK, S. (1968). *Arch. Derm., Chicago*, **98**, 555–557.

RAJAM, R. V. and RANGIAH, P. N. (1952). *Indian J. vener. Dis.*, **18**, 14.

RAJAM, R. V. and RANGIAH, P. N. (1954). Donovanosis, granuloma inguinale, granuloma venereum. *World Health Organisation Monograph*, Series No. 24, Geneva.

RAMA AYYANGAR, M. C. (1961). *J. Indian med. Ass., Calcutta*, **37**, 70–74.

RAMA RAO, N. V. S. and PATNAIK, R. (1966). *Indian J. Derm. Vener.*, **32**, 100.

RANGIAH, P. N. (1962). *Indian J. Derm., Bombay*, **28**, 172–179.

RANGIAH, P. N., SOWMINI, C. N. and VIJAYALAKSHMI, K. V. (1966). *Mediscope, Madras*, **8**, 658–662.

SERMA, J. S. (1957). *Indian J. Derm. venereol.*, **23**, 9.

SERMA, J. S. (1962). *Indian Practit., Bombay*, **15**, 525–532.

SIEBER, P. E. (1965). *Amer. J. Roentgen., Springfield, Ill.*, **95**, 515–516.

STEWART, D. B. (1964). *Med. Clln. N. Amer., Philadelphia*, **48**, 773–786.

THEW, M. A., SWIFT, J. T. and HEATON, C. L. (1969). *J. Amer. med. Ass.*, **210**, 866.

UNITED STATES PUBLIC HEALTH SERVICE (1972). V.D. Fact Sheet, 1971. U.S. Dept. Hlth Education and Welfare, Atlanta, Ga.

VOGEL, L. C. (1965). *Nederl. T. Geneesk.*, **109**, 2425–2426.

WILLCOX, R. R. (1950). *J. roy. Army med. Corps.*, **94**, 167–172.

WILLCOX, R. R. (1951). *Med. Illustr.*, **5**, 67–70.

Part 4
Trichomoniasis

Preamble

The concept of trichomoniasis as the commonest of all sexually transmitted diseases has received growing acceptance over the last 20 years.
Two major conferences, one in Rheims in 1957 and the other in Montreal
in 1959, did much to accelerate agreement that all infested men acquire
the parasite sexually and that a similar mode of transmission applies to
the great majority of affected women. With the exception of possible
neo-natal infection nothing approaching solid evidence of any other
means of transmission has been forthcoming.

The incubation period of trichomoniasis is generally accepted as 4
days to 4 weeks.

Disparity of infestation rates in females and males is partly accounted
for by the natural history of the disease in men. Urination apparently
makes it a short-lived affection in many. There is also the problem of
diagnosis in men, who generally have few parasites. Microscopic
methods are time-consuming and call for great patience. Culture
methods have generally proved to have their limitations too.

One of the few countries to publish any available figures is the U.K.
The figures published annually by the Chief Medical Officer cover only
England nowadays and only those cases attending the 200 special
clinics for the care of the sexually infected. The available figures are as
follows:

	Females	Males	Ratio F : M
1969	12 595	1 001	12·5 : 1
1970	14 491	1 290	12·5 : 1
1971	17 407	1 300	12·9 : 1
1972*	17 356	1 535	11·1 : 1

* Provisional only.

201

In the field of treatment, metronidazole has proved more than a match for all alternatives. Recently it has consolidated its position as the drug of first choice. Husbands or regular consorts of infested women are by no means always or even regularly investigated. Many, however, are treated on the strength of epidemiological evidence. Questionable, on ethical grounds, is the practice of ordering treatment for the husband or consort without seeing him.

18 Epidemiological and Social Aspects

R. S. Morton

It is widely accepted that somewhere approaching one woman in every five is infested at some time during her sexually active years. Some women appear to be more at risk than others, *eg* those in the lower socio-economic strata, the delinquent, the pregnant, the coloured and those with other sexually transmissible disease. The percentage of husbands or regular consorts found infested varies between 13 and 60 per cent and depends largely on the enthusiasm of laboratory workers, the number of sites and methods used and, not least, how often the patient is examined. The great majority of men with trichomoniasis are asymptomatic carriers.

Increasing attention has been paid to detection of the parasite in men. Nhochini (1964) studied 100 men with so-called non-specific urethritis who had consistently failed to respond to treatment. He found eight to be harbouring *T. vaginalis*. Dao (1964) found 24 of 85 husbands of infested women to be similarly affected. He emphasised the need for investigation of the male. This has been a recurring theme in recent years.

The development of the problem of trichomoniasis in France was described by Chappal and Bertrand (1965) and Noreel and Rousseau (1965). Ivankov et al (1966) did the same on behalf of Bulgaria and Okawa et al (1967) for Japan. From South Korea, Kim (1969) reported 19·1 per cent of 298 randomly selected women to have trichomoniasis. In India, Nagesha et al (1970) found the incidence of the infestation to be 14·6 per cent of 2 000 gynaecological patients. It is clear from these and similar papers that there is all over the world a growing awareness of trichomoniasis as an epidemiological problem.

In an invited article Dunlop and Wisdom (1965) reviewed the situation in the U.K. and emphasised the need, not only for investigation of the male, but for his concurrent treatment as a means of preventing reinfection. In a further study Wisdom and Dunlop (1965) found 92 (5·6 per cent) of men with trichomoniasis in a series of 1 645 presenting with non-gonococcal urethritis.

Naguib et al (1966) besides discussing their methods of diagnosis and the need for repetition of tests discuss their patients in a wide variety of social terms, *eg* educational status, marital status, religion, husband's occupation category, etc. The prevalence rate of trichomoniasis in 4 290 women aged 30–45 years was 14·5 per cent. The authors claim that their patients represent a fair sampling of the general population which they serve.

The seasonality of trichomoniasis was studied by Gauderoy and Liefooghe (1966). Their material consisted of 3 504 patients found during 17 238 examinations of smears for cervical cancer. Maximum incidence was in the autumn during each of the 7 years studied. The authors noted a falling incidence from 27·4 per cent of cases in 1960 to 18·6 per cent in 1964 and they attribute this to the more widespread use of metronidazole and other trichomonacides. The association of peak incidence with peak holiday times may have prompted a report by Čatár et al (1966). Writing from the Department of Parasitology in the University of Bratislava they report the survival of *T. vaginalis* in thermal spa water after 72 hours. Although they were unable to find samples in used spa water they call for preventive measures to protect users.

Some idea of the seasonal incidence in England may be gained from recent copies of the quarterly returns made by the Chief Medical Officer.

	1970	1971	1972
1st quarter	3 201	4 114	4 680
2nd quarter	3 773	4 392	4 608
3rd quarter	4 572	5 324	5 075
4th quarter	4 124	4 877	4 628

Thoughts of a means of transmission other than sexual are sometimes prompted by the experience of clinicians with individual patients. Littlewood and Kahler (1966) report the case of a 19 day old female infant with abdominal distension, palpable kidneys and pyuria. *T. vaginalis* was found in both child and mother. Harper (1967) reports the case of a 10 day old boy with a 2-day history of fever, rigors and vomiting in whom the urine revealed trichomonads in large numbers. Like the 19 day old girl, recovery followed the exhibition of metronidazole but the source of the infestation in this latter case was far from clear.

Lang (1967) points out the distress caused to adolescents by vaginal discharge. Trichomoniasis he cites as the commonest cause. O'Sullivan (1967) makes a similar observation and underlines the part played by coitus. Purola et al (1967) writing from Helsinki about 1 335 pregnant women were struck by the high infestation rate in unmarried gravidae. He found associated vaginal thrush in nearly 10 per cent.

Ipsen and Feigl (1970) in the U.S.A. calculated from a basis of 38 000 women in a cancer survey that the risk of infestation among Negroes was three times that among those of Caucasian origin. The authors used a bio-mathematical model. Using old-fashioned counting methods Nicol (1958) in the U.K. calculated ethnic differences as coloured : white — 5 : 1.

Kostein (1964) from Paris found 43 per cent of 1 826 women to have trichomoniasis. He was impressed with the amount of deep distress precipitated by the disease. No less than 255 of the patients were sterile. He cites evidence for trichomoniasis as a possible cause operating either through vaginitis or salpingitis. The latter he sees too as a possible cause of spontaneous abortion. The role of trichomoniasis as an occasional aetiological factor in frigidity and divorce is also noted.

The generally accepted concept that trichomoniasis is commonest in young and sexually active women, is questioned by Valent and Čatár (1967). They found the highest prevalence rate (36·9 per cent) in women aged 46–50 years. A statistically significant higher prevalence rate was found in single women (24·1 per cent), and widows and divorcees (31·2 per cent), than in married women (17·8 per cent). The incidence was higher also in women with gynaecological pathology than in those without. Another finding of interest was that infestation rates varied greatly from place to place throughout Slovakia—from 8·6 per cent to 47·5 per cent; they examined 1 474 women. Of 673 instances of the infestation in men, those named as contacts of infested women gave positive findings in 25·4 per cent as against 2·9 per cent in controls. They also examined 628 girls [sic] and found 3·2 per cent infested.

Trichomoniasis and cervical cancer

Berggren (1969) gave further emphasis to the role of gynaecological pathology. He found the incidence of trichomoniasis in over 13 000 gynaecologically normal Swedish women to be 7·4 per cent. In 348 cases of carcinoma in situ and in 47 of invasive cervical carcinoma the infestation rate was four times greater, ie 29·3 and 29·8 per cent respectively. Apart from this important observation the author discusses the long-term clinical, epidemiological and social significance of the findings without coming to any firm conclusions.

The role of T. vaginalis in pre-cancer of the cervix was examined by Szell et al (1967), Skrocka (1967) and Gray et al (1967) who drew attention to the need for treatment before biopsy. Boqudi (1968) also considered the problem. Bertini and Hornstein (1970a, b) studied the role of trichomoniasis in the development of cervical cancer in different ethnic groups in Israel. They found it to be commoner amongst Western and young Israeli-born women, compared with those originating from Eastern countries. The authors discuss these ethnic differences of incidence in terms of observance of religious laws forbidding extra-marital coitus. No evidence was found that reversible benign dysplasia with trichomoniasis was associated with malignancy. There was evidence however that dysplasia and endocervical hyperplasia were frequently associated with trichomoniasis. A report by De Carneri and Di Re (1970) from Milan takes up this point. They did routine culture tests for *T. vaginalis* in 1 732 adult women attending for screening tests for cervical cancer. The overall positivity rate was 18·2 per cent. There were however striking differences—statistically significant differences—in incidence between the different Papanicolaou cytological classes. In Class I trichomoniasis was 34 per cent less than expected; in Class II, 94 per cent greater; in Class III incidence was 221 per cent greater and in Classes IV and V combined it was 119 per cent greater than expected. Barats (1970) reports similar findings from Russia. He found trichomoniasis in 33 per cent of gynaecological patients as against 69 per cent of those with cervical cancer. In 300 women with cervical erosion but no trichomoniasis, carcinoma was found in 0·7 per cent whereas there was a 3·8 per cent incidence of carcinoma in 300 women with cervical erosion and co-existent chronic trichomoniasis. The highest rate of cervical cancer in the study was found in a group of 100 women with persistent trichomoniasis but nevertheless a clinically healthy cervix. The author concludes that cervical cytology examinations are essential in women with persistent trichomoniasis.

Trichomoniasis as a cause of false positive cancer smears was noted by Tosolini and Gasparini (1968). The association of the two has been discussed by others including Wawrzkiewicz and Kwoczyński (1970).

Other Observations

Asymptomatic infestation with *T. vaginalis* is highlighted by Nagesha (1970). Of 2 000 women under his care 500 had clinical evidence of vaginitis and 58·4 per cent of them had trichomoniasis. The incidence of the disease in the asymptomatic was 14·6 per cent. Persistent and recurrent infestation can generally be blamed on re-infestation by the asymptomatic husband according to Kumar and Sandana (1970). They found 11 of 50 husbands carrying the parasite in the prostatic secretion. Urethral scrapings produced only two positive results and urine deposit was unproductive.

The relevance of these socio-epidemiological observations vis-à-vis trichomoniasis and cervical cancer in an age when the contraceptive pill bids fair to be the most widely used contraceptive cannot be under-estimated.

The concept of sexual transmission of trichomoniasis received further support from a paper by Catterall and Nicol (1969). They demonstrated the parasite in all the sex partners of 56 infested men. This in conjunction with evidence of high infestation rates in male partners of women with trichomoniasis is so suggestive of sexual transmission in both directions as to make it acceptable as the principal mode of dissemination. So much is this so that these considerations can no longer be ignored in diagnostic or therapeutic routines.

Some workers have felt the need is to go further than has been customary in the investigation of males, that is, examination of urethral scrapings, centrifuged urine deposit and prostatic secretion, both microscopically and by culture. Gharse and Deshmukh (1970) investigated 40 consorts of 50 women with apparently resistant trichomoniasis. Each man had his prostatic secretion examined on three occasions. If these tests proved negative a fresh semen ejaculate was examined. In all, 31 (72·5 per cent) of the men gave positive results. This is amongst the highest positivity rates on record.

The common association of trichomoniasis with other forms of sexually transmissible disease is being increasingly recognised as an epidemiological fact. Tsao (1969) in a personal study of 1 335 patients with trichomoniasis found 620 (42 per cent) to have concurrent gonorrhoea. Conversely, he found 46 per cent of patients with gonorrhoea to have associated trichomoniasis. Figures vary from place to place and even from time to time as noted in Russia by Lopatin and Kolesnikova (1971). They found that whereas in 1960–65 only 10·9 per cent of women with gonorrhoea had concomitant trichomoniasis the percentage between 1966–68 was 34·5. Others had made the same point, if less dramatically, so that it has become increasingly clear that the presence of one sexually transmissible disease should prompt repeated tests for others.

The all too seldom stated and reiterated observation that trichomoniasis may masquerade as 'cystitis' was made by Block (1968). He points out that the symptomatology may all too readily prompt a diagnosis of urethritis or cystitis. In a series of 178 such patients, aged 49–87 years [sic], he found no less than 83 per cent harbouring T. vaginalis. The parasite was found in both vagina and in urine deposit in 23 and in the urinary sediment only in 55. The good results of therapy are cited as evidence of trichomoniasis causing the symptoms. The authors used controls matched for age. They also add a note showing how trichomoniasis may present as a family disease.

This last point is taken up by Worwag (1971) in Poland. He suggests the possibility of neo-natal infection. The urine of 110 newborn females and their mothers was examined within a week of the child's birth. The urine deposit was centrifuged and stained with Giemsa's stain and examined by phase contrast microscopy. Of 80 children with infested mothers 44 (55 per cent) were found to be positive in contrast to none of a control group of 30. In a second study by the same author 100 women and their newly born sons were similarly tested. *T. vaginalis* was found in 20 (28·5 per cent) of 70 sons whose mothers were infested. Sons of 30 'TV-negative' mothers were also found free of the parasite. The author concludes that the infants, both female and male, were infested during the course of delivery. These and similar observations made some years ago in Poland remain unconfirmed by work elsewhere. Amongst those who have described cases in the newborn are Glowinski et al (1965), Bonderenko (1966), Grys and Kwadisiewicz (1966), Blattner (1967) and Sander (1967).

Lapchenko (1965) considered the infection in childhood.

Valent (1971) writing from Czechoslovakia calls for widespread curative and preventive measures to control trichomoniasis. Amongst other measures he mentions routine examination of identifiable 'at risk' groups, reliable diagnostic methods, simultaneous treatment of sexual partners and education of both public and all professional health workers.

REFERENCES

BARATS, A. M. (1970). *Sov. Med.*, **33**, 147.
BERGGREN, O. (1969). *Amer. J. Obstet. Gynec.*, **105**, 166.
BERTINI, B. and HORNSTEIN, M. (1970a). *Acta Cytol.*, **14**, 325.
BERTINI, B. and HORNSTEIN, M. (1970b). *Harefauch.*, **77**, 459.
BLATTNER, R. J. (1967). *J. Pediat.*, **71**, 608.
BLOCK, E. (1968). *Nord. med.*, **80**, 921.
BONDERENKO, B. I. (1966). *Pediat. Akush. Ginek.*, **5**, 62.
BOQUDI, E. (1968). *Z. Geburtsh. Gynäk.* **169**, 59.
ČATÁR, G., VALENT, M., GRUNNER, L. and KUTCH, A. (1966). *Waidomšci Parazytologiczne*, **12**, 482.
CATTERALL, R. D. and NICOL, C. S. (1969). *Brit. med. J.* **1**, 765.
CHAPPAL, G. and BERTRAND, P. (1965). *Gynaecologia*, **160**, 17.
DAO, L. (1964). *Gynec. Prat., Paris*, **15**, 25.
DE CARNERI, I. and DI RE, F. (1970). *J. Obstet. Gynaecol. Brit. Commonw.*, **77**, 1016.
DUNLOP, E. M. C. and WISDOM, A. R. (1965). *Brit. J. vener. Dis.*, **41**, 85.
GAUDEROY, M. and LIEFOOGHE, J. (1966). *J. Sci. Med., Lille*, **84**, 409.
GHARSE, R. M. and DESHMUKH, M. A. (1970). *Bombay Hosp. J.* **12**, 113.
GLOWINSKI, M., GOLAB, H. and NORSK, I. (1965). *Wiad. Lek.*, **18**, 825.
GRAY, B., HARPER, W. F. and STILL, R. M. (1967). *J. Obstet., Gynaecol. Brit. Commonw.*, **74**, 98.
GRYS, E. and KWADISIEWICZ, I. (1966). *Pediat. Pol.*, **41**, 969.
HARPER, J. R. (1967). *Proc. roy. Soc. Med.*, **60**, 897.
IANKOV, N., BALTOVA, E. and PARANITEVA, V. (1966). *Akush. Ginek.*, **5**, 188.
IPSEN, J. and FEIGL, P. (1970). *Amer. J. Epidem.*, **91**, 175.
KIM, I. S. (1969). *Korean J. Publ. Hlth*, **6**, 255.
KOSTEIN, P. (1964). *Gynec. Prat., Paris*, **15**, 467.
KUMAR, K. and SANDANA, S. R. (1970). *Indian J. med. Sci.*, **24**, 621.
LANG, W. R. (1967). *J. Amer. Coll. Hlth Ass.*, **15**, 22.
LAPCHENKO, M. L. (1965). *Pediat. Akush. Ginek.*, **5**, 59.
LITTLEWOOD, J. M. and KAHLER, H. G. (1966). *Arch. Dis. Child.*, **41**, 693.

LOPATIN, A. I. and KOLESNIKOVA, N. P. (1971). *Vestn. derm. vener.*, **44**, 78.
NAGESHA, C. N., ANANTHRAKRISHNA, N. C. and SULOCHANA, P. (1970). *Amer. J. Obstet. Gynec.*, **106**, 933.
NAGUIB, S. M., COMSTOCK, G. W. and DAVIS, H. T. (1966). *Obstet. Gynec.*, **27**, 607.
NOREEL, J. and ROUSSEAU, C. (1965). *Rev. Franc., Gynec. Obstet.*, **60**, 557.
NHOCHINI, E. (1964). *Brit. J. vener. Dis.*, **40**, 191.
NICOL, C. S. (1958). *Brit. J. vener. Dis.*, **34**, 192.
OKAWA, T., AZUMA, T. and KODERA, T. (1967). *J. Jap. Obstet. Gynec. Soc.*, **19**, 93.
O'SULLIVAN, J. F. (1967). *Irish J. med. Sci.*, **497**, 207.
PUROLA, E., JAHKALA, M. and ÖSTERLUND, K. (1967). *Ann. Chir. Gynaec. Fenn.*, **56**, 95.
SANDER, C. (1967). *Z. Kinderheilk*, **98**, 364.
SKROCKA, M. B. (1967). *J. Maine med. Ass.*, **58**, 9.
SZELL, I. T., EMBER, G., PALANKAI, H. and SCHMIDT, E. (1967). *Zbl. Geburtsh., Gynak.*, **89**, 312.
TOSOLINI, G. C. R. and GASPARINI, M. (1968). *Friuli. Med.*, **23**, 807.
TSAO, W. (1969). *Brit. med. J.*, **1**, 642.
VALENT, M. (1971). *Bratislavské lekarské., Listy*, **56**, 21.
VALENT, M. and ČATÁR, G. (1967). *Folia. Fac. Med. Univ. Comenianae, Bratislava*, **2**, 101.
WISDOM, A. R. and DUNLOP, E. M. C. (1965). *Brit. J. vener. Dis.*, **41**, 90.
WORWAG, Z. (1971). *Wiad. Parazytol.*, **17**, 351 and 355.
WAWRZKIEWICZ, M. and KWOCZYŃSKI, M. Z. (1970). *Wiad. Parazyt.*, **16**, 195.

19 Clinical Aspects

R. S. Morton

Trichomoniasis affects about 20 per cent of women at some time during their lives. In men, it is variously described as causing between 5 and 15 per cent of cases of non-gonococcal urethritis. Many infested males and females are asymptomatic.

Presenting symptoms

According to Wisdom and Dunlop (1965) there is wide variation in clinical presentation particularly in women where the symptoms may be from mild to acutely severe, from the short-lived to the chronic and from an isolated incident to the persistently recurrent. Symptoms may be either urinary or genital or any combination of these. The confusion with recurrent attacks of cystitis is emphasised. The observation that urinary tract infestation with *T. vaginalis* is commoner in women than in men is made by Glebski (1965). He reported on a urine survey of 47 000 sexually active inhabitants of Lodz in Poland. He found *T. vaginalis* in 10·7 per cent of women and 1·7 per cent of men.

Reviewing a series of 845 patients with leucorrhoea, Gangu and Anjaneyula (1966) found trichomoniasis commonest in the poor, the pregnant, the married and in those aged 21–35 years. Dysuria, vaginal discharge and pruritis were the predominent symptoms. Catterall (1970) stated that trichomiasis was still the commonest cause of pathological vaginal discharge. In a series of 415 consecutive cases he found *T. vaginalis* responsible for 125 (30 per cent); *C. albicans* for 102 (24·0 per cent) and *N. gonorrhoeae* for 95 (22·8 per cent).

The variability of presentation was discussed by Galli and Sylvestre (1965). They found that in females acute and atypical cases form a minority. About 65 per cent of women with the disease may be described as subacutely affected. Of their male patients 41 per cent had prostatitis.

Schapira (1965) makes the point that the more extensive the infestation in the male the more severe the symptoms. In a study involving

94 male partners of women with trichomoniasis he found that cultures made from freshly ejaculated semen were sometimes positive when culture of prostatic material was negative. Zeirz (1966) reiterates this last point. Of 274 men presenting with a fertility problem 7·7 per cent had demonstrable *T. vaginalis* in their semen. In four patients conception followed successful treatment.

With the parasite ever more widely recognised as a cause of urethritis and prostatitis also, it is not surprising to find reports where it is implicated in epididymitis, a condition so often without recognisable cause. Amar (1967) reported three cases associated with positive culture of the protozoan. In each patient there was no response to antibiotic therapy but resolution followed exhibition of a trichomonacide Fisher and Morton (1969) also reported three cases of what they describe as 'subacute' epididymitis. They believed that *T. vaginalis* played a causative role in two cases and was definitely the cause in the third. They gave the following reasons for this view:

(a) the epididymitis of 4 days' duration bore little resemblance to that usually associated with gonorrhoea;

(b) the parasite was identified in the urine by both wet film and culture, and

(c) clinical cure followed treatment with metronidazole and this corresponded with the disappearance of *T. vaginalis*.

Rasul (1970) has described a further three cases.

Walton (1969) drew attention to the phenomenon of haematospermia in trichomoniasis. The role of the disease in male sterility was considered by Argenziano et al (1967). In the female, sterility and abortion as possible associations is mentioned by Carvalho and Baska (1969). 'Adenexitis' due to *T. vaginalis* was described by Pejtsik and Tóth (1969). The possibility that the parasite may play a part in female sterility was also dealt with, somewhat inconclusively, by Nicola and Giarola (1968) and Gaffori and Poggio (1968).

An unusual clinical presentation in a man was cited by Lopatin (1970). The patient had trichomonal urethritis associated with ulceration of the penis. There were seven round ulcers, varying in size from a millet seed to a lentil. The ulcers were covered with a sloughly scale which on removal revealed the ulcers to have steep, soft inflamed edges. They were tender and oedematous with fading, surrounding erythema. Inguinal adenitis was present. Levin and Luseva (1970) also described penile ulcers which they believe due to *T. vaginalis*.

Trichomonal urethritis in males was given a detailed clinical description by Ward (1970). He says there is a history of white, sometimes frothy urethral discharge with associated urethral pruritis, dysuria and occasional urgency. This latter symptom the author associates with prostatic, seminal vesicle and bladder involvement. Haematospermia may occur. Darewicz et al (1970) also described the clinical condition in males.

Trichomoniasis in the female is not infrequently associated with other genito-urinary infections. Of 292 women with gonorrhoea no less than 138 (47 per cent) also had trichomonal vaginitis. From the basis of his presented experience Bungaard (1965) states that the need is to examine all women complaining of dysuria for the presence of *T. vaginalis*.

Association with candidiosis

The co-existence of trichomoniasis and candidiasis has long been recognised. Symptomatic, mixed infections were found in 7·3 per cent of a series reviewed by Gangu and Anjaneyula (1966). In a more detailed study Peterson et al (1967) reported that 12 per cent of 414 pregnant women had positive cultures for the fungus at the same time as trichomonal vaginitis was diagnosed. Jaud (1969) gave the figures for mixed infections as 14·3 per cent. Alteras et al (1965) treated 350 patients aged 15–30 years with metronidozole and found 18·5 per cent had developed candidiasis. Friend (1970) viewed the subject conversely and stated that 20 per cent of patients with vaginal candidiasis had associated trichomonal infestation. Maroudi et al (1966) found that where trichomoniasis, with or without concomitant thrush, was present at confinement a grave danger existed. In a series of 40 such cases requiring suturing, there was wound breakdown in 13.

Other observations

The clinical condition in females as found by photocolposcopy was described by Syrovatko and Kalov (1970). Electron microscope studies of vaginal wall lining before and after metronidazole therapy for trichomoniasis were made by Panaitescu et al (1970).

The most recent detailed review of trichomoniasis is by Catterall (1972). He deals with the wide variety and variable intensity of symptoms and signs. He draws attention to the case of sudden and acute onset and the frequency with which young women develop trichomoniasis a week or more after their first full sexual experience. He gives the complications in females as bartholinitis, infection of Skene's ducts, urethritis and cystitis; and in the males, as prostatitis, cystitis, epididymitis and urethral stricture. He observes how frequently, in both sexes, trichmoniasis is associated with genital warts.

REFERENCES

ALTERAS, I., GRIGORIU, D. and LARA LAZAR, M. (1965). *Dermatologica*, **131**, 309.
AMAR, A. D. (1967). *J. Amer. med. Ass.*, **200**, 147.
ARGENZIANO, G., DE LUCA, M. and ROSSI, A. (1967). *Minerva derm.*, **42**, 388.

BUNGAARD, B. (1965). *Ugeskr. Laeg.*, **127**, 1297.
CATTERALL, R. D. (1970). *Brit. J. vener. Dis.*, **46**, 122.
CATTERALL, R. D. (1972). Venereal diseases, 'The Medical Clinics of North America', **56**, 1203. W. B. Saunders.
CARVALHO, G. and BASKA, B. A. (1969). *Virginia med. month.*, **96**, 444.
DAREWICZ, J., KUCZYŃSKA, K. and CZERNIAWSKI, J. (1970). *Polski Przegl. Chir.*, **42**, Suppl. 6a, 969.
FISHER, I. and MORTON, R. S. (1969). *Brit. J. vener. Dis.*, **45**, 252.
FRIEND, J. R. (1970). *Update*, **2**, 841.
GAFFORI, S. and POGGIO, A. (1968). *Minerva Ginec.*, **20**, 1260.
GANGU, D. and ANJANEYULA, R. (1966). *Hindustan. Antibot. Bull.*, **9**, 69.
GALLI, Z. and SYLVESTRE, L. (1965). *L'Union Medicale du Canada*, **94**, 1628.
GLEBSKI, J. (1965). *Przegl. Derm.*, **52**, 617.
JAUD, M. (1969). *Therapiawoche*, **19**, 2495.
LEVIN, M. M. and LUSEVA, V. A. (1970). *Vestn. derm. vener.*, **44**, 82.
LOPATIN, A. I. (1970). *Vestn. derm. vener.* **44**, 78.
MAROUDI, D., PAPADIMITRIOU, G. and LAPAS, C. (1966). *Ginec. Obstet. Paris*, **65**, 651.
NICOLA, G. and GIAROLA, A. (1968). *Gynec. Prat.*, **19**, 309.
PANAITESCU, D., VOICULESU, R. and IONESU, M. D. (1970). *Microbiologia Parazit. Epidem.*, **15**, 43.
PEJTSIK, B. and TOTH, E. (1969). *Z. Geburtsh Gynäk.*, **170**, 68.
PETERSON, W., HANSEN, F. W., STRAUCH, J. E. and RYDER, C. D. (1967). *Amer. J. Obstet. Gynec.*, **97**, 472.
RASUL, G. (1970). *J. Pakistan med. Ass.*, **20**, 54.
SCHAPIRA, H. E. (1965). *J. Urol.*, **93**, 303.
SYROVATKO, F. A. and KALOV, P. G. (1970). *Akush. Ginek, Sofia*, **9**, 27.
WALTON, H. C. M. (1969). *Brit. med. J.*, **2**, 514.
WARD, J. N. (1970). *Med. Treat., New York*, **7**, 1015.
WISDOM, A. R. and DUNLOP, E. M. C. (1965). *Brit. J. vener. Dis.*, **41**, 90.
ZEIRZ, P. (1966). *Urologe*, **5**, 265.

8

20 Laboratory Aspects

R. S. Morton

There is still widespread discussion as to whether microscopy, culture or other methods are the most productive in the hunt for the trichomonas vaginalis. Transillumination, phase contrast and dark-field microscopy are all in use. Culture media have proliferated. Most contain proteolysed liver, human serum, an antibiotic and a fungicide, all seen as essential ingredients. Many media are used in combination with Stuart's transport medium. It is widely recognised that all these and other methods may be used in concert and that repeated testing, from a multiplicity of sites, especially in males, may be necessary to establish a diagnosis. Repeated testing after treatment is regarded as essential for both males and females.

Chronological review of diagnostic methods

Amies and Garabedian (1965) reported on a fixative slide technique of diagnosis. It revealed T. vaginalis in 38·6 per cent of 1 000 women in contrast to a 47 per cent positive rating by phase contrast microscopy. The new technique is considered useful where specimens have to be mailed. Ethanol mercuric chloride was used as the fixative.

Although many workers favour patiently applied microscopic methods for diagnosis, culture methods are favoured by others. Narang et al (1964) stated that 12 per cent of their cases would have been missed if cultures had not been done. O'Sullivan (1967) also found culture methods superior to wet film examination. Muller (1965) described a new medium for culture of T. vaginalis. It contained casein, peptone, ascorbic acid, cystine chloride and a yeast extract. Oller (1965) found that in 107 patients the Papanicolaou smear was positive for trichomonads in 83 compared with 51 with wet film and 92 with culture. Ruiz-Moreno and Kern-Bontke (1966) in a study of 1 000 female outpatients found trichomonads in the Papanicolaou smear of 201 of whom 62 were asymptomatic. When the smears were grouped according to Papanicolaou's groups I to V classification the results were as follows:

Group I: 91·3 per cent with 84·1 per cent positive for *T. vaginalis*.
Group II ('infected, should be repeated'): 5·3 per cent with 8·9 per cent positive for *T. vaginalis*.
Groups III, IV and V: 3·4 per cent with 7 per cent positive for *T. vaginalis*. There was a decline in the number of suspicious cervical cells after treatment although smears were described only as 'cleaner'.

The application of multiple methods of diagnosis has been applied to males. Fioccardi (1966) found 23 (20 per cent) cases of trichomoniasis in a series of 115 men with non-gonococcal urethritis. The methods of diagnosis were:

3 by wet films,
7 by stained smear, and
13 by culture.

Of the remaining 92 men, four responded promptly to metronidazole given on epidemiological grounds, *ie* the men's wives had trichomonal vaginitis.

Commenting on the difficulty of identifying the protozoan in the urine, Block (1968) recommends that diagnosis may be facilitated by the addition of 10 per cent cresyl blue to the urinary sediment. Cellular and other elements stain blue while tricomonads remain unstained and easily differentiated. Peterson et al (1966) in a survey of 1 001 non-pregnant females with trichomoniasis found the parasite in the catheter urine of 35 per cent. In each instance the urine culture became negative after therapy.

Robinson and Mirchandani (1965) studied 675 women in various stages of pregnancy. They found a mixed flora of vaginal organisms. Micrococci, staphlococci, lactobacilli and enterobacteria were all common. Streptococci occurred only occasionally. In clinically asymptomatic trichomoniasis there was no alteration in respect of vaginal flora or of the pH. Clinically severe cases of trichomoniasis however, showed a move of the pH to the acid and 'almost invariably the presence of streptococci, generally β-haemolytic'.

As in other fields of medicine the exhibition of a specific remedy is not always preceded by scientific diagnosis. Farooki and Sethi (1965) deprecate blind treatment, *ie* prescription based on historical and/or clinical findings only. They put forward evidence to show clearly the advantage to the patient of sound laboratory diagnosis. Hughes et al (1966) compare the efficacy of clinical, cytological and bacteriological methods available for the diagnosis of trichomonal vaginitis. Negative clinical findings were an unreliable guide to the presence or absence of parasites. Positive clinical diagnoses were confirmed only in 75 per cent of cases by laboratory tests. Cytological (staining) methods of examination were found to be superior to wet film examination by direct transillumination microscopy. The cytological method was also thought to be more successful than culture; although culture was markedly more successful in those cases where direct microscopy showed few parasites.

Rayner (1968) added an elucidatory note on this last observation. He determined in the laboratory situation, the minimum number of *T. vaginalis* protozoa required to initiate growth in three different media, the Feinberg and Whittington, the Squires and MacFadzean and a cystine-peptone-liver-maltose (CPLM) compound. For the last of these it was only 1–40 organisms, while for the first, inocula of the order 10^4 to 10^5 were needed. Vaginal secretions from 203 women and urethral scrapings or centrifuged urine deposit from 160 men when applied to both of these media confirmed the CPLM medium as the superior means of detection of *T. vaginalis*.

The discussion on the best diagnostic methods continues. By Gram-staining and using safranine as the counter-stain Cree (1968) had 209 positive smears in contrasts to 249 positive cultures in 916 patients. Eddie (1968) found wet preparations more than 90 per cent as effective as stained smears and cultures. Nagesha et al (1970) in a study of 2 000 women, 500 of whom had clinically apparent vaginitis, found examination of Fontana-stained smears superior to Papanicolaou staining, wet film examination or culture. Taking the Fontana method as giving 100 per cent diagnosis the other methods gave positive findings of the order 82·2 per cent, 54·1 per cent and 68,8 per cent respectively.

Like others, Hulka and Hulka (1967) have cautioned on the diagnosis of trichomoniasis by stained cervical cytology specimens. They reported that 170 women in an extensive cervical cancer survey had atypical smears. Using principally culture methods they found 70·6 per cent of these to have trichomoniasis. They claimed 60 per cent false negative with Papanicolaou staining and wet film methods. Eight weeks after a double blind treatment trial (using metronidazole and a placebo), they found 55·1 and 47·1 per cent of the infested and controls with negative cultures, and cervical smears which had reverted to Papanicolaou cytology of group I and II. The authors concluded that the presence of trichomonads is not a significant factor in the natural history of dysplastic lesions of the cervix. Interpretation of the worth of these observations is blurred by the fact that individuals in the groups may have had sexual intercourse throughout the study period with more than one partner. The problem of dysplasia in cervical cytology specimens, apparently due to vaginal trichomoniasis, is well recognised. Gray et al (1967) studied the cervical biopsy findings before and after treatment of trichomoniasis with metronidazole. Inflammatory and epithelial changes quickly subsided but intracellular oedema and haemorrhage persisted. They recommended that in patients with trichomoniasis with cervicitis and cytological changes, biopsy be delayed till after treatment, when histological interpretation is easier. Cytological changes in the cervix of infested women were also studied by Teras and Kaarma (1969), Gobert et al (1969) and Guerresi (1968).

Serologically based methods of diagnosing trichomoniasis have also been used. In a preliminary report Kramar and Kucera (1966) claimed the ability to demonstrate specific antibiodies against *T. vaginalis* by an indirect immuno-fluorescent reaction. Complement fixation tests were used by Korik (1966). He obtained positive results in 10 per cent. When, however, he used serum from immunised patients and animals the positivity rate in 138 patients was 83 per cent. This aspect was also considered by Krupova (1968) and Iankov et al (1968). A skin test with an antigen prepared from several strains of vaginal trichomonads was evaluated by Lyubimova and Ilyin (1967). They obtained over 60 per cent positive reactions in patients with chronic infestations; 43 per cent positives in those with a past history of trichomoniasis and a 25 per cent positivity rating in fresh cases.

Lumsden et al (1966) writing from Edinburgh, described experiments relating to isolation, cultivation, low temperature preservation and infectivity titration of *T. vaginalis*. They used Feinberg and Whittington's medium. Slow cooling to $-79°C$ in the presence of dimethyl/sulphoxide was an efficient method of preservation. A pH of 5·8–6·8 was found best when few parasites only are available for inoculation of medium. In this last regard Kurnatowska (1968) gives estimates of the trichomonal population of vaginal secretions. Honigberg et al (1966) of Baltimore also sought to define the pathogenicity of inocula by comparing the mean volumes of subcutaneous lesions produced by cultures injected into mice. Excellent correlation was found between the clinical severity of the vaginitis, cervicitis and the mouse assay pathogenicity levels. There was also some degree of positive correlation with spread of inflammation to the patients' urinary tract and pelvis but none at all when such variables as age or phase of menstrual cycle of patients was considered. In a later study Kulda et al (1970), a team including Honigberg of Baltimore, followed up this work by studies of generation times of freshly isolated parasites. They found a high degree of correlation between generation time and pathogenicity levels for each strain and that this applied in both patients and in mice. There was also parallelism in the pathogenicity for both of these hosts.

Over the years under review other trichomonads have been studied. For example Georges and Savill (1968) studied the vaginal implantations of intestinal trichomonads. Results were negative. Trichomonads and other flagellates which have been found in the vagina were described by Dyner (1969).

The behaviour of trichomoniasis in women treated by radiotherapy and by cytotoxic drugs was studied by Zawadszki et al (1967).

The year 1969 showed a renewal of investigations into diagnostic methods. Robertson et al (1969) used culture and phase contrast microscopy of centrifuged and buffered vaginal secretion. This latter they found a more sensitive method of detection than wet films prepared with saline and examined by transillumination microscopy. Thin et al (1969) preferred Papanicolaou staining to other methods of diagnosis of trichomoniasis. Warnings of the high incidence of false positive and false negative findings with the Papanicolaou smear method were given by Perl (1972). Such false findings in his series were as high as 48·4 per cent. He recommends direct microscopy and culture. Nielsen (1969) also offered a cautionary tale. He found that the *T. vaginalis* survived no longer than 24 hours in Stuart's transport medium.

Francechini (1971) offered a new staining method which he claimed was particularly useful in males. A fixed smear of centrifuged urine deposit is further fixed by Boulin's solution of 3 per cent silver nitrate. The preparation is heated to 60°F and kept so in the dark for 1–2 hours. The slide with its fixed silver nitrate film is then 'developed'. The constituents of the necessary solution are given. The author claims that the flagellae, axostyle and undulating membrane all stain well and the cytoplasm little or not at all.

Beck et al (1971) compared wet film, culture and serological methods of diagnosis in 600 consecutive patients. Compared with their culture results, wet film examinations gave 70·7 per cent positives and Papanicolaou staining 63·8 per cent. The complement fixation test used showed antibodies in 75 per cent of the infested. Positive serological tests were recognised as having their limitations as they frequently mean no more than past disease.

The disparity of prevalence of trichomoniasis in males and females has long perplexed investigators. Apart from the tendency to a much shorter natural history in males, due to flushing out of parasites by urination, the difficulty of detecting parasites, albeit often few in number, is widely recognised as a reason. A wide variety of ideas are on offer to overcome this last problem. Ward (1970) recommended microscopy of urethral scrapings and/or centrifuged urine deposit as offering the best yield of parasites in the male contact. This view was also expressed by several speakers during a discussion on the subject at the Jubilee Meeting of the Medical Society for the Study of Venereal Diseases at Glasgow in June 1972. Oates et al (1971) offered a helpful suggestion. He recommended the use of a polyester sponge swab for the taking of specimens. Such swabs are found to be not only gentler on the male urethral mucosa but they have the added advantage of being more absorbent than cotton wool and so are capable of offering larger inocula. Summers and Ford (1972) commenting that Papanicolaou staining had long been well recognised as a diagnostic tool for trichomoniasis in females tried it in males. They applied the method to prostatic fluid and centrifuged midstream urine deposit. Their patients consisted of 46 male contacts. Positive findings were claimed in 33 (71·1 per cent). In the first half of the study positive cytology findings were confirmed in all cases by culture. In view of this, cultures were considered unnecessary thereafter. From these endeavours the authors claim to offer a significant improvement to the armamentarium available for diagnosis of trichomoniasis in the male. Using the Papanicolaou method Bernfeld (1972) found that 10 per cent of his subfertile males harboured *T. vaginalis*.

Such reports clearly challenge culture methods and no doubt have had a hand in leading to studies on the cultural requirements of the protozoan. Christow (1971a, b) studied this with particular reference to vitamin B complex. Farris and Honigberg (1970) studied chick liver cells as a suitable medium while Barrow and Ellis (1970) used tube culture methods. These studies, like earlier work, confirm that culture methods for the detection of *T. vaginalis*, like microscopic methods, leave much to be desired.

REFERENCES

AMIES, C. R. and GARABEDIAN, M. (1965). *J. clin. Path.*, **18**, 27.
BARROW, G. I. and ELLIS, C. (1970). *J. clin. Path.*, **23**, 91.
BECK, K. J., SAATHOFF, M. and MERCKL, H. (1971). *Geburtshilfe Frauenheilkd.*, **31**, 551.
BERNFELD, W. K. (1972). *Brit. J. vener. Dis.*, **48**, 144.
BLOCK, E. (1968). *Nord. med.*, **80**, 921.
CHRISTOW, C. P. (1971a) *Zbl., Bakt., I.* Oreg. Ser. A, **217**, 540.
CHRISTOW, C. P. (1971b). *Ibid.*, **217**, 381.
CREE, G. E. (1968). *Brit. J. vener. Dis.*, **44**, 226.
DYNER, E. (1969). *Wiad. Parazyt.*, **15**, 309.
EDDIE, D. A. S. (1968). *J. med. Microbiol.*, **1**, 153.
FAROOKI, M. A. and SETHI, N. (1965). *Medicus, Pakistan*, **29**, 248.
FARRIS, V. K. and HONIGBERG, B. M. (1970). *J. Parasit.*, **56**, 849.
FIOCCARDI, R. (1966). *Minerva med.*, **57**, 3189.
FRANCECHINI, P. (1971). *Presse. med.*, **79**, 486.
GEORGES, P. and SAVILL, J. (1968). *Amer. Parasit. Hum. Comp.*, **43**, 121.
GOBERT, J. G., GEORGES, P. and SAVILL, J. (1969). *Amer. Parasit. Hum. Comp.*, **44**, 687.
GRAY, B., HARPER, W. F. and STILL, R. M. (1967). *J. Obstet Gynaec. Brit. Commonw.*, **74**, 98.
GUERRESI, E. (1968). *Rev. Ital. Ginek.*, **52**, 819.
HONIGBERG, B. M., LIVINGSTON, M. C. and FROST, J. K. (1966). *Acta Cytol.*, **10**, 353.
HUGHES, H. E., GORDON, A. M. & BARR, G. D. (1966). *J. Obstet. Gynaec. Brit. Commonw.*, **73**, 821.
HULKA, B. S. and HULKA, J. F. (1967). *Amer. J. Obstet. Gynec.*, **98**, 180.
IANKOV, N., BALTOVA, E. and PARENITEV, V. (1968). *Akush. Ginek.*, **7**, 187.
KORIK, L. M. (1966). *Vestn. derm. venerol.*, **40**, 50.
KRUPOVÁ, J. (1968). *Cesk. Epidem.*, **17**, 162.
KRAMAR, J. and KUCERA, K. (1966). *J. Hyg. Epidem.*, **10**, 85.
KULDA, J., HONIGBERG, B. M., FROST, J. K. and HOLLANDER, D. H. (1970). *Amer. J. Obstet. Gynec.*, **108**, 908.

KURNATOWSKA, A. (1968). *Acta med. Pol.*, **9**, 175.

LUMSDEN, W. H. R., ROBERTSON, D. H. H. and McNEILLAGE, G. C. (1966). *Brit. J. vener. Dis.*, **42**, 145.

LYUBIMOVA, L. K. and ILYIN, I. L. (1967). *Vestn. derm. vener.*, **41**, 56.

MULLER, W. A. (1965). *Z. fdg. Hyg. u. chre. Grenzsebieta*, **11**, 75.

NAGESHA, C. N., ANANTHRAKRISHNA, N. C. and SULOCHANA, P. (1970). *Amer. J. Obstet. Gynec.*, **106**, 933.

NARANG, S. S., BHARGAVA, N. C., CHAHAN, B. K., SESHGEIR, I. and RAO, M. (1964). *Indian J. Derm.*, **30**, 150.

NIELSEN, R. (1969). *Brit. J. vener. Dis.*, **45**, 328.

OATES, J. K., SELWYN, S. and BREACH, M. R. (1971). *Brit. J. vener. Dis.*, **47**, 289.

OLLER, L. Z. (1965). *Brit. J. vener. Dis.*, **41**, 304.

O'SULLIVAN, J. F. (1967). *Irish J. med. Sci.*, **497**, 207.

PERL, G. (1972). *J. Obstet. Gynaecol. Brit. Commonw.*, **39**, 7.

PETERSON, W. F., STAUCH, J. E. and RYDER, C. D. (1966). *Amer. J. Obstet. Gynec.*, **94**, 343.

RAYNER, C. F. A. (1968). *Brit. J. vener. Dis.*, **44**, 63.

ROBERTSON, D. H. H., LUMSDEN, W. H. R., FRASER, K. F., HOSIE, D. D. and MOORE, D. M. (1969). *Brit. J. vener. Dis.*, **45**, 42.

ROBINSON, S. C. and MIRCHANDANI, G. (1965). *Amer. J. Obstet. Gynec.*, **91**, 1005.

RUIZ-MORENO, J. A. and KERN-BONTKE, E. (1966). *German. med. Mon.*, **11**, 507.

SUMMERS, J. L. and FORD, M. L. (1972). *J. Urol.*, **107**, 840.

TERAS, J. and KAARMA, H. (1969). *Wiad. Parazyt.*, **15**, 481.

THIN, R. N. T., MELCHER, D. H., TAPP, J. W., NICOL, C. S. and HILL, J. (1969). *Brit. J. vener. Dis.*, **45**, 328.

WARD, J. N. (1970). *Med. Treat., New York.*, **7**, 1015.

ZAWADSZKI, J., HALYS, J. and MATUSZEWSKI, H. (1967). *Wiad. Parazyt.*, **13**, 729.

21 Therapeutic Aspects

R. S. Morton

Metronidazole

The treatment of trichomoniasis was revolutionised by the introduction of metronidazole (Flagyl) by Cosar and Julou (1959) and the first reported clinical trials by Durel et al (1960). The drug is highly specific in trichomoniasis. The recommended dosage for a decade was 200 mg three times per day for 7 days with 400 mg for the same duration for clinical failures. The need for follow-up tests after treatment and for the examination and treatment of infested contacts is seen as essential to permanent cure and epidemiological control. Metronidazole is not generally recommended for use in the first 3 months of pregnancy. Rodin and Hass (1966) have shown that in appropriate dosage it can be given to infants and children with safety.

Narang et al (1964) treated 155 women and 25 men with the recommended course of 200 mg three times per day for the 7 days. There was an immediate failure rate of 3·3 per cent. Of 80 patients followed up for 3 months 91·3 per cent were cured. Most of the recurrences were considered to be re-infections. Simultaneous treatment of the husband was considered essential. Similar cure rates were reported by Peterson et al (1966). Pereyra and Lansing (1964) reviewed the results of identical dosage given over varying periods of 5, 7 and 10 days. Their patients were 2 002 'incarcerated women' in a Californian institution. Cure rates were respectively 97·8, 98·1 and 97·5 per cent. Refractory cases responded to re-treatment with a 5-day course together with 250 mg pessaries of metronidazole daily for the same period. Parapakkham (1967) in a well-planned study of 275 cases came to the conclusion that the addition of vaginal metronidazole offered no benefit to the patient except where oral therapy alone had failed. Baker and Kennan (1967) also found that increasing the number of days of therapy to 10 did not increase the cure rate. They were in agreement with the other workers mentioned about the use of pessaries. Nicol and Evans (1966) used 400 mg three times per day for 7 days and claimed 100 per cent cure rate. Teokharov and

Anikin (1967) reported on the long-term follow-up of 255 women and 154 men. After 4 years 90 per cent were found free of the infestation. The percentage reached 93·9 where oral therapy had been augmented with topical metronidazole.

American studies also took a long view. Gardner and Dukes (1968) noted that reinfection rates in metronidazole-treated women were two and a half times greater if the sex partner was not treated simultaneously. Two and a half years after the publication of this study these findings were more marked. By that time 27 per cent of the women with untreated consorts had had a recurrence as against 8·4 per cent of women whose consorts had originally been treated simultaneously. Shklyar (1967) in a study of 250 husband of infested women found 35·2 per cent positive. He makes the point that simultaneous treatment of the husband whether or not the parasite is found in him, permits of sound evaluation of the therapeutic efficiency of the drug.

Scott-Gray (1964) reported on metronidazole treatment of 300 women at all stages of pregnancy. No side effects were seen in the mothers of their 295 babies. Rodin and Hass (1966) considered that there was now sufficient evidence in the literature to be sure about the safety of prescribing metronidazole in the second and third trimester. They were less certain about the first. An annotation in the *British Medical Journal* (1966) concerned itself with this last point and also warned that the drug should not be used in nursing mothers as it was excreted in breast milk. Baker and Kennan (1967), pointing out that metronidazole was not officially approved for use in pregnancy in their country (U.S.A.), agreed with these findings.

Much has been written about side effects but the overall judgement is that metronidazole is a very safe specific. Beveridge (1964) claimed to reduce the incidence of post-treatment candidiasis from 19 to 7 per cent by concomitant treatment with a vaginal fungicide. She used the standard regimen of metranidazole in 100 consecutive patients. Clark and George (1966) reported similar results. They used an alkaline vaginal douche to reduce the incidence of candidiasis. Oller (1969) used amphotericin B pessaries with similar effect.

Searle Products (15 June 1966) showed the order of frequency of side effects of metronidazole in 4 148 consecutive cases to be as opposite.

In a much smaller series of 277 patients Robinson and Mirchandani (1965) found four cases with nausea and vomiting; two with glossitis; two with dry mouth and burning; two with bad taste; and one patient with a papillary rash. Of the 277 treated pregnant women none had babies showing adverse effects although six babies had congenital anomalies; eight were born prematurely and two were stillbirths. Parker et al (1965) reported that 7·7 per cent of their series of 717 patients mentioned side effects, all of a minor nature. These workers actively looked for trouble. They carried out haematological studies in

Side effects	Number reported	Percentage
Nausea	219	5·28
Taste	157	3·78
Furry tongue	111	2·68
Headache	44	1·06
Diarrhoea	33	0·80
Dizziness	27	0·65
Vaginal burning	21	0·51
Dry mouth	18	0·43
Rash	16	0·39
Vaginal dryness	12	0·29
Gastritis	11	0·27
Drowsiness	11	0·27
Pruritis	11	0·27
Sore tongue	9	0·22
All others*	82	1·97

* None more than 0·2 per cent.

266 of their series of 420 women and 297 of the treated husbands. They found four cases of transient leucopenia. There was no bile in the urine of the 217 tested and of 25 patients subjected to detailed neurological examination before and after a 10-day course of metronidazole, none showed any abnormality. Their cure rate was 97·1 per cent with a recurrence rate of 7·9 per cent of the 189 followed for 2–32 months. Lefebure and Hesseltine (1965) found only 10 of 716 metronidazole-treated patients to have transient leucopenia.

Fagin (1965) described a case of jaundice which he attributed to the exhibition of metronidazole. Lewis and Kenna (1965) described two teenage girls who used metronidazole in suicidal demonstrations. Recovery took place in both within 48 hours. No serious toxic effects occurred in the girl taking the bigger dose—60 tablets each of 200 mg. Powell (1967) writing from the amoeboiasis research unit at the University of Natal, Durban, South Africa, carried out electrocardiographic studies in patients taking metronidazole. The occasional patient showed T-wave changes but the author concluded that the drug is not contra-indicated in cardiac disease.

An interesting observation by Davis (1967) was that doses of metronidazole three to eight times greater than those used in clinical practice had some anti-treponemal activity. Earlier, Yobs et al (1966) showed that the drug had no treponemeicidal action in experimental rabbit syphilis. Wilkinson et al (1967) were prompted to advise clinicians that patients receiving metronidazole should not have blood submitted for the treponemal immobilisation test. An editorial in the *British Medical Journal* (1967) agreed. More recently Ilyin et al (1971) from their clinical observation of 11 patients with both syphilis and trichomoniasis came to the conclusion that metronidazole may have a mild treponicidal effect.

The problem of the *T. vaginalis* developing resistance to metronidazole has been a recurring theme. Nicol et al (1960) in reply to a letter by De Carneri (1966) stated that 200 primary isolates from patients showed sensitivity no different from that of standard reference strains. Diddle (1967) presented details of a case of apparent resistance in a 40 year old woman. Aure and Gjonnesse (1969) also questioned the possibility of growing resistance. They pointed out that in their department the cure rate with metronidazole was 97 per cent in 1962 and 73 per cent in 1968.

De Carneri et al (1969) renewing their earlier suggestion carried out *in vivo* and *in vitro* studies and showed that some degree of resistance could be induced in laboratory strains. They saw such a development as representing a considerable obstacle to the correct evaluation of therapeutic failure. Actor et al (1969) also undertook laboratory studies. They studied the resistance to metronidazole by Trichomonas foetus in hamsters, infested extra-vaginally. They found it possible to promote some degree of drug resistance (8–16 times) by sub-optimal dosage, to infest hamsters with the parasites concerned and note 'clinical' resistance to dosages hitherto considered adequate. Resistance was also considered by Kovács and Galgóczy (1969), Valent et al (1969) and Gobert et al (1969). In contradiction to suggestions of developing resistance is the well-planned study of McFadzean et al (1969). They estimated the metronidazole sensitivy of 25 strains of *T. vaginalis* from patients reported as failing to respond to treatment with the drug. When compared with 55 random isolates no evidence of resistance could be found. The possibility that bacteria in the vagina may be capable of inactivating metronidazole could not be satisfactorily determined by these workers. Catterall (1972) believes this latter to be a possibility and recommends antibiotic treatment before retreatment in cases where resistance appears to be a probability. In this regard, Szanto (1971) described the case of a 66 year old woman with apparent resistance while she was receiving regular oxytetracycline for chronic bronchitis. The author suggests therapeutic antagonism as a possible explanation. In a paper from Russia, Korik (1971) reports some variation in sensitivity between parasites from treatment failure cases and those from untreated patients. He also claimed a 2·5 to 2 000-fold reduction of sensitivity in trichomonads exposed to culture media with gradually increasing concentrations of metronidazole. Similar claims have come from Kurnatowska (1969) in Poland. Absence of similar reports from so much of the rest of the world gives cause for optimism, and this is supported by a very positive report by Keighley (1971). She treated 496 women living in the closed community of London's Holloway

Jail. The cure rate was 98·3 per cent using a bi-daily regime of 400 mg for 7 days. Of the eight failures, five were successfully re-treated. There was no evidence that cure rates had fallen over the preceding decade.

Edward and Mathison (1971) reported experiments to show that metronidazole acts by inhibiting the evolution of hydrogen but not the synthesis of acetyl phosphate. The authors suggest that the drug acts by interfering with the electric transfer of protein ferridoxin.

Other trichomonacides

Perhaps not surprisingly, reports of possible resistance to metronidazole have been associated with trials of other trichomonacides, In 1969 preliminary reports of a new substituted nitromidazole, nitromidazine (naxogen) began to appear. Emanueli and De Carneri (1969) and Moffett et al (1969) claimed 96 per cent cure rates. Gastro-intestinal side effects occurred in 7 per cent of the first of these series. Cantone et al (1969) claimed a 94 per cent cure rate in 176 patients. Cohen (1971) had similar results. In a second series Moffett et al (1971) found no significant therapeutic difference between nitromidazine and metronidazole. Evans and Catterall (1971), however, in a randomised double blind trial compared the two trichomonacides each in the dosage recommended. Nitromidazine cured 39 (68 per cent) of 57 patients while metronidazole cured 51 (89 per cent) of 57. One patient in each series had side effects. The authors concluded that in the recommended dosage nitromidazine is the inferior but it could be useful in patients who prove intolerant to metronidazole. McCann et al (1972) in a similar trial found, after a 3 months follow-up, a 78 per cent cure rate with nitromidazine compared with 90 per cent with metronidazole. A few patients failed to respond to both drugs. The subjects of *in vivo* and *in vitro* resistance as well as the possibility of cross-resistance of the two drugs were discussed by Benazet and Guillaume (1971) and De Carneri and Giannone (1971) in the correspondence columns of the Lancet.

A variety of other drugs have been tried in trichomoniasis. Evans and Catterall (1970) compared the nitrofuron derivative nifuratel (magmilor) in doses of 200 mg three times daily together with pessaries of the same (nightly, for 10 days as recommended) with the standard metronidazole regime. The cure rates were 38 and 85 per cent respectively. This was a much less favourable report than that submitted by Fowler and Hossain (1968) and that of Churcher and Evans (1969). These latter workers suggested that the drug may have masked gonorrhoea in five out of six patients.

There are reports on hamycin by Gangu and Anjaneyula (1966); on pimaricin by De Luca Brunori (1967) and paromomycin by Spitzbart and Wick (1966). Trichopal, a Russian product, was reported on by Potapnev (1968); a di-iodine derivative of oxyquinoline by Arnold

(1968) and a new chlorosulphonamide by Kurnatowska (1969). The latest report on a new drug comes from Singapore and is by Lean and Vengadasalam (1973). The new drug is α-chloromethyl-2-methyl-5-nitro-1-imidazole-ethanol. In a double blind trial with metronidazole there was little to choose between the two trichmonoacides. The numbers concerned were small.

The two main contenders for top trichomonacide have been tried in dosages different from those recommended originally. Campbell (1972) treated 100 women with nitromidazine, 1 g followed after 24 hours by another 1 g dose. The cure rate amongst the 80 patients attending for tests of cure was 91·3 per cent. Giving a third 1 g on the third day raised the cure rate to 97·1 per cent. Jones (1972) treated 195 women with trichomonal vaginitis with a single 2 g dose of nitrimidazine. Of the 159 who attended for follow-up 93·7 per cent were cured. Using a single dose of 1·5 g the cure rate was only 74·1 per cent.

Single dose use of metronidazole

Following reports of the successful treatment of uncomplicated amoeboiasis with a single 2 g dose of metronidazole this schedule was tried by Csonka (1971) in vaginal trichomoniasis. In a controlled trial 29 (82 per cent) of 36 assessed patients were cured, compared with 46 (94 per cent) of 49 treated with 200 mg three times per day for 7 days. Woodcock (1972) in a similar trial had cure rates of 85 and 87·3 per cent. He also tried another shortened regime. He treated 114 women with 400 mg four times per day for 2 days and compared the long term follow-up with that following the standard regime of 200 mg three times per day for 7 days. Recurrence rates at the end of 3 months were 22·7 and 19·1 per cent respectively. He found no evidence of therapeutic antagonism between tetracycline and metronidazole. Morton (1972) treated 16 infested males with a single 2 g dose. Of the 14 who had detailed follow-up tests all were cured. Morton's results in 138 female patients with a single 2 g dose of metronidazole were similar to those of other workers. He tried to differentiate treatment failures from reinfections and came to the conclusion that the true cure rate with a single 2 g dose of metronidazole may be around 90 per cent.

Forgan (1972) reviewed the history of treatment of trichomoniasis.

Coda

A wide variety of work remains to be done in trichomoniasis.

In diagnosis this is particularly true both at the culture level and at the clinic laboratory bench. How, for example, does dark-ground microscopy compare with other wet film examination techniques?

At the epidemiological level the question of neonatal infection requires attention. Polish claims go unconfirmed or unrefuted. And what about trichomoniasis and carcinoma of the cervix? This calls for a carefully planned study along the lines investigating the relationship between herpes genitalis and carcinoma, now being studied.

In how far does the genito-urinary anatomical anomaly, congenital or acquired, prompt treatment failure? Is trichomonal salpingitis a clinical entity? Just how often is so-called cystitis really trichomoniasis? These and other clinical questions still go unanswered.

In the laboratory field the specificity of immunofluorescence requires investigation as does the dynamics of antibody production.

REFERENCES

ACTOR, P., ZIV, D. S. and PACANO, J. F. (1969). *Science*, **46**, 439.
ARNOLD, M. (1968). *Praxis*, **57**, 1663.
AURE, J. and GJONNESSE, H. (1969). *Actor. Obstet. Gynex. Scand.*, **48**, 440.
BAKER, R. M. and KENNAN, A. L. (1967). *Wisconsin med. J.*, **66**, 370.
BENAZET, F. and GUILLAUME, L. (1971). *Lancet*, **2**, 982.
BEVERIDGE, M. M. (1964). *Brit. J. vener. Dis.*, **40**, 198.
BRIT. MED. J. (1966). Editorial, **1**, 907.
BRIT. MED. J. (1967). Editorial, **4**, 4.
CAMPBELL, A. C. H. (1972). *Brit. J. vener. Dis.* **48**, 531.
CANTONE, A. et al (1969). *Giov. mal. Infect. Parasit.*, **21**, 954.
CATTERALL, R. D. (1970). *Brit. J. vener. Dis.* **46**, 122.
CATTERALL, R. D. (1972). *N. Amer. Clin. vener. Dis.*, **56**, 1205.
CHURCHER, G. M. and EVANS, A. J. (1969). *Brit. J. vener. Dis.*, **45**, 149.
CLARK, J. F. J. and GEORGE, T. (1966). *J. nat. med. Ass.*, **58**, 464.
COHEN, L. (1971). *Brit. J. vener. Dis.*, **47**, 177.
COSAR, C. and JULOU, L. (1959). *Ann. Inst. Pasteur.*, **96**, 238.
CSONKA, G. W. (1971). *Brit. J. vener. Dis.*, **47**, 456.
DAVIS, A. H. (1967). *Brit. J. vener. Dis.*, **43**, 197.
DE CARNERI, I. (1966). *Lancet*, **1**, 1042.
DE CARNERI, I., ACHILLI, G., MONTI, G. and TRANE, F. (1969). *Lancet*, **2**, 1308.
DE CARNERI, I. and GIANNONE, R. (1971). *Lancet*, **2**, 1320.
DE LUCA BRUNORI, I. (1967). *Minerva Ginec.*, **18**, 840.
DIDDLE, A. W. (1967). *Amer. J. Obstet Gynec.*, **98**, 583.
DUREL, P., ROIRON, V., SIBOULET, A. and BOREL, L. J. (1960). *Brit. J. vener. Dis.*, **35**, 21.
EDWARD, D. I. and MATHISON, G. E. (1971). *J. gen. Microbiol.*, **63**, 297.
EMANUELI, A. and DE CARNERI, I. (1969). *Sixth International Congress of Chemotherapy*, Tokyo.
EVANS, B. A. and CATTERALL, R. D. (1970). *Brit. med. J.*, **1**, 335.
EVANS, B. A. and CATTERALL, R. D. (1971). *Brit. med. J.*, **4**, 146.
FAGIN, I. D. (1965). *J. Amer. med. Ass.*, **193**, 146.
FORGAN, R. (1972). *Brit. J. vener. Dis.*, **48**, 522.
FOWLER, W. and HOSSAIN, M. (1968). *Brit. J. vener. Dis.*, **44**, 331.
GANGU, D. and ANJANEYULA, R. (1966). *Hindustan. Antibiot. Bull.*, **9**, 69.
GARDNER, H. L. and DUKES, C. D. (1964). *Amer. J. Obstet. Gynec.*, **89**, 990.
GOBERT, J. G., GEORGES, P. and SAVEL, T. (1969). *Amer. Parasit. Hum. Comp.*, **44**, 687.
ILYIN, I. I., ROSTOVA, R. G. & PASECHINK, V. A. (1971). *Vestn. derm. vener.*, **45**, 74.
JONES, J. P. (1972). *Brit. J. vener. Dis.*, **48**, 528.
KEIGHLEY, E. E. (1971). *Brit. med. J.*, **1**, 207.

KORIK, L. M. (1971). *Vestn. derm. vener.*, **45**, 77.
KOVÁCS, E. and GALGÓCZY, J. (1969). *Orv. Hetil.*, **110**, 66.
KURNATOWSKA, A. (1969). *Wiad. Parazyt.*, **15**, 19 and 399.
LEAN, T. H. and VENGADASALAM, D. (1973). *Brit. J. vener. Dis.*, **49**, 69.
LEFEBURE, Y. and HESSELTINE, H. C. (1965). *J. Amer. med. Ass.*, **194**, 15.
LEWIS, B. V. and KENNA, A. P. (1965). *J. Obstet. Gynaec. Brit. Commonw.*, **72**, 806.
MCCANN, J. S., MAHONY, J. D. H. and HARRIS, J. R. W. (1972). *Brit. J. vener. Dis.*, **48**, 387.
MCFADZEAN, J. A., PUGH, I. M., SQUIRES, S. L. and WHELAN, J. P. F. (1969). *Brit. J. vener. Dis.*, **45**, 161.
MOFFETT, M. McGILL, M. I., SCHOFIELD, C. B. S. and MASTERTON, G. (1971). *Brit. J. vener. Dis.*, **47**, 173.
MORTON, R. S. (1972). *Brit. J. vener. Dis.*, **48**, 525.
NARANG, S. S., BHARGAVA, N. C., CHANAN, B. K., SESHAGIR, I. and RAO, M. (1964). *Indian J. Derm.*, **30**, 150.
NICOL, C. S., MCFADZEAN, J. A. and SQUIRES, S. L. (1960). *Lancet*, **1**, 1100.
NICOL, C. S. and EVANS, A. J. (1966). *Lancet*, **2**, 441.
OLLER, L. Z. (1969). *Brit. J. vener. Dis.*, **45**, 163.
PARAPAKKHAM, S. (1967). *Obstet. Gynec., N.Y.*, **29**, 213.
PARKER, R. T., THOMAS, W. L. and JONES, C. P. (1965). *Sth. med. J.*, **58**, 211.
PEREYRA, A. J. and LANSING, D. (1964). *Obstet. Gynec., N.Y.*, **24**, 499.
PETERSON, W. F., STAUCH, J. E. and RYDER, C. D. (1966). *Amer. J. Obstet. Gynec.*, **94**, 343.
POTAPNEV, F. V. (1968). *Ver. V. derm. venor.*, **42**, 55.
POWELL, S. J. (1967). *Amer. J. Trop. Med.*, **16**, 447.
ROBINSON, S. C. and MIRCHANDANI, G. (1965). *Hygiene*, **16**, 447.
RODIN, P. and HASS, G. (1966). *Brit. J. vener. Dis.*, **42**, 210.
SCOTT-GRAY, M. (1964). *J. Obstet. Gynec. Brit. Commonw.*, **71**, 82.
SEARLE PRODUCTS (1966).
SHKLYAR, I. I. (1967). *Vestn. derm. vener.*, **41**, 67.
SPITZBART, H. and WICK, I. (1966). *Zbl. Gynäk.*, **88**, 563.
SZANTO, S. (1971). *Brit. med. J.*, **2**, 467.
TEOKHAROV, B. A. and ANIKIN, A. F. (1967). *Vestn. Avn. vener.*, **4**, 52.
VALENT, M., ČATÁR, G. and JANOŠKA, A. (1969). *Bratisl. Lek. Listy*, **52**, 58.
WILKINSON, A. E., RODIN, P., MCFADZEAN, J. A. and SQUIRES, S. (1967). *Brit. J. vener. Dis.*, **43**, 20.
WOODCOCK, K. R. (1972). *Brit. J. vener. Dis.*, **48**, 65.
YOBS, A. R., CLARK, J. W. JR., SCHROETER, A. L. and POST, W. (1966). *Brit. J. vener. Dis.*, **42**, 122.

Part 5
Candidiasis

22 Introduction, Epidemiology and Social Aspects

J. R. W. Harris

Introduction

Catterall (1971) and Oriel et al (1972) found that *C. albicans* was the commonest infectious agent isolated from female patients attending units for the diagnosis of sexually transmitted disease. This underlines the importance of these organisms to the physicians concerned with the management of such patients.

Organisms belonging to the genus Candida can be sexually transmitted. This was reported as long ago as 1920 by Sigman and was corroborated by Odland and Hoffstaedt (1929). Waisman (1954) pointed out that the candidal infection of the male sexual partner was frequently undiagnosed. Catterall (1966) differentiated between candidal balano-posthitis and balano-posthitis due to hypersensitivity to vaginal candidiasis in the sexual partner. Rohatiner (1966) observed that six out of 28 male consorts of female patients with genital candidiasis were infected with candida organisms. Gilpin (1967) examined the semen from the sexual contacts of women with 'resistant' candidiasis and reported that Candida species were cultured from a high percentage of semen samples. Spitzbart (1968) noted that 18·5 per cent of female patients with candidiasis were initially treatment failures. Only when the husband was also treated did the symptoms subside. Gardner and Kaufman (1969) feel that men are more likely to be recipients than donors of candidal infection. However, they believe that on occasions infection of the male genitalia constitutes a reservoir of reinfection for the sexual partner. Oriel et al (1972) observed that five out of 48 men, who were sexual contacts of women with vaginal yeast infections were found to have mycotic balano-posthitis. Diddle et al (1969) in their series noted that over 10 per cent of the male sexual contacts had candidal balano-posthitis.

REFERENCES

CATTERALL, R. D. (1971). *Brit. J. vener. Dis.*, **47**, 45.

CATTERALL, R. D. (1966). *Lancet* ii, 830.

DIDDLE, A. W., GARDNER, W. H., WILLIAMSON, P. J. and O'CONNOR, K. A. (1969). *Obstet. Gynec.*, **34**, 373.

GARDNER, H. L. and KAUFMAN, R. H. (1969). In 'Benign Diseases of the Vulva Vagina,' 1st ed., pp. 149–167. Mosby, St. Louis.

GILPIN, C. A. (1967). *J. Fla. med. Ass.*, **54**, 337.

ODLAND, H. and HOFFSTAEDT, R. E. (1929). *Arch. Derm. Syph.*, **20**, 335

ORIEL, J. D., PARTRIDGE, B. M., DENNY, M. J. and COLEMAN, J. C. (1972). *Brit. med. J.*, iv, 761.

ROHATINER, J. J. (1966). *Brit. J. vener. Dis.*, **42**, 197.

SPITZBART, H. (1968). *Mykosen*, **II**, 617.

WAISMAN, M. (1954). *Arch. Derm. Syph.*, **70**, 718.

Epidemiology

Infection by Candida species is almost worldwide. The probable association with diets high in fruit and carbohydrate indicate some differences in the frequency of its presence in the intestinal tract of man, in different climatic zones and varied social or economic circumstances (Emmonds et al 1970).

Since mycotic agents are actual or potential pathogens in the genital tract there have been many studies of their distribution in various population groups. These studies frequently give conflicting reports. The correlation of the results is even more confused since various workers have investigated the relative incidences of the different members of the Candida genus. Mrozowski and Thiery (1967) found that while *C. albicans* predominates, *C. krusei* and *C. stellatoidea* were also cultured regularly from genital lesions. Garrido et al (1969) isolated *C. albicans* in 80 per cent of cases and noted that *C. krusei* and *C. parapsilosis* were also common offenders. Giardinelli and Tinetti (1968) while agreeing that *C. albicans* was the most common member of the Candida genus isolated, felt that a similar clinical and symptomatic picture was frequently produced by *Torulopris glabrata*. Gardner and Kaufman (1969) commonly found two species of Candida in the same patient and believed that *C. tropicalis* was more likely to be associated with chronicity and recurrences than *C. albicans*. It is obvious from these reported incidences that there is a geographical variation in the species of Candida producing genital candidiasis. This is not unexpected in view of the importance of diet, climatic and host factors involved. Two recent studies from London by Oriel et al (1972) and Hurley et al (1973) have shown close agreement in the types and isolation rates for yeast species in the vagina of patients attending venereology and ante-natal units. Both groups found *C. albicans* to be the predominant species of Candida isolated and *T. glabrata* to be the fungus next most commonly found.

Obviously many of the series regarding the incidence of genital candidiasis are not directly comparable as the workers involved used different diagnostic criteria. Nevertheless the work of certain groups is comparable. Anyon et al (1971) reported on the prevalence of Candida in the vagina of individuals in an urban community in New Zealand. They isolated Candida in 19·3 per cent of cases. Morris (1969) isolated Candida from 13·5 per cent of female patients attending for their initial examination at a Bristol family planning clinic. Rohatiner (1966) from Guy's Hospital, London, isolated Candida from the vagina and cervix of 29 per cent of patients. Oriel et al (1972) isolated Candida in 26 per cent of patients attending St. Thomas' Hospital, London. Pedersen (1969) found that Candida could be isolated from 11 per cent of patients on the seventh day post-partum.

It has been a long-established fact that the prevalence of genital candidal infection increases in pregnancy. Gardner and Kaufman (1969) emphasise that this rate increases as pregnancy progresses. Thus no two series will be completely comparable as the patients will have been seen at differing stages of pregnancy. Pedersen (1969) isolated Candida from the vagina of 32 per cent of pregnant women, while Garrido and his colleagues (1969) cultured the genus from 46·5 per cent of pregnant women. Carroll et al (1973) in a prospective study of 303 women found an incidence of only 16·5 per cent.

Species of Candida are recovered frequently from the stools, oral cavity, nails and intertriginous areas. De Sousa and van Uden (1960) found that of 55 women whose vaginal cultures were positive for *C. albicans* 75 per cent harboured the organism in the faeces, while only 25 per cent of normal females had positive faecal cultures. Rohatiner (1966) noted that 48 per cent of patients with vaginal candidiasis had positive rectal cultures. Anyon et al (1971) found that 17·2 per cent of patients in an urban community in New Zealand had positive rectal cultures and Pedersen (1969) isolated the organism from the rectum in 69 per cent of pregnant women. These observations indicate the importance of the rectum as a potential source of infection. Gardner and Kaufman (1969) feel that the oral cavity could be an important source of infection depending on the sexual habits of the patient.

REFERENCES

ANYON, C. P., DESMOND, F. B. and EASTCOTT, D. F. (1971). *N.Z. med. J.*, **73**, 9.
CARROLL, C. J., HURLEY, R. and STANLEY, V. C. (1973). *J. Obstet. Gynaec. Brit. Comm.*, **80**, 258.
EMMONDS, C. W., BINFORD, C. H. and UTZ, J. P. (1970). In 'Medical Mycology', 2nd ed., p. 177, Lea and Feibiger, Philadelphia.
GARDNER, H. L. and KAUFAMN, R. H. (1969). In: 'Benign Diseases of the Vulva and Vagina', 1st ed., pp. 149–167, Mosby, St. Louis.
GARRIDO, R. N., BARROETA, S. and DE MONTILVA, A. (1969). *Mycopathologia, Den Haag*, **37**, 39.

GIARDINELLI, M. and TINETTI, E. (1968). *Minerva Ginec.*, **20**, 709.

HURLEY, R., LEASK, B. G. S., FAKTOR, J. A. and DE FONSEKA, I. (1973). *J. Obstet. Gynaec. Brit. Comm.*, **80**, 252.

MROZOWSKI, J. and THIERY, M. (1967). *Bull. Soc. roy. Belge. Gynéc. Obstét.*, **37**, 225.

MORRIS, C. A. (1969). *J. clin. Path.*, **22**, 488.

ORIEL, J. D., PARTRIDGE, B. M., DENNY, M. J. and COLEMAN, J. C. (1972). *Brit. med. J.*, iv, 761.

PEDERSEN, G. T. (1969). *Dan. med. Bull.*, **16**, 207.

ROHATINER, J. J. (1966). *Brit. J. vener. Dis.*, **42**, 197.

DE SOUSA, H. M. and VAN UDEN, N. (1960). *Amer. J. Obst. Gynec.*, **80**, 1096.

23 Predisposing Factors

J. R. W. Harris

More than the mere presence of Candida is necessary for development of the clinical disease. It would appear that the host factors controlling susceptibility are of importance. These have been summarised by Catterall (1971). In early infancy and during pregnancy physiological factors predispose towards candidiasis. In some patients low renal threshold for glucose results in glycosuria. Climatic factors, obesity and maceration provide ideal growth conditions. Certain endocrine disorders are associated with both superficial and systemic infections. This has been observed with diabetes mellitus, hypoparathyroidism, hypothyroidism, Addison's disease and pancreatitis. Candidiasis frequently accompanies malnutrition and debilitation. It can be a severe and fatal complication in a patient whose resistance has been reduced because of chronic disease or its treatment. It may appear as a late infection in patients in the last stages of a terminal illness. The alteration in role from commensal to pathogen frequently occurs following therapy with antibiotics, corticosteroids and anti-trichomonal agents. There has been controversy over the predisposing role of oral contraceptives.

Pregnancy is one of the most common predisposing factors. The high hormone levels lead to a pronounced increase in the glycogen content of the vagina producing a favourable environment for the growth of the Candida genus. While many believe that Candida frequently behaves as a commensal in these conditions, Beare et al (1968), Bourg (1964) and Carroll et al (1973) feel that the isolation of C. albicans from the vagina of pregnant women indicates a need for specific antifungal therapy. Janovski and Douglas (1973) advise scrupulous hygiene of the vulva as preventative measure and also feel that treatment is essential in the presence of fungal infection. Undoubtedly the reduced glucose tolerance and increased incidence of glycosuria renders some patients more susceptible. Pedersen (1969) demonstrated the rapid decrease in vulvo-vaginal candidal infection following delivery when he noted that only 11 per cent of patients had positive vaginal cultures on the seventh day post-partum, as opposed to 42 per cent in the last trimester. This is to be expected from the precipitous drop in oestrogen and progesterone levels after delivery. The use of large doses of oestrogen to inhibit engorgement of the breasts can alter the post-partum sequence of events.

The use of antibiotics is clearly related to the prevalence and severity of candidal infections (Seelig, 1966a). Several theories have been advanced to explain this (Seelig, 1966b). Some workers believe that the organisms multiply more rapidly because of the reduction in bacterial competition, or that the antibiotic alters the host immunological mechanisms. Loh and Baker (1955) reported increases of 1 000-fold in intestinal Candida among patients who were taking oxytetracycline and chlortetracycline. Silverman and Okun (1971) showed that these stool counts could be significantly reduced if the patient took oxytetracycline and nystatin concurrently as opposed to oxytetracycline alone. Meneghini et al (1966) noted that 7–8 per cent of 5 000 patients who had been treated with antibiotics had evidence of balano-posthitis or vulvo-vaginitis due to *C. albicans*. They felt that antibiotic treatment given to susceptible patients greatly increased the possibility of candidiasis.

There was some controversy as to whether metronidazole therapy predisposed to candidal infection. Keighley (1962), Beveridge (1962) and Csonka (1963) were all of the opinion that there was an increased rate of candidiasis among patients treated with this drug. Rees (1960) and Rodin et al (1960) had previously stated that this did not happen. Oller (1969) observed that patients treated with metronidazole and concurrent amphotericin B pessaries were less likely to develop infection with candida species than those treated with metronidazole alone.

Winner and Hurley (1964) established the association between candidiasis and abnormal metabolic states especially steroid imbalance. Many investigators would agree that systemic corticosteroid therapy reduces the host resistance to candidal infection. Thompson (1966) showed in laboratory studies the susceptibility of animals to infection with Candida is increased after corticosteroid therapy. Yet at the same time, some workers believe that topical corticosteroid does not have an adverse effect on vulvo-vaginal candidiasis (Gardner and Kaufman, 1969). Obviously the full implications of the relationship between corticosteroids and candidiasis are not yet fully understood. Several of the diseases in which there are therapeutic indications for corticosteroid therapy may themselves predispose towards infection with the organisms.

Bourg (1964) suggested that progestational steroids, by causing changes similar to those in pregnancy, might be responsible for an increased incidence of candidiasis among patients taking oral contraceptives. Francis (1964), Yaffee and Grots (1965), Catterall (1966a), Porter and Lyle (1966) and Walsh et al (1968) also felt that there was an increased incidence of candidiasis among women taking oral contraceptives. However, Grimble (1966), Rohatiner and Grimble (1967) and Morris (1969) were unable to confirm these observations. Jackson and Spain (1968) felt that the type of oral contraceptive being used was significant. They found the chances of a patient having vaginal candidiasis were significantly less among those using a sequential regimen than among those using a combination regimen. Gardner and Kaufman (1969) were not entirely in agreement with this view while Diddle et al (1969) believed that the incidence of candidiasis was not related to the type of oral contraceptive used. Rohatiner and Grimble (1970) in their paper stated that the majority of workers were of the opinion that the incidence of candidal vulvo-vaginitis is no greater in women who take oral contraceptives than in those who do not. They believe that in the combined type of oral contraceptive the dose of oestrogen or convertible progesterone is more important than the relative amounts. Catterall (1971) concluded that a review of the literature indicated a probable relationship between the use of gestogenic contraceptive pills and the development of candidiasis. Spellacy et al (1971) carried out a cross-sectional prospective study to determine the relationship between combined and sequential type oral contraceptives and vaginal candidiasis. While the results showed an increased incidence of Candida on culture from patients on combination type oral contraceptives relative to both patients on sequential type drugs and patients with intrauterine devices, the differences were not of statistical significance. Oriel et al (1972) cultured *C. albicans* from 29 per cent of patients taking oral contraceptives and 14·5 per cent of patients who were not using such medication. Dugois et al (1971) were not convinced that oral contraceptives increased the incidence of genital candidiasis but postulated that oestrogen/progesterone preparations increased the virulence of *C. albicans* through pseudogestational changes induced in the vaginal epithelium. Oriel et al (1972) while noting the increase in the occurrence of *C. albicans* in the general tract of patients on oral contraceptives did not observe an increase in the signs and symptoms of genital infection. This is in complete variance with the views expressed by Dugois and his colleagues (1971).

Oral contraceptives generally promote changes similar to those seen in the luteal phase of the menstrual cycle and in early pregnancy. Javier et al (1968) observed that the fasting blood sugar was raised and the glucose tolerance decreased in 40 per cent of patients. Taft et al (1969) concluded that the impairment in carbohydrate tolerance was due to oestrogens alone. They did not observe an exaggerated insulin response to glucose in patients taking tablets containing only a low dose of progestogen. Wynn (1969) noted that progestogens derived from 19-norsteroids may be partly metabolised into oestrogens. Plasma cortisol levels were elevated to levels comparable with those observed in late pregnancy in patients who were on the combined type of oral contraceptive (Daly et al 1969). Assuming that oral contraceptives affect glycogen metabolism sufficiently to result in increased susceptibility to Candia infection such an effect will depend either on the total amount of corticosteroid present or on the relative amounts of oestrogen. This oestrogen can either be ingested or metabolised from 19-norsteroid. The degree of this susceptibility is more marked in certain individuals. These, according to Spellacy (1969), appear to be women of older age, high parity, with a positive family history of diabetes mellitus who have delivered large infants, and who gain excessive weight while taking the drugs.

Kudelko (1971) published a very interesting paper on chronic candidal vaginitis. He studied a group of 70 patients who had had unsatisfactory results on conventional therapy. These women were evaluated to find evidence for an allergic diathesis. *C. albicans* allergens were included in the hyposensitisation injections and 63 patients had both subjective and objective improvement. He advocates that specific hyposensitisation may be indicated in certain patients with resistant genital candidiasis.

REFERENCES

BEARE, J. M., GENTLES, J. C. and MACKENZIE, W. R. (1968). In: 'Textbook of Dermatology', 1st ed., p. 872, Blackwell, Oxford and Edinburgh.
BEVERIDGE, M. M. (1962). *Brit. J. vener. Dis.*, **38**, 220.
BOURG, R. (1964). *Bull. Soc. roy. belge Gynéc Obstét.* **34**, 97.
CARROLL, C. J., HURLEY, R. and STANLEY, V. C. (1973). *J. Obstet. Gynaec. Brit. Comm.*, **80**, 258.
CATTERALL, R. D. (1966a). *Lancet*, ii, 830.
CATTERALL, R. D. (1971). *Brit. J. vener. Dis.*, **47**, 45.
CSONKA, G. W. (1963). *Brit. J. vener. Dis.*, **39**, 258.
DALY, J. R., ELSTEIN, M. and MURRAY, J. (1969). In: 'Chlormadinone Acetate', p. 63, Symposium held in Cambridge, 1968. Excerpta Medical Foundation.
DIDDLE, A. W., GARDNER, W. H., WILLIAMSON, P. J. and O'CONNOR, K. A. (1969). *Obstet. Gynec.*, **34**, 373.
DUGOIS, P., AMBLARD, P., MANENT, J. and DE BIGNICOURT, B. (1971). *Sem. Hop, Paris*, **47**, 2803.
FRANCIS, W. G. (1964). *Arch. App. Ther.*, **6**, 523.
GARDNER, H. L. and KAUFMAN, R. H. (1969). In: 'Benign Diseases of the Vulva and Vagina', 1st ed., pp. 149–167. Mosby, St. Louis.
GRIMBLE, A. (1966). *Lancet*, ii, 1029.
JACKSON, J. L. and SPAIN, W. T. (1968), *Amer. J. Obst. Gynec.*, **101**, 1134.
JANOVSKI, N. A. and DOUGLAS, C. P. (1973). In: 'Diseases of the Vulva', 1st ed., p. 109. Haper and Row, London.
JAVIER, Z., GERSHBERG, H. and HULSE, M. (1968). *Metabolism*, **17**, 443.
KEIGHLEY, E. E. (1962). *Brit. med. J.*, ii, 93.
KUDELKO, N. M. (1971). *Ann. Allergy*, **29**, 266.
LOH, W. P. and BAKER, E. E. (1955). *Arch. intern. Med.*, **95**, 74.
MENEGHINI, C. L., COZZA, G. and GHISLANZONI, G. (1966). *Derm. Int.*, **5**, 163.
MORRIS, C. A. (1969). *J. clin. Path.*, **22**, 488.
OLLER, L. Z. (1969). *Brit. J. vener. Dis.*, **45**, 163.
ORIEL, J. D., PARTRIDGE, B. M., DENNY, M. J. and COLEMAN, J. C. (1972). *Brit. med. J.*, iv, 761.

PEDERSON, G. T. (1969). *Dan. med. Bull.*, **16**, 207.

PORTER, P. S. and LYLE, J. S. (1966). *Arch. Derm.*, **93**, 402.

REES, E. (1960). *Brit. med. J.*, ii, 906.

RODIN, P., KING, A. J., NICOL, C. S. and BARROW, J. (1960). *Brit. J. vener. Dis.*, **36**, 147.

ROHATINER, J. J. and GRIMBLE, A. (1967). *J. Obstet. Gynaec. Brit. Comm.*, **74**, 575.

ROHATINER, J. J. and GRIMBLE, A. (1970). *J. Obstet. Gynaec. Brit. Comm.* **77**, 1013.

SEELIG, M. S. (1966a). *Amer. J. Med.*, **40**, 887.

SEELIG, M. S. (1966b). *Bact. Rev.*, **30**, 442.

SILVERMAN, A. G. and OKUN, R. (1971). *Amer. J. obstet. Gynaec.*, **111**, 398.

SPELLACY, W. N., ZAIAS, N., BUHI, W. C. and BIRK, S. A. (1971). *Obstet. Gynec.*, **38**, 343.

SPELLACY, W. N. (1969). In: 'Metabolic Effects of Gonadal Hormones and Contraceptive Steroids', p. 126, Plenum, London.

TAFT, P., WINIKOFF, D., TAYLOR, K. and PAGE, D. (1969). In: 'Chloramadinone Acetate', p. 60. Symposium held in Cambridge, 1968. Excerpta Medical Foundation.

THOMPSON, R. E. M. (1966). 'Symposium on Candida Infections', p. 68, Livingstone, Edinburgh and London.

WALSH, W., HILDEBRANT, R. J. and PRYSTOWSKY, H. (1968). *Amer. J. Obstet. Gynec.*, **101**, 991.

WINNER, H. I. and HURLEY, R. (1964). 'Candida Albicans', pp. 74, 135. Churchill, London.

WYNN, V. and DOAR, J. W. H. (1969). In: 'Metabolic Effects of Gonadal Hormones and Contraceptive Steroids, p. 157. Plenum, New York.

YAFFEE, H. S. and GROTS, I. (1965). *New Engl. J. Med.*, **272**, 647.

24 Clinical Aspects

J. R. W. Harris

In the male the glans penis, prepuce and urethra can be infected with *C. albicans*. Genito-crural candidiasis also occurs and several workers have noted hypersensitivity or toxic reactions of the glans penis following intercourse with patients who have vulvo-vaginal candidiasis. Perianal candidal infection is usually secondary to broad spectrum antibiotic therapy but can also occur in susceptible persons and is occasionally observed in homosexual patients.

Urethritis in the male due to *C. albicans* is a relatively uncommon occurrence. It has been reported by Castellani (1962), Siboulet (1963), Catterall (1966b), Rohatiner (1966) and Parker (1970). Catterall (1966b) noted that symptoms were often mild and the condition was asymptomatic. Urethral discharge, dysuria, frequency and pruritus at the external meatus or along the urethra were the most frequent complaints. Balano-posthitis occurs in uncircumcised males, the most frequent symptom being soreness at the tip of the penis associated with pruritus. Patients will sometimes notice discharge from underneath the prepuce and believe that this is a urethral discharge. Occasionally the patient is unable to retract the foreskin due to phimosis. The main symptom of both intertriginous and perianal candidiasis is pruritus (Blaylock et al, 1971). Catterall (1966b) felt that the incubation period was probably between 5 and 21 days.

Forman (1966) observed that patients who had been in contact with individuals suffering from genital candidiasis had on occasions noticed low-grade dermatitis of the penis. Scrapings and cultures from these lesions showed no candidal organisms and he felt that this phenomenon was due either to the instant toxic action of the Candida or possibly to a specific sensitivity. Catterall (1966) reported that four patients complained of soreness and ulceration of the glans penis commencing from 6 to 24 hours after intercourse. He postulated that this was a hypersensitivity phenomenon.

On examination Catterall (1966) noted that the urethritis was usually subacute and that the discharge was small in amount. Frequently it was necessary to take an early morning smear and culture to make the diagnosis. Both he and Siboulet (1963) observed that a number of patients had had the urethritis for some considerable time. The candidal balanitis can be erosive, membranous or consist of erythematous plaques studded with small pustules. If it is erosive there is frequently associated oedema of the prepuce. In severe cases the entire mucous membrane surface is covered with a confluent white cheesy material on an underlying red base. The intertriginous candidiasis is seen on opposing surfaces of the scrotum and thighs. It is characterised by an early vesicular or pustular eruption. The centre of the lesion is well defined, the borders are round, extension is peripheral and there is usually scaling at the border. The patch may be rimmed by satellite lesions. Perianal candidiasis appears as a white, macerated, confluent area which is on occasions fissured and frequently there are secondary excoriation marks (Blaylock et al, 1971). The patients believed to have a hypersensitivity reaction had multiple small circular erosions of the glans penis unassociated with oedema (Catterall, 1966).

Pruritus of the vulva is the cardinal symptom of *C. albicans* in the female. It varies in degree from patient to patient but can be slight or intolerable preventing the patient resting or working (Dewhurst, 1972). It is more severe at night. Gardner and Kaufman (1969) have noted that burning is a common complaint. This is more marked after micturition and may be related to the urine coming in contact with the inflamed vulva. They call this 'vulvular dysuria'. Both the patient and the clinician may interpret this symptom as being due to cystitis. Barr (1971) notes that dysparunia is a frequent complaint and patients also notice burning and itching immediately after intercourse. Certain workers have believed that this is an allergic reaction to candidal organisms in the ejaculate. Some patients notice excessive vaginal discharge while others complain of dryness.

The clinical spectrum is varied and may be altered if the patient is pregnant or has already been partially treated. Gardner and Kaufman (1969) believe that erythema of the vulva is the most common clinical finding in female genital candidiasis. This may be localised to the mucocutaneous surface between the labia minora or may extend on to the labia majora, perineum and perianal tissues. Involvement of a larger area is uncommon unless the patient is pregnant, obese or has a predisposing factor such as diabetes. Cutaneous vesicopustules or satellite lesions rarely occur in the uncomplicated case. Oedema of the labia minora occurs on occasions although this is a much more common finding in the pregnant patient (Janovski and Douglas, 1973). If pruritus has been severe, excoriations and abrasions may be found between the labia minora and majora. The patient may have received some medication before examination. Frequently this is some preparation containing topical corticosteroids. These tend to alleviate the pruritus and to alter, to some extent, the clinical picture. Lichen simplex and lichenification occurs in patients with chronic candidiasis. On the labia majora thickening is apparent and pigmentation is common. On the labia minora the lesions have a greyish-white appearance and may be diffuse or localised with associated thickening of the tissues (Wilkinson, 1968).

In the pregnant patient the vaginal discharge will be white or yellow and contain curds. Plaques, which are usually white, are loosely adherent to the vaginal wall (Dewhurst, 1972). These plaques vary in size, number and physical characteristics. Janovski and Douglas (1973) note that when the plaques are removed the underlying vaginal wall shows marked erythema with tiny superficial ulcers. Carroll et al (1973) believe, as a result of their investigations, that the clinical diagnosis of genital candidiasis in pregnancy can be firmly based on the presence of such plaques. Gardner and Kaufman (1969) feel that vaginal secretions containing Candida in most non-pregnant women are essentially normal in consistency, colour, volume and odour. They only found typical vaginal plaques in 20 per cent of non-pregnant patients. This would be the experience of many other workers in the field (Nicol, 1971; Oriel et al, 1972). Occasionally the vagina may be partially covered by a grey pseudo-membrane (Emmonds et al, 1970).

REFERENCES

BARR, W. (1971). In 'Clinical Gynaecology', 1st ed., p. 59, Churchill Livingstone, Edinburgh and London.

BLAYLOCK, W. K., SHADOMY, H. J. and SHADOMY, S. (1971). In 'Dermatology in General Medicine', 1st ed., p. 1791, McGraw-Hill, New York.

CARROLL, C. J., HURLEY, R. and STANLEY, V. C. (1973). *J. Obstet. Gynaec. Brit. Comm.*, **80**, 258.

CASTELLANI, A. (1962). *Ann. N.Y. Acad. Sic.*, **93**, 162.

CATTERALL, R. D. (1966). 'Symposium on Candida Infections', p. 113, Livingstone, Edinburgh and London.

DEWHURST, C. J. (1972). In: 'Integrated Obstetrics, and Gynaecology for Postgraduated', 1st ed., p. 580. Blackwell, Oxford and London.

EMMONDS, C. W., BINFORD, C. H. and UTZ, J. P. (1970). 'Medical Mycology', 2nd ed., p. 177. Lea and Feibiger, Philadelphia.

FORMAN, L. (1966). In: 'Symposium on Candida Infections', p. 117. Livingstone, Edinburgh and London.

GARDNER, H. L. and KAUFMAN, R. H. (1969). In: 'Benign Diseases of the Vulva and Vagina', 1st ed. pp. 149–167. Mosby, St. Louis.

JANOVSKI, N. A. and DOUGLAS, C. P. (1973). In: 'Diseases of the Vulva', 1st ed., p. 109. Harper and Row, London.

NICOL, C. S. (1971). *Brit. med. J.*, ii, 507.

ORIEL, J. D., PARTRIDGE, B. M., DENNY, M. J. and COLEMAN, J. C. (1972). *Brit. med. J.*, iv, 761.

PARKER, J. D. T. (1970). *Brit. J. vener. Dis.*, **46**, 43.

ROHATINER, J. J. (1966). *Brit. J. vener. Dis.*, **42**, 197.

SIBOULET, A. (1963). *Presse med.*, **71**, 2779.

25 Laboratory Aspects

J. R. W. Harris

It is apparent from the clinical descriptions above that a firm diagnosis of genital candidiasis cannot be made from consideration of the symptoms and signs alone. Whitehouse and Porteous (1962) advised that the female patient who is not pregnant should be examined during the pre-menstrual phase as the specimens taken at this time are most likely to demonstrate the fungus. Catterall (1966, 1970) advised repeated examinations of both male and female patients and Oriel et al (1972) remarked that the patients with the most florid clinical manifestations frequently showed evidence of candidiasis only on culture. In the clinic situation specimens can be examined either by wet mount preparation, potassium hydroxide preparation or by staining. Peeters et al (1970) feel that none of these methods is sufficiently reliable and that the diagnosis must be established by the mycological laboratory. Eddie (1968) noted that only half of the patients who yielded candidal organisms on culture showed organisms on direct microscopy. Becker and Schweisfurth (1971) found that 60 per cent of the infections were diagnosed on culture alone. The potassium hydroxide preparation is widely used in dermatology but is little used in departments for sexually transmitted diseases. Gardner and Kaufman (1969) feel that this is the most efficient method for the rapid diagnosis of candidiasis. Wet mount preparations must be relatively thin and the egg-shaped budding yeast cells can be confused with the nuclei of epithelial cells or obscured by excessive vaginal debris. In Gram-stained films the spores are strongly Gram-positive and the hyphae have large Gram-positive granules. However, they can be so overstained or so shrunken that they are difficult to identify (Emmonds et al 1970).

Specimens for culture should be taken from the vulva, vagina, cervix, perianal area and where appropriate the oral cavity. Emmonds et al (1970) suggest that specimens for culture should be inoculated on to Sabouraud's modified agar medium with chloramphenicol and incubated at either 30°C or room temperature. If two or more species of Candida are present they should be separated before any specific

243

identification is attempted. Species identification by Oriel et al (1972) and Hurley et al (1973), using the techniques formalised by Lodder and Kreger-van Rij (1952) and reviewed by Lodder (1970) can be carried out if desired. Initial testing for germ tube production in inoculated horse serum and mycelium formation and chlamydospore production in corn meal agar, is followed by fermentation tests using carbon and nitrogen auxanograms. Denny and Partridge (1968) have recently found growth and colour change on triphenyltetrazolium chloride medium to be of value. Cacciapuoti et al (1969) published an alternative method of sugar fermentation which they believed reduced the laboratory time for the identification of the various members of the genus Candida. Fribourg-Blanc (1970) found that direct fluorescent antibody technique was as efficient as flazo orange dye to suppress non-specific fluorescence. A total of 700 specimens were investigated and compared. Both direct fluorescent antibody technique and culture were superior to examination of wet mount preparation or Gram-staining. As many normal individuals are hypersensitive or have agglutinins to Candida antigens, the presence of antibodies may relate to present or past illness or to superficial colonisation of a commensal nature. Hence cutaneous and serological tests are not specific enough or sufficiently related to a present illness to be useful in the diagnosis of candidiasis (Emmonds et al, 1970). Rohatiner and Grimble (1967) reviewed serological tests in the diagnosis of genital candidiasis and came to the conclusion that flocculation, agglutination and precipitation tests were of little value but that there was a correlation between the presence of genital candidiasis and significantly positive titres on fluorescent testing (Vogel and Padula, 1958). However, Lehner (1970) found no correlation between fluorescent antibody titre of a particular immunoglobulin class and the corresponding immunoglobulin concentration and Taschdjian et al (1972) found fluorescent antibody titres ranging from 0 to 1 : 320 in patients who were free of candidal infection.

REFERENCES

BECKER, H. and SCHWEISFURTH, R. (1971). *Mykosen,* **14**, 127.

CACCIAPUOTI, B., BORRE, E. and RIGOLI, E. (1969). *Ann. Inst. Sup. Sanit.,* **5**, 54.

CATTERALL, R. D. (1966). 'Symposium on Candida Infections', p. 113. Livingstone, Edinburgh and London.

CATTERALL, R. D. (1970). *Brit. J. vener. Dis.,* **46**, 122.

DENNY, M. J. and PARTRIDGE, B. M. (1968). *J. clin. Path.,* **21**, 383.

EDDIE, D. A. S. (1968). *J. med. Microbiol.,* **1**, 153.

EMMONDS, C. W., BINFORD, C. H. and UTZ, J. P. (1970). 'Medical Mycology', 2nd ed., p. 177. Lea and Feibiger, Philadelphia.

FRIBOURG-BLANC, A. (1970). *Ann. Biol. Clin.,* **28**, 269.

GARDNER, H. L. and KAUFMAN, R. H. (1969). In: 'Benign Diseases of the Vulva and Vagina', 1st ed., pp. 149–167. Mosby, St. Louis.

HURLEY, R., LEASK, BG. S., FAKTOR, J. A. and DE FONSEKA, I. (1973). *J. Obstet. Gynaec., Brit. Comm.*, **80**, 252.

LEHNER, T. (1970). *J. med. Microbiol.*, **3**, 475.

LODDER, J. and KREGER-VAN RIJ, N. J. W. (1952). In: 'The Yeasts: A Taxonomic Study', p. 459. N. Holland Pub., Amsterdam.

LODDER, J. (ed.) (1970). 'The Yeasts'. N. Holland Pub., Amsterdam.

ORIEL, J. D., PARTREIDGE, B. M., DENNY, M. J. and COLEMAN, J. C. (1972). *Brit. med. J.*, iv, 761.

PEETERS, H., GANTOIS, A. and SOETEWAY, F. (1970). *Ned. T. Geneesk*, **114**, 1401.

ROHATINER, J. J. and GRIMBLE, A. (1967). *J. Obstet. Gynaec. Brit. Comm.*, **74**, 575.

TASCHDJIAN, C. L., KOZINN, P. J., GUESTA, M. B. and TONI, E. F. (1972). *Amer. J. clin. Path.*, **57**, 195.

VOGEL, Z. A. and PADULA, J. F. (1958). *Proc. Soc. exp. Biol., N.Y.*, **98**, 135.

WHITEHOUSE, W. L. and PORTEOUS, C. R. (1962). *Lancet*, i, 506.

26 Therapy

J. R. W. Harris

The initial treatment following diagnosis is local application of nystatin compounds, symptomatic therapy and examination and treatment of the sexual partner. Patients should be questioned and investigated as necessary for any predisposing factor, and should be treated if possible. Those who have recurrent or chronic candidiasis will require special management.

The urethritis due to candidal organisms was treated by Catterall (1966) with urethral instillation of antifungal agents. He used a suspension of nystatin 100 000 units per ml and found equally satisfactory results using phenylmercuric disulphonate (Penotrane) urethral jelly at regular intervals for 2 weeks. Parker (1970) found that urethral instillation with amphotericin B (Fungizone) on two occasions was satisfactory. He used a suspension of 12·5 mg of the powder in 5 ml sterile water and 2·5 ml 5 per cent dextrose solution. Tests for cure were carried out by both workers using stained films and cultures following treatment.

Candidal balano-posthitis responds to careful washing of the external genitalia twice daily with soap and water and application of nystatin ointment containing 100 000 units per g (Catterall 1966). Scott (1966) believes that soap containing antiseptics such as hexachlorophene should not be used and that isotonic saline should be used instead. The hypersensitivity form of balano-posthitis which occurs within 24 hours of intercourse is usually transient and clears up without treatment within 1 or 2 days. Genito-crural and perianal candidiasis respond well to local applications of nystatin 100 000 units per g or amphotericin B, 2 per cent cream or ointment (Blaylock et al, 1971). Occasionally it may be necessary to give oral nystatin to prevent re-infection from the gastro-intestinal tract.

Nystatin continues to be the drug of choice in the treatment of vulvovaginal candidiasis (Nicol, 1971). It was discovered in 1950 by Hazen and Brown and its use vaginally was initially reported by Sloane in 1955. Alternative drugs such as amphotericin B were compared with nystatin in pessary form by Csonka (1967). He concluded that nystatin was somewhat more effective based on *in vitro* studies, but felt that amphotericin B had a place in the treatment of patients who failed to respond to nystatin. Gardner and Kaufman (1969) felt that candicidin was of some value although it had not proved superior to nystatin in clinical practice. Lemire (1968) reported on the use of chlordantoin and noted that it appeared to produce more local reaction than nystatin. Shklyar and Reznichenko (1971) and Nekachalov and Lenartovich (1971) found levorin in either foam pessary or 1 per cent alcohol solution to be effective. Thiery et al (1972) reported that 2 per cent miconazole applied twice daily for 14 days resulted in a 100 per cent cure rate 2 months after therapy. Gentian violet is one of the oldest and most reliable of all forms of treatment. It has the disadvantages that it stains clothing and that chemical vulvo-vaginitis often develops. Despite these it has been recommended as a second line of treatment in recurrent Candida infections (*Brit. med. J.*, 1967). The author of this article also recommended that really intractable cases should be treated with di-iodohydroxyquinolone pessaries.

Nicol (1971) advises that nystatin vaginal pessaries should be inserted morning and evening for 2 weeks. Nystatin ointment should be applied, if necessary, to the vulva and perineum. The male sexual partner should receive treatment with ointment only. Seale (1970) advises that the couple be encouraged to have intercourse during this period as the pessary *in situ* will also treat the male glans penis. Gardner and Kaufman (1969) feel that it is justifiable to apply topical steroids to relieve the pruritus and reduce the inflammatory reaction until the candidacidal agent has had time to take effect. Local applications of corticosteroids do not appear to stimulate the growth of Candida although systemic therapy with these drugs certainly does stimulate mycotic proliferation.

Patients with chronic or recurrent candidiasis require special management and this has been discussed by Gardner and Kaufman (1969). While most cases are probably caused by autogenous re-infection in patients who have predisposing host factors a proportion will be the result of further sexual transmission. Initially the predisposing factors must be evaluated and if possible removed. If this is impracticable all efforts must be made to ensure that the patient becomes asymptomatic and that the relapse rate is kept to a minimum. The therapy with nystatin pessaries should be prolonged for up to 4 weeks, without interruption during the menstrual flow (*Brit. med. J.*, 1967). Oral nystatin 500 000 units either three or four times a day should be taken for 2 weeks (Nicol, 1971). Nystatin ointment 100 000 units per g should be liberally applied to vulva, perineum and perianal areas. Scott (1966) believed that this should also be rubbed underneath the hood of the clitoris. Care should be taken to keep the area as dry as possible; washing with antiseptic soaps should be avoided and the wearing of clothes which promote sweating, such as tights should be prohibited (Tann, 1968). The male sexual contact should be considered as a source of re-infection and nystatin ointment should be applied to the glans penis twice daily for 10 days. It may be necessary to advise the use of protective sheaths during intercourse for some months in view of Gilpin's observation (1967) that frequent recurrence is associated with infected ejaculate. The sexual contact should have other carrier sites such as the perianal region, gastro-intestinal tract, nails and the oral cavity examined to exclude residual foci of infection. Should oro-genital contact take place it may be necessary to prescribe nystatin 100 000 units per ml in aqueous suspension as a mouthwash for some days for both partners.

Finally, it is important to remember that the discovery of candidal organisms in patients with predisposing factors, who do not manifest any signs and symptoms, does not constitute an indication for therapy.

REFERENCES

BLAYLOCK, W. K., SHADOMY, H. J. and SHADOMY, S. (1971). In: 'Dermatology in General Medicine', 1st ed., p. 1791, McGraw-Hill, New York.

BRIT. MED. J. (1967). ii, 297.

CATTERALL, R. D. (1966). 'Symposium on Candida Infections', p. 113, Livingstone, Edinburgh and London.

CSONKA, G. W. (1967). Brit. J. vener. Dis., 43, 210.

GARDNER, H. L. and KAUFMAN, R. H. (1969). In: 'Benign Diseases of the Vulva and Vagina', 1st ed., pp. 149–167. Mosby, St. Louis.

GILPIN, A. (1967). Quoted in 'Benign Diseases of the Vulva and Vagina', 1st ed., pp. 149–167. Mosby, St. Louis.

LEMIRE, S. (1968). Canad. med. Ass. J., 99, 211.

NEKACHALOV, V. Y. and LENARTOVICH, V. A. (1971). Vestn. derm. vener., 45, 50.

NICOL, C. S. (1971). Brit. med. J., ii, 507.

PARKER, J. D. T. (1970). Brit. J. vener. Dis., 46, 43.

SCOTT, J. S. (1966). Quoted by Gardner and Kaufman. (1969). In: 'Benign Diseases of the Vulva and Vagina', 1st ed., pp. 152, 161. Mosby, St. Louis.

SEALE, J. (1970). M.S.S.V.D. Spring Meeting, Belfast.

SHKLYAR, I. I. and Reznichenko, A. I. (1971). Vestn. derm. vener., 45, 81.

TANN, L. (1968). Brit. med. J., iv, 776.

THIERY, M., MROZOWSKI, B. J. and VAN KETS, H. (1972). Mykosen, 15, 35.

Part 6
Non-specific Genital Infection

Preamble

Of all cases of non-gonococcal urethritis (NGU), identification of a cause has proved possible in only 5–10 per cent. The absence of a discernible or specific cause in most cases has led to the term non-specific urethritis, or more simply, NSU. With greater recognition that other non-specific conditions may occur in genito-urinary organs, *eg* cervix, prostate, bladder and rectum, and may in some way be associated with NSU the term non-specific genital infection has come into current usage.

During the last decade, search for a cause or causes of the condition has intensified, and largely overshadowed observations in the epidemiological, social and clinical areas. The two principal contenders as causal agents are the mycoplasmas, particularly T- (for 'tiny') mycoplasmas; and members of the genus Chlamydia*, particularly those in subgroup A. Currently available findings favour the latter as a cause; but it may well be that more than one cause will eventually be found.

In spite of so much laboratory and other research, non-specific genital infection continues to be the venereologist's most perplexing daily problem, clinically, diagnostically and therapeutically.

*These in the past were called Tric agent or Tric virus or Bedsonia.

27 Epidemiological and Social Aspects

R. S. Morton

Introduction

There is general agreement that non-specific genital infection is acquired by sexual intercourse. This view is largely based on epidemiological evidence, for example, the observation that gonorrhoea and non-gonococcal urethritis have increased *pari passu* for more than 20 years, and that both conditions show the same seasonal variation.

Few countries produce incidence figures. Numbers of cases of non-gonococcal urethritis in men were first notified in England and Wales in 1951 when 10 794 were reported. The number in 1972 was 62 498. In countries and areas where gonorrhoea is well managed and where its control is most effectively pursued non-specific urethritis (NSU) becomes commoner in men than the gonococcal variety. No clinical condition comparable to NSU in men has been described in women.

Reiter's syndrome or disease occurs in about 1 per cent of men with non-specific urethritis (*qv*).

Csonka (1965) reviewed non-specific genital infection. He pointed out that a significant proportion of married men with NSU, in contrast to those with gonorrhoea, deny extra-marital intercourse. He emphasises the absence of a comparable condition in women and notes the great variability of incubation period. Graphs plot the quarterly returns for gonorrhoea and NSU in males in England and Wales and show a periodic increase in both conditions in summer and a decrease in winter. The most plausible explanation is that both conditions are sexually transmitted. Csonka also notes that NSU is much commoner in the indigenous population than in immigrants. No explanation is offered. The role of psychological factors is also dealt with.

The epidemiological riddle

Ambady (1965) lists 13 common causes of urethritis including gonorrhoea. He notes the clinical entity of post-gonococcal urethritis

(PGU). Hutfield (1965) listed the causes of non-gonococcal urethritis and included bacterial and abacterial infections and intra-urethral lesions, including syphilis, chancroid, herpes genitalis, lymphogranuloma venereum, genital warts, stricture, foreign bodies, neoplasm, trauma and chemicals, exogenous and endogenous. Heinz-Dieter Jung (1966) writing from Germany, gives another classification. He notes the worldwide increase in the condition, calls for more exacting investigations and generally emphasises the problems of NSU.

Seale (1966) noted that more than half of 36 wives of men with NSU were severely depressed or anxious at some time during their attendance for investigation. The proportion suffering severe symptoms was not as great as when gonorrhoea was the reason for the attendance of wives. On the other hand the marriage was considered to be more disturbed by NSU than by gonorrhoea in the husband. Guilty feelings in husbands varied little whatever their infection.

Noting that NSU not infrequently occurred in men denying extra-marital exposure Weston (1965) suggested that some men developed an allergic response to their regular partners after months or years. The high degree of consort specificity and the high recurrence rate of the condition was felt to support this view. Using a cellular acetate in a bi-dimensional immuno-diffusion technique he found marked reaction, even in high titre, between urethral discharge, serum of affected men and the vaginal secretion of their consorts. The findings were not consistent, but do in Weston's view warrant further investigation.

Teokharov (1967) found *Haemophilus vaginalis** in 12 (9·3 per cent) of 129 men with NSU. He used Gram-stained smears and cultures. He described short pleomorphic bacilli lying outside and on epithelial cells which he called clue cells. The findings are said to be so charac-teristic as to lead the author to a belief that the diagnosis need not be verified by culture. Eight of the wives of the 12 men showed *H. vaginalis* in vaginal smears. In parallel with this study 304 women were tested. Positive findings of *H. vaginalis* in them were associated with the presence of clinical symptoms. The author believes the condition sexually transmissible and that most affected men are asymptomatic. Davidson and Layton (1968) and Donkelberg et al (1970) also comment on *H. vaginalis* and its potential to cause vaginitis. In 1971, Furness et al (1971) investigated 56 patients (32 with NSU, 15 with prostatitis and nine with non-specific epididymitis) and 25 controls. They cultured washings from the bulbous urethra. Corynebacteria† were isolated from 17 men (15 with NSU, two with prostatitis and none with epididymitis). Only one control patient gave positive findings. A modified blood agar

---

* According to Zimmerman and Turner (1963) the organism does not belong to the genus Haemophilus but is probably a Corynebacterium and, taxonomically, should be so classified.

medium was used. The authors suggest that these organisms may have a role to play in NSU.

Post-gonococcal urethritis (PGU) was studied by Holmes et al (1967) in 88 men on board an aircraft-carrier. At 20 days after treatment for gonorrhoea 37 of 58 men treated with penicillin and probenecid had signs of PGU as against eight of 30 whose gonorrhoea was treated with tetracycline. Of the 45 men diagnosed as having PGU, 31 had a urethral discharge; only one had symptoms. It was noted that the dosage of penicillin used was likely to be too great for L forms of gonococci to have played a part in the epidemiology of PGU. PGU was also considered by Lopatin (1967) and by Mahony (1969) who regarded the two conditions, gonorrhoea and PGU, as being acquired concomitantly.

Furness and Csonka (1966) noted the presence of diphtheroids in cases of NSU, their disappearance with successful treatment, their persistence with treatment failure and their re-appearance with relapse. One similar epidemiological point was made by Morrison (1967). He showed that men continuing to associate with the same consort and suffering a recurrence of NSU usually responded to the same antibiotic which cleared their original NSU. Men with a new consort more often found a different antibiotic effective.

Osoba (1972) writing from Ibadan, Nigeria, reported that NSU was nearly twice as common as gonorrhoea in males in spite of a random testing of 130 women showing that 5 per cent had gonorrhoea. The widespread practice of self-treatment with freely available antibiotics was given as the main reason.

In women with persistent irritative urinary symptoms and 'negative' urine cultures, non-specific urethritis should be considered as a possibility according to Marshall et al (1970). They suggest a two-glass urine test as a means of differentiating urethritis from cystitis. There is no hint that they associate the condition with non-specific genital infection in the consorts.

Seventeen children aged 5–15 years with NSU were described by Williams and Mikhael (1971). Some had blood-stained discharge and two developed stricture of the bulbous urethra.

Morrison (1969) considered the possible epidemiological role of the smegma bacillus in NSU. He stained 110 urethral scrapings from men and 89 labia minora and vestibule scrapings from women. He used Ziehl–Nielsen's staining method and made positive findings in 45 per cent of the men and 46 per cent of the women. He was unable to demonstrate that these organisms play any part in NSU.

Archer (1968) makes a point which may be of epidemiological and social import. He sought to estimate the prevalence of T-mycoplasma in the urine of 100 pregnant women; 94 women attending an infertility clinic; 98 women in a geriatric unit and 105 nuns of an enclosed order.

Positive findings were made in 58, 51, 29 and 8 per cent respectively. In discussing his findings he draws attention to recent observations on the epidemiology of carcinoma of the cervix that early marriage and multiple sex partners appear to play a part. In seeing the presence of T-myco-plasma in women as a mark of sexual experience he says 'If there is a factor transmitted during coitus then the role of T-mycoplasmas [in carcinoma of the cervix] should be considered.'

Ravic (1971) notes that recent findings of viruses in human smegma and semen in association with cancers of prostate, cervix and bladder and strongly suggests a concept that these organisms are sexually trans-missible. He surveyed a series of white, middle class, private patients seen between 1930–41 and showed a 1·7 per cent incidence of prostatic cancer in the more or less sexually segregated Jewish members of the group; as against a 20 per cent prostatic cancer incidence amongst the generally uncircumcised non-Jews. Cancers of other organs, susceptible to sexually transmitted disease, such as the bladder and the rectum, also showed a lower incidence in Jews.

REFERENCES

AMBADY, B. A. (1965). *Indian J. Derm.*, **31**, 211.
ARCHER, J. F. (1968). *Brit. J. vener. dis.*, **44**, 232.
CSONKA, G. W. (1965). *Brit. J. vener. Dis.*, **41**, 1.
DAVIDSON, A. J. L. and LAYTON, K. B. (1968). *Med. J. Aust.*, **1**, 759.
DONKELBERG, W. E. JR., SKAGGS, R. and KELLOG, D. S. JR. (1970). *Amer. J. clin. Path.*, **53**, 370.
FURNESS, G. and CSONKA, G. W. (1966). *Brit. J. vener. Dis.*, **42**, 185.
FURNESS, G., KAMAT, M. H., KHAMINSK, Z. and SEEBODE, J. J. (1971). *J. Urol.*, **106**, 557.
JUNG, H.-D. (1966). *J. Urol.*, **59**, 865.
HOLMES, K. K., FLOYD, D. W., JOHNSON, D. W., FLOYD, T. M. and KVALE, P. A. (1967). *J. Amer. med. Ass.*, **202**, 467.
HUTFIELD, D. C. (1965). *Clin. Med.*, **72**, 1639.
LOPATIN, A. I. (1967). *Soviet. Med.*, **30**, 113.
MAHONY, J. D. H. (1969). *Ulster med. J.*, **38**, 148.
MARSHALL, S., LYON, R. P. and SCHIEBLE, J. (1970). *Calif. Med.*, **112**, 9.
MORRISON, A. I. (1967). *Brit. J. vener. Dis.*, **43**, 170.
MORRISON, A. I. (1969). *Brit. J. vener. Dis.*, **45**, 55.
OSOBA, O. A. (1972). *Afr. J. med. Sci.*, **3**, 187.
RAVIC, A. (1971). *Cancer*, **27**, 1493.
SEALE, J. R. (1966). *Brit. J. vener. Dis.*, **42**, 31.
TEOKHAROV, B. A. (1967). *Vestn. Derm. vener.*, **41**, 63.
WESTON, T. E. T. (1965). *Brit. J. vener. Dis.*, **41**, 107.
WILLIAMS, D. I. and MIKHAEL, B. R. (1971). *Proc. roy. Soc. Med.*, **64**, 133.
ZINNERMAN, K. and TURNER, G. C. (1963). *J. Path. Bact.*, **82**, 213.

28 Clinical Aspects

R. S. Morton

Introduction

The bulk of clinical observations concerning non-specific genital infection have been principally related in recent years to research concerned with the possible causative agents, the mycoplasmas and members of the genus Chlamydia. The clinical aspects will now be dealt with and will be followed immediately by a clinician's appreciation of recent advances in the laboratory (see section 29). Some overlap has been inevitable. Emphasis varies. But first, those clinical aspects not concerned with the organisms mentioned.

General clinical observations

Urethroscopy was carried out in 284 of 598 men treated for non-specific urethritis by Morrison (1965). Four men were found to have a stricture. Two had symptoms.

Non-specific urethritis is the commonest presenting form of non-specific genital infection. Scepticism about the reality of prostatic involvement led Morton (1968) to attempt putting its diagnosis on a more scientific basis. He was discontented with the haphazard nature of prostatic massage and low-power microscopy of the beads obtained. Firstly, he defined the range and upper limit of normality of the total white cell counts in human semen by examination of the total ejaculate of apparently normal men and men with a history, or overt evidence, of genito-urinary infection. He then applied the method to 35 young adult males with acute anterior uveitis, a condition claimed to be commonly associated with prostatitis. Twenty (57 per cent) of the men were found to have prostatitis as defined by the finding that they had more than 5 million white cells per ml of total semen ejaculate (Dark and Morton, 1968).

Oates (1969) gave a detailed review of non-specific prostatitis. Messent (1970) studied 25 cases of NSU with persistent threads in the urine following treatment with oxytetracycline. He found that such findings were frequently associated with prostatic involvement. This was so in 13 patients.

Lagerholm and Lodin (1966) contrasted the cytology of urethral pus from men with NSU and men with urethral gonorrhoea. There were possibly more lymphocytes in the NSU cases. The number of epithelial cells was the same.

Nicolai and Hines (1966) described their newly recognised syndrome of pre-menstrual urethritis.

NSU has been described when mild or asymptomatic as a diagnosis of inclination, that is, some clinicians are more inclined to diagnose the condition than others and vice versa. Early morning examination before urination is a well-tried method of coming to a supportable conclusion one way or the other. Rodin (1971) took this technique a step further. He applied it to a group of 88 asymptomatic men attending a V.D. clinic and according to his criteria found that 11 (12·5 per cent) of them had non-specific urethritis. He concludes, 'It is likely that the true incidence of NSU is much greater than is indicated by reported figures'.

King (1972) gives a detailed clinical description of non-specific genital infection in men and women. In men he lists urethritis, acute abacterial or haemorrhagic cystitis, prostatitis, vesiculitis, epididymitis (said to occur in 2 per cent of NSU cases) and urethral stricture. In women he lists abacterial pyuria, cervicitis, Bartholinitis and pelvic infection. Amongst general complications he lists acute follicular conjunctivitis, Reiter's disease and anterior uveitis. He gives ankylosing spondylitis as a possible complication.

THE MYCOPLASMAS

Shepard and Calvy (1965) stated that most mycoplasmas play no part in NSU but that the T-mycoplasma (T for 'tiny', ie tiny culture colonies) was still suspect.

Csonka et al (1966) found *Mycoplasma hominis* equally distributed in men with NSU and controls, whereas they found T-mycoplasma in 70·2 per cent of men with NSU and in only 12·6 per cent of controls. There was no clinical difference between the NSU found in positive and in negative culture cases, although therapeutic response was generally better in culture positive patients. A group of 545 men including 313 with NSU was studied. Also studied was a group of 304 women including consorts of men with NSU. They had specimens of urine, and urethra and endocervix secretions, submitted for culture of *M. hominis* and T-mycoplasma. Positive culture rates in female consorts were highest in those with clinically obvious cervicitis. Female controls were culture negative. The authors conclude that T-mycoplasmas and their close association with clinical events suggests that these organisms play an important role in the aetiology of so-called non-specific genital infection.

In regard to Csonka's observation about treatment response, Shepard et al (1966) described selective inhibition of T-mycoplasma by erythromycin. They also found T-mycoplasma associated with 70–80 per cent of their men with NSU.

The role of mycoplasmas in clinical conditions in cattle and humans was reviewed by Hirth et al (1966), Moustardier (1966) and Ludwick et al (1967). Jones (1967) considered that spontaneous abortion may on occasion be due to *M. hominis*. The causal role of mycoplasmas in NSU was questioned by Black and Rasmussen (1968) in Denmark. They believed that resolution of the problem will depend on serological typing of mycoplasmas found in men with NSU and in controls.

Of 250-new born babies, 10 per cent developed infected eyes. Eight, according to Jones and Tobin (1968), yielded positive cultures of *M. hominis* as did 20 per cent of ante-natal patients.

The clinical aspects of mycoplasmas in non-specific genital infection were reviewed by Dunlop et al (1966a). They found these organisms in the genital tract of most women, in the rectum of a few and in the urethra of a modest proportion of men. They found little or no evidence that mycoplasmas were the cause of clinical conditions. Hare et al (1969) also found no evidence to implicate any form of mycoplasma in disease processes. The same conclusion was reached in France by Sepetijian et al (1969). Shepard (1970) renewed his efforts to implicate T-mycoplasma. He reviewed the literature and reported hitherto unpublished work. T-mycoplasma he found in 70–84 per cent of men with NSU. He noted that where the organism was not eliminated by tetracycline early relapse could be expected. He also brought evidence to show that treatment of wives minimised the chances of recurrence of NSU in the husband. These and other observations led Shepard to the view that T-mycoplasma is one of the major etiological agents in NSU.

Foy et al (1970) found *M. hominis* to be twice as common in the cervices of Negroes as compared with Caucasians. They also studied the acquisition of mycoplasmas by 100 neonates, 47 females and 53 males. Specimens were taken from the throat, genitals, umbilical stump, urine and conjunctivae on first, second and third days of life and again at intervals at up to two years, when 47 infants were still available. T-mycoplasma was isolated from 38 per cent of females and 6 per cent of males. These positive findings were generally made shortly after birth. Positive isolations fell sharply after 3 months of age. Other mycoplasmas were also found. The authors conclude that the role of *M. hominis* and T-mycoplasma in abortion, pathological delivery and neonatal conjunctivitis must be viewed with caution. Mendel et al (1970) came to a similar conclusion after studying 88 gynaecological and

32 obstetrical patients with vaginitis. Positive cultures were of *M. hominis* only. Its presence was unconnected with abortion or other obstetric complications. This and its common association with the presence of the trichomonas vaginalis and haemophilus vaginalis led the authors to the conclusion that *M. hominis* may be a commensal or parasite of low virulence.

Gregory and Payne (1970) found *M. hominis* in the cervices of 92 per cent of 300 women attending a venereal diseases clinic, and only in 38 per cent of women attending a family planning clinic. Mårdh and Weström (1970) in Sweden examined 247 women for T-mycoplasma. The group consisted of pregnant and non-pregnant patients. Seventy had clinical evidence of genital infection. Positive isolations of T-mycoplasma were made in 45·8 per cent of the clinically healthy and 55·4 per cent of those with evidence of genital infection. Few positive cultures were found in the pre-pubertal or post-menopausal patients. In the pregnant and healthy, the isolation rate was 68·4 per cent and in the pregnant and infected, 85·7 per cent. In 90 per cent of those with positive urethral cultures the organism was also recovered from the cervix. The high incidence in the urethra was viewed as very significant and these workers recognised a clinical entity which they called 'T-mycoplasma-uria'. Positive isolations were also made from the Fallopian tubes at laproscopy in two cases of acute salpingitis. These authors conclude that hormonal influences such as sexual maturity, pregnancy and oral contraceptives, rather than sexual activity, are more important factors in converting the organism from a commensal to a pathological role.

Bashmakova and Soldova (1969) reported a case of intra-uterine infection due to mycoplasma. Hardwick et al (1970) and Knudsin and Driscoll (1970) considered the possible role of mycoplasmas in abortion. Braun et al (1971), starting from reports of positive blood cultures of *M. hominis* in cases of fever after abortion, and positive tissue culture in material from aborted foetuses and still births, sought evidence of pathogenicity of the organism. They were able to demonstrate a relationship between the presence of T-mycoplasma in the genital tract of pregnant women and subsequent low birth weights. Whether the relationship is one of cause and effect could not be determined. Caspi and Hertzek (1971) describe a case of amnionitis associated with T-mycoplasma. There was generalised infection in the mother. Her twins and the sperm donor (the babies were conceived by AID), but not the husband, yielded T-mycoplasma also. The authors conclude that these organisms are potentially virulent. Caspi and Hertzek (1972) followed up this observation by a detailed study. They compared the incidence of positive mycoplasma cultures from the crevices and the foetuses after 81 induced and 100 spontaneous abortions. The great majority of isolations were of T-mycoplasmas rather than *M. hominis*. After induced abortion 28 per cent of cervices gave positive cultures; after spontaneous abortion the figure was 37 per cent. The products of conception gave positive culture in 5 and 31 per cent respectively. Whether the foetuses were infected directly through the placenta or via amnionitis is not clear. The most recent report along these lines comes from McCormack et al (1973). They carried out cultures for *M. hominis* and T-mycoplasma in 388 consecutive women who delivered themselves in Boston City Hospital. Cultures of blood and urine were made in those women who developed post-partum fever. *M. hominis* was found in the blood of two of 27 such women. It was also found in the blood of one of 31 afebrile controls. Yhu-Hsiung Lee et al (1972), McCormack's co-workers, describe the culture methods used.

Meanwhile the isolation of mycoplasmas from NSU cases has been further explored. Altucci and Varone (1971), Sveltmann et al (1971), Haas et al (1971) and Jansson et al (1971), approaching the problem from a variety of angles, came to the conclusion that there is little difference in the incidence of mycoplasmas in men with NSU and those without. Sveltmann et al believe that T-mycoplasmas form part of the normal genital flora of sexually active young people. Jansson et al included haemagglutination tests for men with NSU and mycoplasmas. They found serological evidence of recent infection in 24 per cent. They conclude that only some of the 10 serotypes identified are pathogenic. Their second conclusion is that the time has now come for human inoculation experiments as a means of resolving the many problems involved.

Some of the highest positive rates of isolation in infected men have been made by Markham et al (1972). They found the incidence of T-mycoplasma to be 83 per cent of men with gonorrhoea; 85 per cent of men with NSU and 52 per cent of healthy control. Men with gonorrhoea and T-mycoplasma were found to be more likely to develop PGU. A high percentage of female partners harboured the T-myco-plasma. The exhibition of tetracycline and erythromycin was associated with cure of the NSU and elimination of the organism. McCormack et al (1972) showed a positive correlation between isolation of T-mycoplasma from the vaginae of 183 nurses and their number of sex partners. This, and all the evidence accumulated by McCormack et al, leads them to the belief that more evidence of pathogenicity must be forthcoming before T-mycoplasma can be implicated in NSU, abortion or subfertility.

Gnarpe and Friberg (1972) have tried to meet at least one of these challenges. They investigated 55 couples attending on account of primary sterility and compared the findings with those in couples where the wife was pregnant. One of the interesting observations was that T-mycoplasmas were commonly found attached to spermatozoa and it was thought that this might well inhibit fertilisation. Gnarpe and

Friberg (1973) treated their subfertile couples with doxycycline in a course lasting 10 days and sometimes repeated. Most mycoplasmas were inhibited. They were eradicated in 10 men and nine of 11 women. After only 5 months follow-up 29 per cent of 52 couples were pregnant. Gnarpe and Friberg take the view that some T-mycoplasma strains are important pathogens.

Ford (1973) points out that one of the problems in NSU is that T-mycoplasma and the TRIC agent (Chlamydia) may both be present in the same patient. He isolated both in 11 of 16 cases of NSU. A further problem is that the disease and both the alleged causes are sensitive to tetracyclines and erythromycin. He notes that both organisms are resistant to lincomycin.

THE CHLAMYDIA GROUP

In a well-illustrated report, Jones (1964) has described the clinical and historical background of trachoma, neonatal inclusion blennorrhoea and the inclusion conjunctivitis of the adult. The latter was seen to occur in a series of stages comparable with those of trachoma. The intermediate stage is newly described as 'TRIC virus punctate kerato-conjunctivitis'. Jones suggests that the virus involved in all these eye conditions may be the same, with variable pathogenicity. He also suggests that some eye conditions may arise from the patient's own genitals. It is suggested that virus isolation techniques, used for eye conditions, should be applied to so-called non-specific genital infections; and that clinical assessment methods, used by ophthalmologists and as mentioned above, might with profit be applied to genital infections also. Jones suspects that such methods would reveal TRIC virus infection as one of the commonest of all sexually transmitted diseases.

In a series of collaborative studies with Jones (Jones et al, 1964; Khalaf Al-Hussaini et al, 1964: Dunlop et al, 1964) the association of genital infection and eye disease was reported in detail. Viral inclusions were found in conjunctival scrapings in five babies with ophthalmia neonatorum. The infecting agent was isolated by culture in three of them. Inclusions were found in cervical scrapings from one mother whose cultures were also positive. Four of the five fathers were found to have urethritis. Of three fathers from whom urethral scrapings were taken, inclusions were found in all and culture was positive in one. This is the first definite report of isolations from a case of 'non-specific urethritis'. Cultures in these studies were by inoculation of the yolk sac of embryonated hens' eggs. These authors also produced evidence suggesting that genital infection by TRIC agent occurs in association with trachoma and with other forms of eye infection due to this agent. Moore et al (1965) showed that TRIC agent was the cause of a follicular conjunctivitis in many parts of the world. Dunlop et al (1969a) reported further findings, starting from a total of 20 babies with neonatal conjunctivitis and their parents. They suggested the terms 'TRIC agent urethritis and cervicitis'. Mordhorst (1965) in a series of new-born babies and their mothers confirmed the above findings. Babies with TRIC agent conjunctivitis they describe as 6–9 days old, with profuse purulent conjunctival discharge, pronounced palpebral oedema, infiltration of conjunctival epithelium and pseudo-membrane formation.

Pasieczny and Sommerville (1966) tested serum from NSU patients by complement fixation for antibody to the LB4 agent of the TRIC group. Positive reciprocal titres of 32 or greater were found in 25 per cent of NSU patients, 15 per cent of controls, 22 per cent of men with gonorrhoea and 6 per cent of a few men with syphilis. Morton et al (1964) had no success with culture in embryonated hens' eggs of material from cases of NSU. Specimens were taken from the first inch of the urethra. This group also failed to grow virus or agent in human amnion cells or kidney cells. Haemagglutination and haemabsorption tests on tissue culture fluid were negative.

Jones et al (1966) described the clinical appearance produced in the eyes of adults by TRIC agent, ie in trachoma and inclusion conjunctivitis. Freedman et al (1966) did the same concerning ophthalmia neonatorum due to TRIC agent. Dunlop et al (1966b) described and illustrated the clinical appearance of the cervices of mothers of such babies. Twenty-four of 28 mothers had cervical follicles and 20 had a purulent cervical discharge. TRIC agent was grown from eight of 19 fathers seen; 17 had NSU and seven showed TRIC agent. Of 39 patients with trachoma, punctate kerato-conjunctivitis, or inclusion conjunctivitis the TRIC agent was isolated from the genitals of 11. In San Francisco, Dawson and Schachter (1967) saw these clinical manifestations in a similarly numbered group. They also found much the same laboratory evidence of TRIC agent. This was probably the most encouraging confirmatory evidence of the London group's work. Ford and McCandlish (1969) isolated the TRIC agent from 15 (11·3 per cent) of 133 men with NSU.

Dunlop et al (1969b) completed the transition of terminology change from 'TRIC agent' to 'Chlamydia (Bedsonia)'. Their report describes 25 persons with proven or suspected chlamydial infection. Some of the cases could be grouped, for example:

1. A baby suffering from Chlamydial ophthalmia neonatorum had a mother with the agent in cervix and rectum and a father with it in the urethra.
2. Two women, one with follicular conjunctivitis and the other with punctate kerato-conjunctivitis each had Chlamydia isolated from the eye, the genital tract and the rectum. The husband of one had urethritis, from which Chlamydia was isolated.

3. Seven men with N.S.U. all had positive Chlamydia isolates as did the female consort of one of them.

Such findings, in conjunction with the previous studies, point clearly to the possibilities of social, sexual and auto-infections.

In a group of women with a history of non-specific vaginitis, leucor-rhoea and cervical erosion Agarwal and Dhir (1969) isolated Chlamydia from 10 of 115 vaginal swabs and from seven of 56 cervical scrapings.

Mordhorst and Dawson (1971) report a long-term follow-up of 16 babies with chlamydial ophthalmia neonatorum. After $4\frac{1}{2}$ years, pelvic inflammatory disease had occurred in four of 12 mothers seen and Reiter's disease had occurred in two of the fathers. The need for long-term clinical follow-up is said to be clear.

Until recently the only methods available for the detection of Chlamydia in NSU were Giemsa or immunofluorescent staining and culture by inoculation of the yolk sac of fertile hens' eggs. All those are now seen as having marked limitations. Philip et al (1971) reported the use of irradiated McCoy cell cultures. They grew a Chlamydia from three of 12 patients with lymphogranuloma venereum, 10 of 47 patients with NSU and PGU and five of 59 patients with gonorrhoea. A Chlamydia was also isolated from two consorts of men with Chlamydia positive NSU. This promising new laboratory tool has proved to be a much more sensitive culture medium than fertile hens' eggs. Dunlop et al (1972a) developed 44 isolates of Chlamydia from 99 men with NSU. Positive cultures were also obtained from the genital tract and rectum of 10 of 34 sex partners of these men. Using the same basic technique similar findings have been made by Richmond et al (1972) and Oriel et al (1972). These consistent findings suggest a cause for NSU. Richmond and her colleagues have reservations about this, although they noted that patients with gonorrhoea and positive Chlamydia cultures were more liable to develop PGU. The association of Chlamydia and NSU was reviewed by Dunlop et al (1972b). All writers insist that to gain high culture 'yields', specimens from men should be taken from the *whole* anterior urethra.

Shaaban et al (1972) showed a high incidence of genital Chlamydia isolations from a series of Egyptian women. Ten genital isolations were made from 41. The authors suggest that because three isolates came from 11 women with no evident gynaecological lesions the Chlamydia may be a commensal (*vide infra*).

Summary

The diagnosis of NSU is made not only by exclusion of gonorrhoea but by exclusion of all known causes of non-gonococcal urethritis (NGU). On present evidence there is less support from the clinical field for mycoplasmas, than for organisms of the genus Chlamydia, as a cause. What evidence is there from the laboratory? What tests are available to the clinician who seeks to reduce the high percentage of NSU cases amongst those he sees with NGU? Recent laboratory advances go some way to answering these questions.

REFERENCES

AGARWAL, L. P. and DHIR, S. P. (1969). *Orient. Arch. Ophthal.*, **7**, 68.
ALTUCCI, P. and VARONE, G. L. (1971). *Path. Microbiol.*, **37**, 89.
BASHMAKOVA, M. A. and SOLDOVA, V. M. (1969). *Vop. Okhr. Materin Detst.*, **14**, 69.
BLACK, F. T. and RASMUSSEN, O. G. (1968). *Brit. J. vener. Dis.*, **44**, 324.
BRAUN, P., YHU-HSIUNG LEE et al. (1971). *New. Engl. J. Med.*, **284**, 167.
CASPI, E. and HERCZEK, E. (1971). *Amer. J. Obstet. Gynec.*, **111**, 1102.
CASPI, E and HERCZEK, E. (1972). *Israel J. med. Sci.*, **8**, 122.
CSONKA, G. W., WILLIAMS, R. E. O. and CORSE, J. (1966). *Lancet*, **1**, 1292.
DARK, A. J. and MORTON, R. S. (1968). *Brit. J. Ophthal.*, **52**, 907.
DAWSON, C. R. and SCHACHTER, J. (1967). *Amer. J. Ophthal.*, **63**, 1288.
DUNLOP, E. M. C., JONES, B. R. and KHALAF AL-HUSSAINI, M. (1964). *Brit. J. vener. Dis.*, **40**, 33.
DUNLOP, E. M. C., KHALAF AL-HUSSAINI, M. et al. (1966a). *Trans. ophthal. Soc. U.K.*, **86**, 321.
DUNLOP, E. M. C., HARPER, I. A. et al. (1966b). *Brit. J. vener. Dis.*, **42**, 77.
DUNLOP, E. M. C., HARE, M. J. and JONES, B. R. (1969a). *Brit. J. vener. Dis.*, **45**, 274.
DUNLOP, E. M. C., HARE, M. J. and DAROUGAR, S. et al. (1969b). *J. infect. Dis.*, **120**, 463.
DUNLOP, E. M. C., VAUGHAN-JACKSON, J. D. et al. (1972a). *Brit. J. vener. Dis.*, **48**, 425.
DUNLOP, E. M. C., JONES, B. R., and DAROUGAR, S. (1972b). *Brit. med. J.*, **2**, 575.
FREEDMAN, A. et al. (1966). *Trans. ophthal. Soc. U.K.*, **86**, 313.
FORD, D. K. and MCCANDLISH, L. (1969). *Brit. J. vener. Dis.*, **45**, 44.
FORD, D. K. (1973). *J. infect. Dis.*, **127**, Suppl., p. 66.
FOY, H. M., KENNY, G. E. et al. (1970). *J. infect. Dis.*, **121**, 579.
GNARPE, H. and FRIBERG, J. (1972). *Amer. J. Obstet. Gynec.*, **114**, 727.
GNARPE, H. and FRIBERG, J. (1973). *Nature, Lond.*, **242**, 120.
GREGORY, J. E. and PAYNE, F. E. (1970). *Amer. J. Obstet. Gynec.*, **107**, 220.
HAAS, H., DOREMAN, M. L. and SACK, S. (1971). *Brit. J. vener. Dis.*, **47**, 131.
HARDWICK, H. J., PURCELL, R. H. and IUPPA, J. B. (1970). *J. infect. Dis.*, **121**, 260.
HARE, M. J., DUNLOP, E. M. C. and TAYLOR-ROBINSON, D. (1969). *Brit. J. vener. Dis.*, **45**, 282.
HIRTH, R. S., PLASTRIDGE, W. N. and TOURTELLOTTE, M. E. et al. (1966). *J. Amer. vet. med. Ass.*, **148**, 277.
JANSSON, E., LASSUS, A. et al. (1971). *Brit. J. vener. Dis.*, **47**, 122.
JONES, B. R. (1964). *Brit. J. vener. Dis.*, **40**, 3.
JONES, B. R., KHALAF AL-HUSSAINI, M. and DUNLOP, E. M. C. (1964). *Brit. J. vener. Dis.*, **40**, 19.
JONES, B. R., KHALAF AL-HUSSAINI, M. et al. (1966). *Trans. ophthal. Soc. U.K.*, **86**, 291.
JONES, D. M. (1967). *Brit. med. J.*, **1**, 338.
JONES, D. M. and TOBIN, B. (1968). *Brit. med. J.*, **3**, 467.
KHALAF AL-HUSSANI, M., JONES, B. R. and DUNLOP, E. M. C. (1964). *Brit. J. vener. Dis.*, **40**, 25.

KING, A. J. (1972). 'Clinics of North America, Venereal Diseases', **56**, 1193. Saunders.

KNUDSIN, R. B. and DRISCOLL, S. G. (1970). *Surg. Gynec. Obstet.*, **131**, 89.

LAGERHOLM, B. and LODIN, A. (1966). *Acta derm.-venereol., Stockh.*, **46**, 457.

LUDWICK, W., SACHDEU, K. S. et al (1967). *Wien. Klin. Wschr.*, **79**, 180.

MCCORMACK, W. M., ALMEIDA, D. C. et al. (1972). *J. Amer. med. Ass.*, **221**, 1375.

MCCORMACK, W. H. et al (1973). *J. infect. Dis.*, **127**, 193.

MARKHAM, N. P., MARKHAM, J. G. and SMITH, E. R. (1972). *Brit. J. vener. Dis.*, **48**, 200.

MÅRDH, P. A. and WESTRÖM, L. (1970). *Acta path. microbiol. scand.*, **78**, 367.

MENDEL, E. B., ROWAN, D. F. et al (1970). *Obstet. Gynec.*, **35**, 104.

MESSENT, J. J. (1970). *Brit. J. vener. Dis.*, **46**, 469.

MOORE, M. C., HOWARTH, W. H. et al (1965). *Med. J. Aust.* **2**, 441.

MORDHORST, C. H. (1965). *Acta path. microbiol. scand.*, **64**, 277.

MORDHORST, C. H. and DAWSON, C. R. (1971). *Amer. J. Ophthal.*, **71**, 861.

MORRISON, A. I. (1965). *Brit. J. vener. Dis.*, **41**, 132.

MORTON, R. S., GILLESPIE, E. H. and WILSON, M. A. (1964). *J. clin. Path.*, **17**, 114.

MORTON, R. S. (1968). *Brit. J. vener. Dis.*, **44**, 72.

MOUSTARDIER, G. (1966). *J. Med. Bordeaux*, **143**, 713.

NICOLAI, C. H. and HINES, D. W. (1966). *Amer. J. Obstet. Gynec.*, **95**, 137.

OATES, J. K. (1969). *Brit. J. Hosp. Med.*, **2**, 556.

ORIEL, J. D., REEVE, P. et al (1972). *Brit. J. vener. Dis.*, **48**, 429.

PASIECZNY, I. and SOMMERVILLE, R. G. (1966). *Brit. J. vener. Dis.*, **42**, 191.

PHILIP, R. N., HILL, D. A. et al (1971). *Brit. J. vener. Dis.*, **47**, 114.

RICHMOND, S. J., HILTON, A. L. and CLARKE, S. K. L. (1972). *Brit. J. vener. Dis.*, **48**, 437.

RODIN, P. (1971). *Brit. J. vener. Dis.*, **47**, 452.

SEPETIJIAN, M., THIVOLET, J. et al (1969). *Path. et Biol.*, **17**, 953.

SHAABAN, M. M. et al (1972). *J. Obstet. Gynaec. Brit. Commonw.*, **79**, 360.

SHEPARD, M. C. and CALVY, G. L. (1965). *New Engl. J. Med.*, **272**, 848.

SHEPARD, M. C., LUNCEFORD, C. D. and BAKER, R. L. (1966). *Brit. J. vener. Dis.*, **42**, 21.

SHEPARD, M. C. (1970). *J. Amer. med. Ass.*, **211**, 1335.

SVELTMANN, S., ALLEN, V. et al (1971). *Hlth Lab. Sci.*, **8**, 62.

YHU-HSIUNG LEE et al (1972). *Appl. Microbiol.*, **23**, 824.

29 Laboratory Aspects

E. M. C. Dunlop

THE GENITAL MYCOPLASMAS

The possible relationships of the mycoplasmas that produce large colonies and those that produce tiny colonies ('T-strains') to non-gonococcal urethritis were reviewed by King (1964) under the heading of pleuropneumonia-like organisms (PPLO). He considered that the weight of the confusing evidence then available was against the large-colony-forming mycoplasmas being primary causes of urethritis and that the evidence for 'T-strains' being a new type of mycoplasma was not proven.

The space available does not permit a detailed account here of the many publications that have appeared on this subject since 1964; these include reviews (Ford, 1968, 1970; Taylor-Robinson and others, 1969; Sharp, 1970; McCormack and others, 1973).

Biological characteristics

Since 1964 the characteristics of T-strains (or T-mycoplasmas) have been established and these have shown that these organisms are members of the genus Mycoplasma: thus electron-microscopy studies have shown that, although they produce small colonies on agar, the size and structure (Williams, 1967), including the presence of a triple-layered limiting membrane, of individual organisms are the same as those of individual large-colony mycoplasmas; like them their growth in liquid medium is inhibited by antibody. They grow on the same kinds of medium with minor variations, as do larger mycoplasmas. There are certain differences. Thus T-mycoplasmas require urea; they metabolise it (Purcell and others, 1966; Shepard, 1966) to produce ammonia by means of a urease enzyme. Hence, phenol red may be used as an indicator in the medium to detect the rise in pH due to ammonia; such colour-change (Taylor-Robinson and Purcell, 1966) may be used as the basis of techniques for isolation, serotyping, estimation of the numbers of organisms in clinical specimens and for the detection of specific antibody. *M. hominis* metabolises arginine causing the release of ammonia with a resultant rise in pH; *M. fermentans* ferments glucose to produce lactic acid so that the pH is lowered. The actions of these large-colony mycoplasmas on specific metabolites can be detected by the colour-change technique. T-mycoplasmas have a more rapid growth cycle than that of the large-colony mycoplasmas; they are relatively more sensitive to the inhibiting effects of erythromycin and of thalium acetate; they are relatively unaffected by lincomycin; they do not metabolise glucose or arginine. No mycoplasma is affected by antibiotics (such as penicillin), that act upon the cell wall.

Nomenclature

The nomenclature of the mycoplasmas has been amended (Taylor-Robinson and others, 1969). Because there are an unknown number of serotypes (or strains) of 'T-strain mycoplasmas' it seems better that the term T-mycoplasmas should be used for these organisms. The term 'mycoplasmas' has come to be used generally and accepted rather than the strictly correct plural word mycoplasmata.

Association with non-specific urethritis in men

There is still no definite evidence to incriminate large-colony myco-plasmas as a cause of 'non-specific' urethritis; it is still possible that particular subtypes (Nicol and Edward, 1953; Purcell and others, 1967; Razin, 1968) might be capable of producing disease while a majority cannot. *M. fermentans* is rarely found in material from healthy men or from inflamed areas other than from balanitis (Ruiter and Wentholt, 1952) so it is unlikely that this organism can cause NSU. In those studies in which the mycoplasmas that were isolated were not identified, it is likely that they were *M. hominis*. There were marked disagreements between the results of different early studies (King, 1964); also between later studies summarised by Taylor-Robinson and others (1969). These authors pointed out that the differences between controlled studies stemmed largely from the use of different control groups.

The men selected for a control group for patients suffering from NSU should have similar sexual behaviour to that of the patients. It is relevant that a higher incidence of genital infection by mycoplasmas has been found in men who gave a history of recent sexual intercourse than in those who did not (Holmes and others, 1967; Shepard, 1954). Not surprisingly then, T-mycoplasmas were more seldom isolated from healthy men over 45 years of age than from healthy men under 45 years of age (Haas and others, 1971). In women the incidence of infection by mycoplasmas (particularly T-mycoplasmas) has been related to previous sexual intercourse and increased with the number of partners with whom intercourse had taken place (McCormack and others, 1972).

Apart from the selection of control groups it seems that the method of testing is important. Thus the rates of isolation of mycoplasmas from men suffering from urethritis were similar when the results of cultures of urine and of urethral material were compared, according to Csonka and others (1966); but Serpetjian and others (1969) found that cultures of urine were less effective for the detection of *M. hominis* in such cases. It is significant that cultures of urethral material were more likely to yield T-mycoplasmas (Black and Rasmussen, 1968) when men, free from obvious urethritis, were tested. This is probably due to the association of mycoplasmas with desquamated epithelial cells (Shepard and Calvy, 1965). *M. hominis* is less commonly isolated from circumcised than uncircumcised men. This factor does not affect the isolation rate of T-mycoplasmas (Hare and others, 1969).

In studies of NSU in which control groups of varying degrees of comparability have been tested there have been similar rates of isolation of *M. hominis* from control subjects and from patients suffering from NSU that suggest that the agent is not a cause of the disease. This applies to early studies (King, 1964) and later studies (Ford and Du Vernet, 1963; Csonka and others, 1966; Black and Rasmussen, 1968). Post-gonococcal urethritis (PGU) may be diagnosed after a suitable interval has elapsed following the treatment of gonococcal urethritis. The diagnosis is made in those cases in which the gonococcus has been eliminated by treatment but urethritis persists, or recurs, and is apparently 'non-specific'. Csonka and others (1966) grew *M. hominis* from urethral material from five of 50 men suffering from gonorrhoea alone but not from 13 men suffering from gonorrhoea who developed PGU. Holmes and others (1967) found a relationship between PGU and the isolation of mycoplasmas from urethral material: thus of 17 men from whom mycoplasmas were isolated 16 developed PGU compared with 41 men from whom mycoplasmas were not isolated, of whom 21 (51 per cent) developed PGU. Hare and others (1969) regarded those patients who did not develop PGU as a suitable control group for those that did. Of 120 men treated for gonorrhoea, 35 were observed to develop PGU during observation lasting for 4 weeks. The incidence of urethral infection by *M. hominis* was 43 per cent in this group compared with 40 per cent in the remainder and 41 per cent in the 29 men who were known to have remained free from PGU during observation for 4 weeks. This study was repeated with the addition of tests for chlamydial infection (Vaughan-Jackson, 1974): *M. hominis* was isolated with similar frequencies from those who developed PGU and from those who did not. In contrast, Chlamydia was isolated only from those who developed PGU or defaulted before that condition could be diagnosed.

If *M. hominis* were a cause of urethritis it would seem likely that the incidence of urethritis would be highest in the cases of patients with high concentrations of organisms in urethral material. This was not the case (Hare and others, 1969); thus, of 26 patients with high concentrations of organisms in the urethra six developed PGU, of 24 with low concentrations nine developed PGU. The rises or falls in the concentrations of organisms were similarly unrelated to PGU. Thus four patients developed PGU after rises in concentrations of *M. hominis*; five after the concentrations had not changed; six after the concentrations had declined and 20 in the absence of *M. hominis*.

It seems that *M. hominis* is unlikely to be a significant cause of NSU, so attention recently has been focused upon the T-mycoplasmas. These organisms have been isolated from urethral material in up to 93 per cent of selected cases of NGU (Shepard, 1970). They have been isolated more commonly from patients suffering from NGU than from controls in a number of studies (Ford and others, 1962; Ford and Du Vernet, 1963; Shepard, 1966; Csonka and others, 1966; Ruys and others, 1967; Holmes and others, 1967; Shipley and others, 1968; Sueltmann and others, 1971). In view of the relationship of the finding of T-mycoplasmas to recent sexual intercourse noted above, some of these control groups, for example, prisoners and hospital in-patients (Ford and others, 1962; Ford and Du Vernet, 1963), might be expected to have low incidences of infection; the hospital staff members (Csonka and others, 1966) were tested only by means of urine culture.

In contrast, T-mycoplasmas have been isolated with similar frequencies from control subjects and from patients suffering from NSU in a number of studies (Ingham and others, 1966; Fowler and Leeming, 1969; Haas and others, 1971; Jansson and others, 1971; Lassus and others, 1971). In each of two studies (Catalano and others, 1968; Black and Rasmussen, 1968) the incidence of infection detected in control subjects was higher than in the patients.

PGU was related to T-mycoplasmas by Csonka and others (1966) who cultured that organism from urethral material from 10 of 13 men who developed PGU and from only 14 of 50 who did not develop PGU following treatment with penicillin. Hare and others (1969) studied 120 men suffering from gonorrhoea. In contrast they found T-mycoplasmas in 21 (60 per cent) of 35 who developed PGU, in 59 (69 per cent) of the remainder and in 24 (83 per cent) of 29 men who were known to have remained free from PGU during observation for 4 weeks following treatment. Vaughan-Jackson (1974) made a similar study with the addition of tests of urethral material for Chlamydia. Tests for T-mycoplasmas gave results as before, in contrast to tests for Chlamydia which were positive only in those cases in which PGU developed or in the cases of patients who defaulted before PGU could be excluded.

Hare and others (1969) also estimated the numbers of T-mycoplasmas in specimens. If the mycoplasmas were causing urethritis it would be likely that the incidence of PGU would be higher in the cases of patients with high concentrations of organisms. This was not so. Thus, of 42 men with high concentrations of organisms in urethral material 10 developed PGU; this compared with 38 men with low concentrations of T-mycoplasmas of whom 11 developed PGU. A rise in concentration of T-mycoplasmas was not particularly associated with PGU. Thus eight patients developed PGU after rises in the concentration, two after the concentration had remained unchanged, 11 after falls in concentration and 14 in the absence of the organism. Fowler and Leeming (1969) found no evidence to connect T-mycoplasmas with PGU.

The detection of antibody to a mycoplasma in association with signs of inflammation does not prove that the mycoplasma is the primary cause of the inflammation. Most studies have not shown significant formation of antibody. However, Jansson and others (1971) used an indirect haemagglutination test and found that 13 (24 per cent) of 54 patients suffering from NSU showed an antibody response, to one of the two isolates tested, that was compatible with recent infection. The highest titre of antibody obtained was in the case of a symptom-free sailor who had had several attacks of NSU.

The sensitivities of T-mycoplasmas to antibiotics are compatible with their being a cause of NSU. They are sensitive to tetracyclines and to erythromycin (Shipley and others, 1968; Braun and others, 1970; Shepard and others, 1970) and these antibiotics are effective against NSU (Willcox, 1955, 1968; Grimble, 1968) although erythromycin is less effective than the tetracyclines and does not inhibit *M. hominis*. They are insensitive to lincomycin (Shipley and others, 1968; Braun and others, 1970a; Csonka and Corse, 1970) which is ineffective against NSU (Csonka and Spitzer, 1969) but does inhibit *M. hominis* (Csonka and Corse, 1970).

T-mycoplasmas and *M. hominis* are commonly found in genital material from sexually active women (Csonka and others, 1966; Archer, 1968; Braun and others, 1970b, 1971; Mård and Weström, 1970c. McCormack and others (1972), in a study of 156 student and graduate nurses not receiving tetracyclines, showed that of the girls who denied genital contact only a few were harbouring T-mycoplasmas compared with 38 per cent of those who had had one sexual partner, 55 per cent of those who had had two and 75 per cent of those who had had three or more. *M. hominis* was less commonly found but isolation rates followed a similar pattern.

If NSU is due to T-mycoplasmas why is it that the condition is not even more common than it is?

It is possible that only certain strains are pathogenic in the urethra of the male. This possibility seems unlikely because, although Purcell and others (1969) tested only a few strains, they found that serologically the T-mycoplasmas isolated from patients suffering from NSU 'did not differ significantly' from those isolated from healthy subjects. This should be investigated further as there are many strains of T-mycoplasma. Thus Ford (1967) tested 32 isolates from the genital tract against antisera prepared in rabbits against six different isolates: 17 isolates were typable with these antisera, the remainder were not. Black (1970) tested 12 isolates obtained from men suffering from NSU: 10 were typable, two were not, indicating that there were at least seven serotypes in the 12 isolates tested. Purcell and others (1969) tested 12 isolates and found that all were different.

There is no convincing evidence as yet to incriminate T-mycoplasmas as a cause of non-specific urethritis in man.

Mycoplasmas (*M. hominis* and T-mycoplasmas) have been isolated from other inflammatory conditions affecting men. They have been incriminated in para-urethral abscesses and prostatitis. *M. fermentans* has been isolated in cases of balanoposthitis.

Reiter's disease was ascribed by some workers to *M. hominis* and then to T-mycoplasmas (*vide infra Reiter's disease*).

In the cases of women, mycoplasmas have been considered to cause Bartholin's abscesses, vaginitis, non-specific cervicitis and pelvic inflammatory disease. The work of Mård and Weström (1970a) on the last condition is of particular interest. They studied 50 women in whose cases salpingitis was diagnosed at laparoscopy when tubal material was obtained for culture; 13 control subjects were also examined by the same means. *M. hominis* was grown from tubal material from four patients suffering from salpingitis and T-mycoplasma from two. No isolate was obtained from tubal material from the 13 control subjects nor from 21 women suffering from infections of the lower genital tract. In one case of salpingitis Coxsackie B5 and in another ECHO 6 virus were isolated. *M. hominis* was isolated from the lower genital tract in the cases of 31 of the 50 patients suffering from salpingitis and from only two of the non-infected controls.

Indirect haemagglutination (IHA) was used by these authors (Mård and Weström 1970b) to study antibody response to *M. hominis* in the cases of 52 women suffering from salpingitis diagnosed at laparoscopy. *M. hominis* was isolated from the cervix, or from a Fallopian tube and cervix, in 36 cases, in 25 of which (69 per cent) there was an IHA titre of 1 in 16 or greater. In 29 cases in which more than one specimen of serum was tested there was such a level of antibody in 16 (55 per cent). *M. hominis* was isolated from the lower genital tract in the cases of all 16. Six of the 16 showed a four-fold or greater rise in titre; *M. hominis* was isolated from tubal material from two of these six. It is noted that *M. hominis* was isolated from 27 (38·6 per cent) of 70 women suffering from infections of the lower genital tract, 19 of these 70 had IHA titres of 1 in 16 or greater but the percentage of isolate-positive cases in which there was a significant titre is not recorded as it is for the salpingitis patients. Mård (1970) found an increase in immunoglobulin IgM in 34 per cent of cases of salpingitis. This increase was associated with the isolation of *M. hominis* and with the presence of indirect haemagglutinating antibody against that agent. Earlier Lemcke and Csonka (1962) had shown an antibody response in 30 (58·8 per cent) of 51 cases of salpingitis by means of complement-fixation tests using three strains of *M. hominis* as antigens; the incidence of positivity related to severity of the salpingitis: of the 19 severe cases 12 gave positive results. Melén and Gotthardson (1955) found high titres in five of 27 cases. Mård and Weström (1970c) reported also that one of the two patients suffering from salpingitis, from whom T-mycoplasma was isolated from tubal material, showed an increase of antibody to that agent as measured by metabolic inhibition. Kundsin (1970) reported the isolation of T-mycoplasma from a Fallopian tube affected by chronic inflammatory changes.

It is possible that *M. hominis* and T-mycoplasma may have a primary role in some cases of salpingitis. On the other hand these agents are commonly found in the genital tract particularly in women with multiple sexual partners (McCormack and others, 1972); in such women the chance of infections by other agents, such as members of the Chlamydia, would also be increased. The presence of antibodies to an agent, in serum from a patient, does not necessarily prove that that agent is the primary cause of an inflammatory process in that patient.

Mycoplasmas have also been related to septic abortion, puerperal infections, infertility, spontaneous abortion, stillbirth, premature delivery and to the low birth-weight of infants; it is of interest that chromosomal aberrations have occurred in cell cultures infected by *M. hominis* (see McCormack and others, 1973; *Nature* Editorial, 1973).

Ophthalmia neonatorum has been ascribed to *M. hominis*. Jones and Tobin (1968) isolated this agent from eight of 250 clinically infected eyes of newborn babies. Tyrrell and Taylor-Robinson (1968) commented on this report of ophthalmia neonatorum 'due to' *M. hominis*: they considered that the inference that the conjunctivitis was 'due to' *M. hominis* was not a legitimate deduction.

The colonisation of infants by genital mycoplasmas has been studied (Klein and others, 1969; Foy and others, 1970; Braun and others, 1971). Foy and others (1970) reported a 2-year study of 100 babies starting on the first or second day of life. T-mycoplasma was isolated from 38 per cent of female babies and *M. hominis* from 6 per cent. T-mycoplasma was isolated from 6 per cent of male babies. Examination of the infants (including two from whom *M. hominis* was isolated from conjunctival material) revealed no sign of disease. Only one infant had conjunctivitis, TRIC agent was isolated from conjunctival material in that case but no mycoplasma was cultured. Like *M. hominis*, T-mycoplasma was usually isolated directly after birth and the rate of isolation declined sharply after 3 months. Colonisation of babies has been related to the mycoplasmas present in the genital tracts of the mothers (Foy et al, 1970).

REFERENCES

ARCHER, J. F. (1968). *Brit. J. vener. Dis.*, **44**, 232.

BLACK, F. T. (1970). 'Proceedings of Fifth International Congress of Infectious Diseases', p. 407.

BLACK, F. T. and RASMUSSEN, O. G. (1968). *Brit. J. vener. Dis.*, **44**, 324.

BRAUN, P., KLEIN, J. O. and KASS, E. H. (1970a). *Appl. Microbiol.*, **19**, 62.

BRAUN, P., KLEIN, J. O. and LEE, Y.-H. (1970b). *J. infect. Dis.*, **121**, 391.

BRAUN, P., LEE, Y.-H., KLEIN, J. O., MARCY, S. M., KLEIN, T. A., CHARLES, D., LEVY, P. and KASS, E. H. (1971). *New Engl. J. Med.* **284**, 167.

CATALANO, G., VARONE, G. L. and ARGENZIANO, G. (1968). *G. mal. infett.*, **20**, 1009.

CSONKA, G. and CORSE, J. (1970). *Brit. J. vener. Dis.*, **46**, 203.

CSONKA, G. W. and SPITZER, R. J. (1969). *Brit. J. vener. Dis.*, **45**, 52.

CSONKA, G. W., WILLIAMS, R. E. O. and CORSE, J. (1966). *Lancet*, **1**, 1292.

FORD, D. K. (1967). *Ann, N.Y. Acad. Sci.*, **143**, 501.

FORD, D. K. (1968). *Canad. med. Ass. J.*, **99**, 900.

FORD, D. K. (1970). 'The Role of Mycoplasmas and L Forms of Bacteria in Disease', ed. by T. T. Sharp, p. 137. Charles C. Thomas, Springfield, Illinois.

FORD, D. K. and DU VERNET, M. (1963). *Brit. J. vener. Dis.*, **39**, 18.

FORD, D. K., RASMUSSEN, G. and MINKEN, J. (1962). *Brit. J. vener. Dis.*, **38**, 22.

FOWLER, W. and LEEMING, R. J. (1969). *Brit. J. vener. Dis.*, **45**, 287.

FOY, H. M., KENNY, G. E., LEVINSOHN, E. M. and GRAYSTON, J. T. (1970). *J. infect. Dis.*, **121**, 579.

FOY, H. M., KENNY, G. E., WENTWORTH, B. B., JOHNSON, W. L. and GRAYSTON, J. T. (1970). *Amer. J. Obstet. Gynec.*, **106**, 635.

GRIMBLE, A. (1968). *Brit. J. vener. Dis.*, **44**, 230.

HAAS, H., DORFMAN, M. L. and SACKS, T. G. (1971). *Brit. J. vener. Dis.*, **47**, 131.

HARE, M. J., DUNLOP, E. M. C. and TAYLOR-ROBINSON, D. (1969). *Brit. J. vener. Dis.*, **45**, 282.

HOLMES, K. K., JOHNSON, D. W., FLOYD, T. M. and KVALE, P. A. (1967). *J. Amer. med. Ass.*, **202**, 467.

INGHAM, H. R., MACFARLANE, W. V., HALE, J. H., SELKON, J. B. and CODD, A. A. (1966). *Brit. J. vener. Dis.*, **42**, 269.

JANSSON, E., LASSUS, A., STUBB, S. and TUURI, S. (1971). *Brit. J. vener. Dis.*, **47**, 122.

JONES, D. M. and TOBIN, B. (1968). *Brit. med. J.*, **3**, 467.

KING, A. J. (1964). 'Recent Advances in Venereology', p. 359. Churchill, London.

KLEIN, J. O., BUCKLAND, D. and FINLAND, M. (1969). *New Engl. J. Med.*, **280**, 1025.

KUNDSIN, R. B. (1970). *New Engl. J. Med.*, **282**, 928.

LASSUS, A., PURKO, R.-L., STUBB, S., MATTILA, R. and JANSSON, E. (1971). *Brit. J. vener. Dis.*, **47**, 126.

LEMCKE, R. and CSONKA, G. W. (1962). *Brit. J. vener. Dis.*, **38**, 212.

MÅRD, P.-A. (1970). *Acta path. microbiol. scand.*, **78B**, 726.

MÅR, DP.-A. and WESTRÖM, L. (1970a). *Brit. J. vener. Dis.*, **46**, 179.

MÅRD, P.-A. and WESTRÖM, L. (1970b). *Brit. J. vener. Dis.*, **46**, 390.

MÅRD, P.-A. and WESTRÖM, L. (1970c). *Acta path. microbiol. scand.*, **78B**, 367.

McCORMACK, W. M., ALMEIDA, P. C., BAILEY, P. E., GRADY, E. M. and LEE, Y.-H. (1972). *J. Amer. med. Ass.*, **221**, 1375.

McCORMACK, W. M., BRAUN, P., LEE, Y.-H., KLEIN, J. O. and KASS, E. H. (1973). *New Engl. J. Med.*, **288**, 78.

MELÉN, B. and GOTTHARDSON, A. (1955). *Acta path. microbiol. scand.*, **37**, 196.

NATURE Editorial (1973). *Nature Lond.*, **242**, 83.

NICOL, C. S. and EDWARD, D. G. (1953). *Brit. J. vener. Dis.*, **29**, 141.

PURCELL, R. H., CHANOCK, R. M. and TAYLOR-ROBINSON, D. (1969). 'The Mycoplasmetales and the L-phase of Bacteria', ed. L. Hayflick, p. 221. Appleton-Century Crofts, New York.

PURCELL, R. H., TAYLOR-ROBINSON, D., WONG, D. and CHANOCK, R. M. (1966). *J. Bact.*, **92**, 6.

PURCELL, R. H., WONG, D., CHANOCK, R. M., TAYLOR-ROBINSON, D., CANCHOLA, J. and VALDESUSO, J. (1967). *Ann. N.Y. Acad. Sci.*, **143**, 664.

RAZIN, S. (1968). *J. Bact.*, **96**, 687.

RUYS, A. C., HERDERSCHEË, D. and WALDMAN, J. (1967). *Ann N.Y. Acad. Sci.*, **143**, 390.

RUITER, M. and WENTHOLT, H. M. M. (1952). *J. invest. Dermat.*, **18**, 313.

SERPETJIAN, M., THIVOLET, J., MONIER, J.-C. and SALUSSOLA, D. (1969). *Path. et Biol.*, **17**, 953.

SHARP, J. T. (1970). 'The Role of Mycoplasmas and L Forms of Bacteria in Disease', ed. J. T. Sharp, Charles C. Thomas, Springfield, Illinois.

SHEPARD, M. C. (1954). *Amer. J. Syph.*, **38**, 113.

SHEPARD, M. C. (1966). *Hlth Lab. Sci.*, **3**, 163.

SHEPARD, M. C. (1970). *J. Amer. med. Ass.*, **211**, 1335.

SHEPARD, M. C. and CALVY, G. L. (1965). *New. Engl. J. Med.*, **272**, 848.

SHEPARD, M. C., LUNCEFORD, C. D. and BAKER, R. L. (1960). *Brit. J. vener. Dis.*, **42**, 21.

SHIPLEY, A., BOWMAN, S. J. and O'CONNOR, J. J. (1968). *Med. J. Aust.*, **1**, 794.

SUELTMANN, S., ALLEN, V., INHORN, S. L. and BENFORADO, J. M. (1971). *Hlth Lab. Sci.*, **8**, 62.

TAYLOR-ROBINSON, D., ADDEY, J. P., HARE, M. J., JONES, B. R. and DUNLOP, E. M. C. (1969). *Brit. J. vener. Dis.*, **45**, 265.

TAYLOR-ROBINSON, D. and PURCELL, D. (1966). *Proc. roy. Soc. Med.*, **59**, 1112.

TYRRELL, D. A. J. and TAYLOR-ROBINSON, D. (1968). *Brit. med. J.*, **3**, 801.

VAUGHAN-JACKSON, J. D. (1974). In preparation.

WILLCOX, R. R. (1955). *Brit. J. vener. Dis.*, **31**, 186.

WILLCOX, R. R. (1968). *Brit. J. vener. Dis.*, **44**, 157.

WILLIAMS, M. H. (1967). *Ann N.Y. Acad. Sci.*, **143**, 397.

THE GENUS CHLAMYDIA

The history of urethritis has been linked with that of conjunctivitis (Dunlop, 1965; Thygeson, 1971; Dunlop and others, 1972a) ever since Neisser (1879) described the gonococcus in discharge from the eye and from the genital tract. Thus both conjunctivitis and genital infection may be gonococcal or non-gonococcal; if they are the latter they may be bacterial or abacterial ('non-specific') in origin. The Chlamydia group of agents has been proven to be responsible for much infectious disease of the eye; in the light of recent studies it seems likely that a considerable proportion of 'non-specific' infection of the genital organs and of the rectum is also due to Chlamydia.

Culture in yolk sac

Fifty years after Chlamydia had first been found in smears from the eye (Halberstaedter and Prowazek, 1907) and then from the genital tract, the agent was first cultured (T'ang and others, 1957). Until it had been cultured the significance of the agent had remained controversial despite many studies, including those reviewed by Harkness (1950).

T'ang and others (1957) succeeded in culturing the causative agent of trachoma in the yolk sacs of fertile hens' eggs. The conjunctiva of volunteers was inoculated with the agent and trachoma resulted (Collier and others, 1958, 1960). Chlamydia was isolated from the eyes of babies suffering from ophthalmia neonatorum (Jones and others, 1959; Hanna and others, 1960). The agent was isolated from the cervix of a mother of twins suffering from ophthalmia neonatorum; this mother was suffering from trachoma and one of the twins developed that condition (Collier, 1960). Jones and Collier (Jones and Collier, 1962; Jones, 1964) produced trachoma experimentally by inoculating

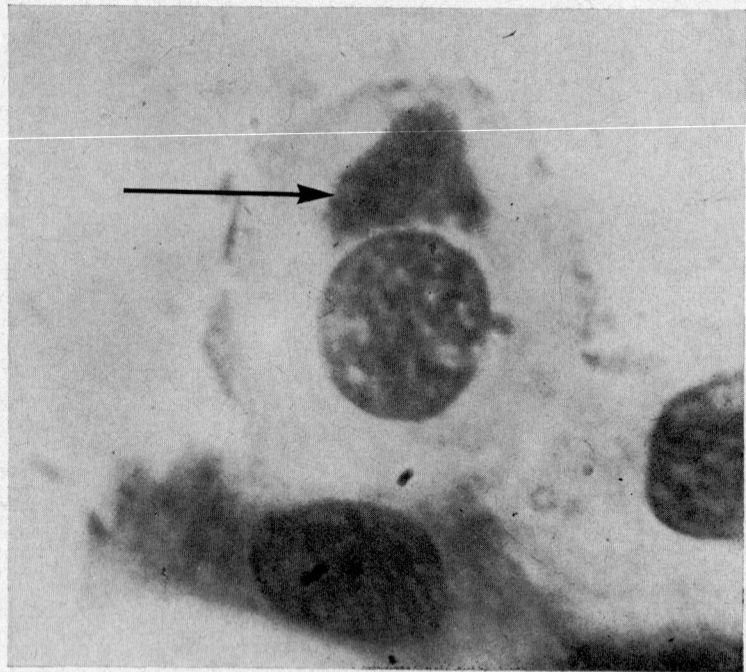

Fig. 21. Halberstaedter–Prowazek inclusion body; Giemsa-stained scraping (× 2,250) from the conjunctiva of a baboon with conjunctivitis due to inoculation of TRIC agent 10L-9/Gu from the urethra of Mr. H. (Jones, Al-Hussaini and Dunlop (1964) *Brit. J. vener. Dis.*, **40**, 1). Baby H. was suffering from ophthalmia neonatorum due to TRIC agent and his father from urethritis due to the same cause. (Reproduced with permission of the authors and the Editor of the *British Journal of Venereal Diseases*.)

the conjunctiva of an adult volunteer with agent isolated from the eye of a baby suffering from ophthalmia neonatorum; this agent was of genital origin because the baby had acquired the infection from the genital tract of its mother; another inoculation of this volunteer with an isolate from the cervix of the mother of such a baby had produced inclusion conjunctivitis only. Chlamydia was isolated from babies suffering from ophthalmia neonatorum, from their mothers who were suffering from genital infection and from their fathers who were suffering from 'non-specific' urethritis (NSU) (Dunlop and others, 1964, 1967) (see Figs. 21, 22).

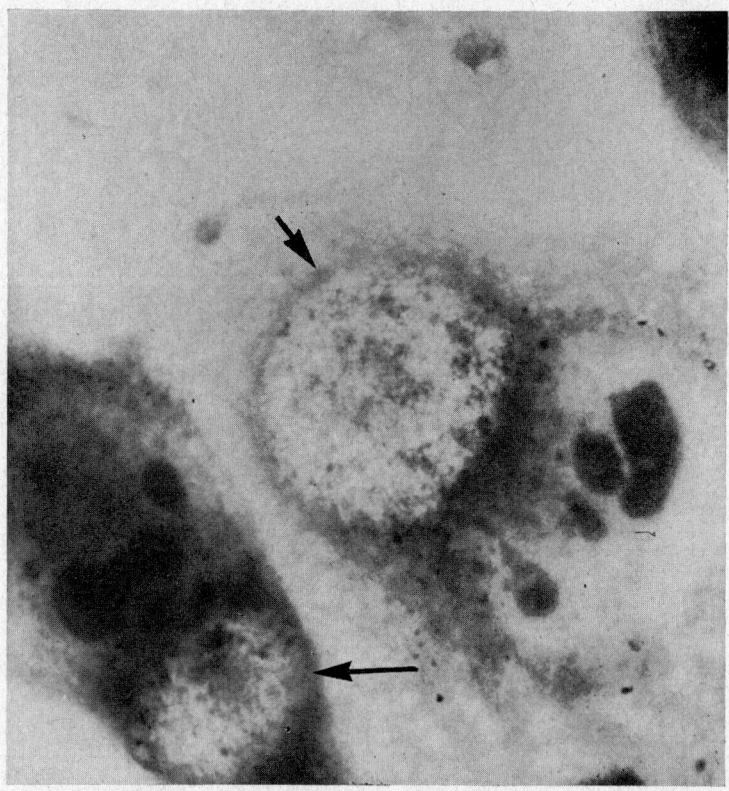

FIG. 22. Isolate (×2,400 approx.) from urethral material from Mr. J.C. (Gordon et al (1969) *J. infect. Dis.*, **120**, 451; Dunlop et al (1969) ibid., **120**, 463). Mr. J.C. was suffering from NSU. The isolate was Giemsa-stained after 48 hours in irradiated McCoy-cells. (Reproduced with permission of the authors and the Editor of the *Journal of Infectious Diseases*.)

Chlamydia was isolated from the urethra in the cases of two of nine men who had presented at a clinic because of NSU (Dunlop and others, 1965a). Chlamydia isolated from the urethra of an additional such patient was used to inoculate the conjunctiva of three baboons and produced conjunctivitis typical of TRIC agent in all. Subsequently Chlamydia was isolated from up to 21 per cent of men who presented with NSU and up to 35 per cent of the female contacts of such men (Dunlop and others, 1967); also Chlamydia was isolated from the genital tract in the cases of men and of women presenting in London, Copenhagen and San Francisco because of fresh infection of the eye by TRIC agent, and from sexual contacts of persons so presenting. In each case studied, the isolate from the eye and that from the genital tract were the same. It seems that in these groups of patients infection was more likely to be spread by sexual contact than by eye-to-eye transmission. In them the infection of the eye (including trachoma) probably arose as a complication of such genital infection (Dunlop and others, 1965b, 1966, 1967; Jones and others, 1965; Mordhorst, 1967; Dawson and Schachter, 1967). This contrasts with the situation in developing areas with conditions in which eye-to-eye transmission of trachoma in early childhood is extremely common.

Chlamydia has been isolated from genital material obtained from patients presenting in different parts of the world including the United Kingdom, France, the United States of America, Canada, Denmark, Russia (Pukner and Kozlova, 1965; Pukner and others, 1966), Egypt (Shabaan and others, 1972) South Africa (Scott, 1968) and Taiwan (Chiang and others, 1968).

Terminology

Because an isolate from the eye of a patient suffering from trachoma was indistinguishable, even by inoculation of volunteers (Jones and Collier, 1962; Mitsui and others, 1962; Jones, 1964), from an isolate from the eye of a baby suffering from ophthalmia neonatorum, such an isolate was named TRIC agent; the *TR*– standing for trachoma and the –*IC* for inclusion conjunctivitis (Gear and others, 1968). The term 'agent' is now used because members of the Chlamydia group are neither viruses nor bacteria (Moulder, 1964, 1966). Thus, although they are restricted to an obligate intracellular growth, they have a characteristic development cycle, multiplying by binary fission. They contain both DNA and RNA, they have cell walls of the bacterial type, ribosomes and enzyme systems, including those that permit the catabolysis of certain substances (Weiss, 1967); they are inhibited in varying degrees (Jawetz, 1969; Storz, 1971) by sulphonamides (McCallum and Findlay, 1938) and by antibiotics that affect bacterial multiplication including tetracyclines; they are inhibited by rifampicin, erythromyciu and by trimethoprim (Becker and others, 1971) and to some degree by penicillin and by chloramphenicol (T'ang and others, 1957); they are not affected by the aminoglycosides (streptomycin, neomycin, kanamycin) that do not enter cells readily. One bovine strain has been shown to be sensitive to lincomycin (Shipley and others, 1968).

This group of agents has been called Bedsonia (after the late Sir Samuel Bedson who isolated and characterised the agent of psittacosis), and by many different names which resulted in increasing confusion. Applying the taxonomic rules of nomenclature, Page (1966) re-proposed the name Chlamydia for the genus. The term TRIC agent is suitable for a Chlamydia isolated from an eye affected by characteristic disease; but an isolate from an extra-ocular site should be designated by the genus name (Chlamydia) only, unless there is strong clinical evidence that it is TRIC agent or the agent of lymphogranuloma venereum (LGV) or another chlamydial agent. The uses of the micro-immunofluorescence (micro-IF) test (see below) are not yet known; however, it seems that an agent may be identified by it as one of the different serotypes of TRIC agent or of LGV, or as another of the Chlamydia; it is not yet known whether there may be variations in pathogenicity (to the eye or to other tissues) between the individual members of each serotype, between the different serotypes of TRIC agent, or between the serotypes of LGV.

Isolates of Chlamydia are either members of subgroup A whose inclusions contain glycogen and so stain with iodine (this subgroup includes TRIC agent and most isolates of LGV), or of subgroup B whose inclusions do not contain glycogen and so do not stain with iodine; subgroup B is mainly of avian (for example, psittacosis) or of animal origin (Gordon and Quan, 1965).

Isolates of subgroup B Chlamydia (as well as the more commonly found subgroup A) have been obtained in yolk sac from specimens from patients suffering from LGV (Schachter, 1967, Schachter and Meyer, 1969) and from Reiter's disease (Schachter, 1967; Harper and others, 1967; Dunlop and others, 1967); the matter was reviewed by Jones (1972). Such isolates have also been obtained from abortion specimens (Schachter, 1967) and one with some subgroup B properties has been obtained in cell culture from ocular material from a patient suffering from trachoma (Dwyer and others, 1972).

The term Chlamydia (with a capital C) is a genus name. Its use in the plural (Lancet Editorial, 1973) is incorrect as this would imply the existence of a number of such genuses. The different members of this genus may be referred to as chlamydiae (without a capital C); similarly the term chlamydial may be used as an adjective.

The use of the term TRIC agent has stemmed from the fact that the term Chlamydia oculogenitale, as opposed to Chlamydia trachomatis, is outmoded by present knowledge and should no longer be used. Further extensions of nomenclature at this time, including the revival of the term paratrachoma (of Lindner) and its application to the D to I serotypes of Chlamydia and for infections caused by them (Dwyer and others, 1972) are probably undesirable in the present state of knowledge.

New tests for chlamydial infection

(a) Isolation in cell culture. Isolation in yolk sac is an insensitive method for the diagnosis of chlamydial infection. This was shown by the fact that TRIC agent was isolated by this method from cervical material from only seven of 28 mothers of babies suffering from ophthalmia neonatorum due to that agent (Dunlop and others, 1967). Also it was open to cross-contamination in the laboratory which could result in spurious isolation (Harper and others, 1967).

Culture in irradiated McCoy-cells (Magruder and others, 1963; Gordon and others, 1967) provided the first alternative method to culture in yolk sac for the primary isolation of Chlamydia. Comparisons have shown that it is significantly more sensitive for the detection of Chlamydia in clinical specimens from different sites than the detection of inclusions and isolation in yolk sac (Gordon and others, 1969; Dunlop and others, 1969; Darougar and others, 1971a, d; Philip and others, 1971).

A sensitive but simplified one-passage technique of culture in irradiated McCoy-cells has been developed; serum was added to the transport medium and specimens were stored in liquid nitrogen instead of in a mechanical refrigerator (Darougar and others, 1971b, 1972). High-speed centrifugation increases the sensitivity of the method (Darougar and others, 1974). Using cell culture, isolates were obtained from urethral material obtained with an endourethral curette and a meatal swab from 18 of 41 (44 per cent) of men who had presented because of NSU and from the genital tract in the cases of five of 21 of their female sexual contacts (Dunlop and others, 1971a). This study was extended: valid tests were obtained of urethral material from 99 men; Chlamydia was isolated from 44 (44·5 per cent). Thirty-four of their female sexual partners were tested; Chlamydia was isolated from 10, all of whose male consorts were Chlamydia-positive (Dunlop and others, 1972). Using bacteriological loops and cotton-tipped applicators to obtain urethral material Philip and others (1971) grew Chlamydia from eight of 35 men suffering from non-gonococcal urethritis (NGU), two of 11 men with post-gonococcal urethritis and from five of 32 men with gonorrhoea. Cervical and urethral specimens were also tested from nine female contacts of men suffering from NGU; isolates were obtained from two. Using swabs to collect urethral material Richmond and others (1972) isolated Chlamydia from 40 of 103 men suffering from NGU (39 per cent). Oriel and others (1972) obtained uncontaminated specimens by means of an endourethral curette from 98 men suffering from NSU; they isolated Chlamydia in 35 cases (36 per cent). This compared with 14 isolates from 37 uncontaminated specimens (38 per cent) obtained by swabbing the urethral meatus and distal urethra; the contamination-rate for the specimens obtained with the curette was only 7 per cent compared with 18 per cent for those obtained by swabbing. Ford and McCandlish (1971) isolated Chlamydia from urethral material obtained with a curette from only eight of 151 men with NGU. In 44 cases isolation was also attempted in yolk sac; in two of these cases isolates were obtained by both methods. In their hands the two methods appeared of similar sensitivity although the cell-culture method was quicker and cheaper.

Earlier studies have been extended using the cell-culture technique which is more sensitive than the methods used previously. Thus, of 23 women presenting because of proven infection of the eye by TRIC agent, isolates were obtained from cervical material from 19 of the 21 in whose cases the cervix was tested, and from rectal material from 11 of 21. Eleven male sexual contacts of these women were tested; isolates were obtained from urethral material from six, all of whom were suffering from 'NSU'. Twenty-two men who presented because of ocular infection, due to TRIC agent, were tested; isolates were obtained from urethral material from 10, all of whom had 'NSU'; 19 female sexual partners of these men had tests of the genitalia and rectum; isolates were obtained from eight (Vaughan-Jackson and others, 1972). Isolates were obtained from cervical material from 11 of 15 mothers of babies suffering from ophthalmia neonatorum due to TRIC agent (Darougar and others, 1972) compared with seven of 28 such mothers, when material was cultured in yolk sac (Dunlop and others, 1967).

The sensitivity of the cell-culture technique and the resistance of the McCoy-cell culture to bacterial contamination permitted the isolation of Chlamydia from the rectum (Gordon and others, 1969; Dunlop and others, 1969; Darougar and others, 1971c; Dunlop and others, 1971b) whereas culture from that site had previously been unsuccessful.

Controls showed that cross-contamination in the laboratory did not occur using culture in cell-culture (Gordon and others, 1969; Darougar and others, 1971a, c). The simplified technique of culture in irradiated McCoy-cells is now a sensitive and practicable diagnostic method (Darougar and others, 1971b; 1972) that can be used generally for diagnosis, epidemiological studies and assessment of the results of treatment.

(b) Micro-immunofluorescence (micro-IF) test. Until recently the distinction between TRIC agent and LGV agent in the laboratory has had to be made by the detection of the different but somewhat irregular patterns of pathogenicity to animals of the two agents; hence the designation of an isolate as LGV agent rather than TRIC agent (or the converse) usually has been made because of its clinical origin (Treharne and others, 1972).

The micro-IF test (Wang, 1971) has so far proved to be the best method of immunological classification; up to now it has shown the existence of nine main serotypes (A to I) of TRIC agent and three serotypes (I, II, III) of LGV agent (Wang and Grayston, 1970, 1971; Treharne and others, 1971, 1972, 1973; Dwyer and others, 1972; Dunlop and others, 1973; Gordon and others, 1973; Wang and others, 1973). Serotypes A, B and C were isolated from the eyes of patients suffering from endemic trachoma in the Middle East, Africa and Asia, where the presumed method of spread of infection is by eye-to-eye transmission. Only two such isolates were type D (Jones, 1972). With few exceptions, serotypes D to I were isolated from the eye, rectum or the genital tract of patients seen in London, Copenhagen and the USA in whose cases the presumed route of transmission of infection was genital.

The precision of the micro-IF test makes it a valuable method for studying infection by Chlamydia: it can be used to distinguish TRIC agent from LGV agent and to identify serotypes of Chlamydia in epidemiological studies and for the preparation of intradermal tests; intradermal tests may prove useful because the Frei test and the use of so-called specific acid-extracts for intradermal tests have given some positive but confusing results in studies of chlamydial infections other than LGV (Barwell and others, 1967). The Frei test was positive in only four of 11 cases of LGV (Schachter and others, 1969); a complement-fixation test (LGVCFT) for group antibody was positive at a titre of 1 in 32 or more in seven of 12 cases.

Measurement of anti-chlamydial group antibody by means of a complement-fixation test using chlamydial group antigen is insensitive and of limited use particularly in chlamydial infections other than LGV (Barwell and others, 1967). The micro-IF test is more sensitive; moreover it detects antibodies to individual chlamydial serotypes (Dwyer and others, 1972).

Dwyer and others (1972) reported that sera in 14 of 17 isolate-positive NSU cases gave titres of 1 in 16 or more, compared with only four of 24 isolate-negative cases; 14 of 18 sera from 11 patients suffering from Reiter's disease and 34 of 36 isolate-positive cases of oculogenital chlamydial infection. Clear-cut responses to single chlamydial serotypes occurred more commonly in sera from patients suffering from hyperendemic trachoma (due to TRIC serotypes A, B and C) than in sera from patients infected by serotypes D, E, F and G. It is probable that early convalescent sera would be more likely to show monospecific reactions; experimental work with animals (Treharne and others, 1971) suggests that the specificity would be greatest in the IgM response, which could be detected separately in the micro-IF test.

However, fractionation of the serum might be necessary before the test to obviate the masking effect of anti-chlamydial IgG (Juchau and others, 1972).

As yet the results of micro-IF tests for the detection of antibody must be interpreted with caution. This must continue until the performance of the test in control groups free from chlamydial infection has been outlined, and until the range of subgroup B Chlamydia definable by the test has been established, so that representative subgroup B serotypes are included in the test. Further results of this test in the cases of patients suffering from the various forms of chlamydial infection and from Reiter's disease are particularly required, as are sensitivity tests to antibiotics and to chemotherapentic agents of different isolates of Chlamydia that have been precisely identified by the micro-IF test.

(c) **Radio-isotope precipitation (RIP) test.** This test (Gerloff and Watson, 1967; Philip and others, 1971; Dwyer and others, 1972) and the LGVCFT measure antibody to chlamydial group antigen. The RIP test is more sensitive than the LGVCFT. It would seem to be of less value than the micro-IF test which measures type-specific antibody. Markedly lower titres in the micro-IF test for type-specific antibody than in the RIP test for antibody to chlamydial group antigen may suggest that the patient has been infected by a serotype of Chlamydia not included in the micro-IF test (Dwyer and others, 1972).

Pathogenicity of Chlamydia

Chlamydia is a pathogen in the eye. It is likely to be a pathogen in the genital tract (and the rectum) where a reservoir of chlamydial infection exists (Dunlop and others, 1966); thus Chlamydia from the genital tract produces disease of the eye as shown by each baby suffering from TRIC ophthalmia neonatorum, and as shown by the inoculation of the conjunctiva of man (Jones and Collier, 1962; Jones, 1964; Mitsui and others, 1962) and of experimental animals (Dunlop and others, 1965; Mordhorst, 1967; Darougar and others, 1971c). Also an isolate from the rectum of the mother of a baby suffering from TRIC ophthalmia neonatorum produced typical follicular conjunctivitis in two baboons and established urethral infection in a male baboon from which the agent was re-isolated (Darougar and others, 1971c). The association of the presence of Chlamydia in the genital tract with local inflammatory change is close; for example, in the parents of babies suffering from TRIC ophthalmia neonatorum and in adults presenting with fresh ocular infection by TRIC agent. Moreover the inflammatory changes associated with the presence of TRIC agent may be found in the sexual partners of such patients (Dunlop and others, 1967; Vaughan-Jackson and others, 1972). For the rectum (Dunlop and others, 1971b), as for other sites, there is an association between the presence of inflammatory changes and the isolation of Chlamydia. Furthermore, examination with an operating microscope shows that the clinical signs associated with the presence of Chlamydia in the conjunctiva, genital tract and rectum may resemble each other closely.

Inflammatory changes are found in biopsy specimens taken from the clinically affected marginal areas of the cervix in the cases of women from whom isolates have been obtained from that site; electron microscopy has shown the agent within the inflamed tissue (Ashton and others, 1974).

Of 318 men tested by the group at The London Hospital and Institute of Ophthalmology (Dunlop and others, 1967, 1972b; Vaughan-Jackson and others, 1972) Chlamydia was detected in urethral material from 100, all of whom had urethritis. Thirteen men did not have urethritis. Chlamydia was not detected in urethral material from any of them. There was an association between urethritis and the presence of Chlamydia.

In early studies using insensitive tests (culture in yolk sac, examination of smears) large amounts of the urethral epithelial cells to be tested were obtained by means of a curette (Dunlop and others, 1964, 1965a). This made the study of a control group impracticable according to these workers. However, Oriel and others (1972) used a curette to obtain uncontaminated material, for culture in cell culture, from a control group of 31 men shown not be be suffering from urethritis; no isolate was obtained compared with 35 isolates from 98 men suffering from NSU from whom uncontaminated specimens were obtained. A miniature endourethral swab has been devised (Dunlop and others, 1972c) that can be passed to the bulb of the urethra in the male. Results using this non-traumatic method to collect material for culture in irradiated McCoy-cells are as good as those using a urethral curette (Dunlop and others, 1972c). This method has been used in the study of a 'control' group by Vaughan-Jackson (1974). Men suffering from gonorrhoea were tested initially before treatment for gonorrhoea and then during follow-up after treatment with either kanamycin 2 g by intramuscular injection or with procaine penicillin 2·4 mega units by intramuscular injection together with 2 g of probenecid by mouth. Chlamydia was isolated only from those men who developed post-gonococcal urethritis (PGU) or from those who defaulted before the diagnosis of PGU could be made; no isolate was obtained from the 'control' group comprised of men who did not develop PGU. In contrast to this finding, and confirming the work of Hare and others (1969), T-mycoplasmas were detected with similar frequency in urethral material from those men who developed PGU and those who did not. The choice of such a 'control' group ensures that all the patients have been exposed to sexually transmitted infection as shown by the initial gonorrhoea. If Chlamydia were a non-pathogenic organism transmitted by sexual intercourse the incidence in the 'controls' and in men suffering from PGU should be much the same, as has proved to be the case for mycoplasmas (Hare and others, 1969; Vaughan-Jackson, 1974).

Philip and others (1971) isolated Chlamydia from urethral material obtained with bacteriological loops and cotton-tipped applicators from eight of 35 men suffering from NGU, two of 11 suffering from PGU and from five of 32 suffering from gonorrhoea; they concluded that a causal relationship of Chlamydia to NGU could not be established. Gordon and Quan (1971) using a loop, which is an insensitive method for obtaining urethral material, obtained no isolate from 10 controls, compared with 19 isolates from 84 men suffering from NSU from whom urethral material was obtained by a number of different methods.

Richmond and others (1972) obtained urethral material with a swab passed into the distal urethra. Chlamydia was isolated in cell culture from 40 of 103 men suffering from NGU (39 per cent); 32 of 99 men suffering from gonorrhoea (32 per cent) and from five of 92 controls (5 per cent). PGU was detected in 21 cases after follow-up for 1 week or more; Chlamydia had been isolated in 17 of these (81 per cent); so PGU was more likely in the cases of patients from whom Chlamydia had been isolated. Chlamydia was isolated more commonly from those men with long-standing NGU than from those who presented early. The authors suggest that Chlamydia is not the primary cause of NGU but that urethritis from any cause may 'reactivate' quiescent chlamydial infection (they consider that it can then cause urethral discharge). If the overnight urethral secretion had been tested it is possible that the 'controls' and the patients, passed as 'clear' after treatment of gonorrhoea, but from whom Chlamydia was isolated, might have been proved to be suffering from low-grade urethritis (Rodin, 1971). The control series of Oriel and others (1972) in which Chlamydia was not isolated from uncontaminated urethral scrapings from 31 men without urethritis suggests that this agent is not commonly present unless the patient has urethritis. After culture of 98 uncontaminated urethral specimens obtained with a curette from men suffering from NSU these authors obtained isolates from 35 (36 per cent).

Furthermore, the isolation of Chlamydia from the urethra in the cases of men suffering from 'non-specific' urethritis, who had presented because of ocular infection by TRIC agent in themselves or in their sexual partners (Dunlop, 1967; Mordhorst, 1967), demonstrates that Chlamydia is a primary pathogen in the urethra of the male and does not necessarily require additional infection such as gonorrhoea to make it pathogenic. Thus, Vaughan-Jackson and others (1972) studied 33 such men using cell culture. Chlamydia was isolated from the urethra in the cases of five of the nine in which there was a history of urethritis; in 10 of the 12 in which there were signs of marked urethritis and in six of 15 in which there was mild urethritis. No isolate was obtained in the six in which there was no urethritis. In only one patient was there an associated infection (candidiasis) and in that case no isolate was obtained.

Shaaban and others (1972) working in Egypt, isolated Chlamydia in yolk sac from cervical material from 10 of 41 women of poor socio-economic status who came from a population with a high incidence of trachoma. An isolate was obtained from a woman suffering from carcinoma of the cervix; three isolates were obtained from 11 patients without evidence of genital disease so the authors considered that Chlamydia might have been a 'commensal' in the female genital tract. No details were given of any investigation for inflammatory change by means of an operating microscope, by smears or of any tests for bacteria, trichomomonads, candida, herpes virus or for syphilitic infection. Presumably such tests were not carried out and the changes described were those seen by the naked eye; nor were the findings related to the presence of absence of urethritis in the male sexual partners of these women. The results of micro-IF typing of these isolates would have been of particular interest. Hyperendemic trachoma, which is spread by eye-to-eye transmission in early life, is due to TRIC agent types A, B and C; trachoma in developed countries is due to types D to I that may be isolated from the genital tract as well as from the eye. If culture in irradiated McCoy-cells had been used no doubt the incidence of chlamydial infection detected would have been even higher.

Hanna and her co-workers (Hanna and others, 1968; Jawetz and others, 1967) have drawn attention to the fact that the highly pathogenic Chlamydia agents that cause psittacosis, ornithosis and lymphogranuloma venereum produce episodes of subclinical infection in man during which the agent persists. Using fluorescent-antibody staining they produced evidence to show that infection of the eye by TRIC agent may also produce latent infection at that site during the incubation of disease, during and after treatment and after apparent healing. It would be surprising if this state of affairs did not also obtain in the genital tract, but if it does this would not of course imply that Chlamydia was non-pathogenic in this site. Meyer (1967) stressed the importance of latent or attenuated infection due to this group of pathogenic agents in animals and in man. The trauma from repeated tests of the eye may reactivate infection so that the agent is more readily detected (Darougar, 1973). It is likely that gonorrhoea produces a similar Koebner phenomenon in chlamydial infection and perhaps vice versa; it is possible also that the urethra, already inflamed as a result of chlamydial infection, may be more susceptible to gonococcal infection than when not inflamed. It would seem that the frequency of PGU and the high isolation-rate of Chlamydia in gonorrhoea and in PGU are compatible with Chlamydia being pathogenic in the urethra.

REITER'S DISEASE AND THE GENUS CHLAMYDIA

An unidentified agent that was pathogenic to mice was isolated in yolk sac from material from the urethra and the conjunctiva of a patient suffering from Reiter's disease (Dunham and others, 1947). Siboulet and Galistin (1962) cultured, in yolk sac, urethral and conjunctival material from three such patients. Inclusions had been found in urethral scrapings from all three. Agent was isolated in each case but the isolates were not maintained so could not be identified.

Schachter (1967b) gave further details of the findings first reported by Schachter and others (1966). In 13 definite cases of Reiter's disease material had been cultured in yolk sac, and isolates had been obtained in six as follows: from synovial fluid in two of six; synovial membrane in four of five; conjunctiva in two of seven and urethra in the same number. In three culture-positive cases, the LGVCFT gave titres of greater than 1 in 16. Isolates were also obtained from synovial fluid or synovial membrane from two patients suffering from rheumatoid arthritis both with an LGVCFT titre of 1 in 16. The isolates in this study (and probably those from at least two of four abortion specimens from which isolates were obtained) were subgroup B Chlamydia.

This group of workers later reviewed their findings in a total of 23 cases of Reiter's disease (Ostler and others, 1971). They considered then that Chlamydia had been demonstrated in smear, cultured in yolk sac, or both, in 12 cases. In six cases the agent had been isolated in yolk sac. An isolate was obtained in one of 22 cases from the conjunctiva; in five of 23 from the genital tract and in two of 11 from joints. (These findings should be compared with those given by Schachter, 1967b.) In seven of the 23 cases the LGVCFT gave a titre of 1 in 16 or more.

When Harper and others (1967) reported the possibility of spurious isolations if yolk sac was used for culture, they had cultured genital material from 20 patients (Dunlop and others, 1967) suffering from Reiter's disease and isolates had been obtained in two cases. Synovial material had been cultured in eight cases; isolates had been obtained in four including one in which synovial fluid was cultured on two occasions with negative results although an isolate was obtained from excised synovial tissue. As none of these six isolates was obtained at first pass there was the possibility that they were spurious due to contamination in the laboratory.

The results of culture in irradiated McCoy-cells of material from a further 29 men suffering from Reiter's disease were reported by this group (Vaughan-Jackson and others, 1972). Isolates were obtained from urethral material from three of ten previously untreated patients but not from 19 who had received treatment prior to testing. No isolate was obtained from conjunctival material from 12 (four of whom had not received treatment) or from synovial fluid from nine (three of whom were untreated). An isolate was obtained from genital material from one of the three women who were sexual contacts of men with positive tests, but not from 11 sexual contacts of men with negative tests. It is relevant that one isolate from synovial fluid in the series cultured in yolk sac (Dunlop and others, 1967) by these workers proved to be a subgroup B Chlamydia like those reported by Schachter (1967b).

Apart from cross-contamination in the laboratory it is possible that agent apparently isolated in yolk sac may have been already there in the eggs due to latent chlamydial infection of chickens. However, Schachter (1967a) isolated subgroup B Chlamydia from material from a bubo due to clinical LGV and quoted Arnstein as reporting that this agent appeared incapable of surviving in the tissues of chickens. Whether this applies to all subgroup B Chlamydia isolated in yolk sac is uncertain. The isolation of an agent (10L-207) with certain properties of subgroup B Chlamydia from eye material from a patient suffering from trachoma, reported by Dwyer and others (1972), was made in cell culture and would not have been due to spurious isolation.

Despite the negative findings so far in cell culture it may be that isolates of Chlamydia from joints are not due to spurious isolation in yolk sac. This is because some were obtained at first passage (Schachter, 1967b); because members of subgroup B Chlamydia are not readily recognisable in cell culture and because they may not grow as well in irradiated McCoy-cells as do members of subgroup A.

There is serological evidence, particularly from the micro-IF test, to suggest chlamydial infection in a considerable proportion of patients with Reiter's disease, and this test shows a high level of antibody reacting with 10L-207, an agent with certain properties of subgroup B Chlamydia (Dwyer and others, 1972).

Significant fixation (titre 1 in 16 or more) was found in the LGVCFT in the cases of 18 of 77 patients (28·4 per cent) suffering from Reiter's disease (Schachter, 1971) and in seven of the 23 patients in whose cases Schachter and his colleagues had demonstrated the presence of Chlamydia (Ostler and others, 1971). Similar fixation was found in the cases of 9·1 per cent of 154 men suffering from gonorrhoea, 5·2 per cent of 154 men suffering from NGU and 2·4 per cent of 'normal' persons (Schachter, 1971). Barwell and others (1967) found fixation to a titre of 1 in 32 or more in the case of only one of 19 patients suffering from Reiter's disease; the titre was 1 in 32 in this case in which no isolate was obtained. A titre of 1 in 32 or more was found in the case of only one man (in which Chlamydia was isolated) of 87 men suffering from NSU. A titre of 1 in 32 or more was also found in the cases of two of 40 female contacts of men suffering from NSU. In both cases Chlamydia was isolated.

Also, intradermal tests with chlamydial antigens gave positive findings in Reiter's disease (Barwell and others, 1967). The LGV acid-extract gave positive results in eight of 13 cases; the TRIC acid-extract in nine of 13. In the cases of men suffering from NSU these tests each gave positive results in nine of 50. In the cases of sexual contacts of men suffering from NSU the LGV acid-extract was positive in two of 26; the TRIC acid-extract in one of 26. This group of workers reported the results of cell culture in a further series of cases of Reiter's disease (Vaughan-Jackson and others, 1972): the LGVCFT was negative (titre less than 1 in 16) in the cases of all 28 patients tested, including the three in which Chlamydia was isolated from urethral material. It was negative also in the cases of 14 female contacts of these men, including one case in which Chlamydia was isolated. In contrast, the micro-IF test was positive (titre 1 in 16 or more) in eight of the 10 cases of Reiter's disease in which the test was carried out. The titres in the two in which Chlamydia had been isolated were 1 in 32 and 1 in 128. Dwyer and others (1972) reported from the same laboratory that sera in 14 of 17 isolate-positive NSU cases gave titres of 1 in 16 or more with the micro-IF test. This compared with only four of 24 isolate-negative cases and 14 of 18 sera from 11 patients suffering from Reiter's disease. In cases of Reiter's disease there was a relatively high level of antibody reacting with '10L-207', an agent with certain properties of subgroup B Chlamydia.

Ford (1968) cultured material in yolk sac from 12 patients suffering from Reiter's disease with negative results. However, he reported an LGVCFT titre of 1 in 16 or more in the cases of 20 of 50 patients (40 per cent) and in those of 17 of 100 male patients attending a VD clinic in Canada.

Kinsella and others (1968) found titres of 1 in 8 or greater in nine of 24 cases of Reiter's disease (37 per cent); 61 of 168 other men attending a VD clinic (36 per cent) mostly because of urethritis; in none of 46 cases of ankylosing spondylitis and in three of 39 'normal controls' (8 per cent) seen in Texas. Schachter and others (1969) reported that a patient suffering from Reiter's disease developed buboes suggestive of LGV; they regarded LGV as a clinical entity that might be due to different members of the Chlamydia genus including members of subgroup B as well as the more usual subgroup A.

Mordhorst and Dawson (1971) reported that Reiter's disease had previously affected two fathers of babies suffering from ophthalmia neonatorum due to TRIC agent.

The isolation of Chlamydia in cell culture from a patient suffering from Reiter's disease has been confirmed by the late Francis Gordon and others (1973). They isolated subgroup A Chlamydia (micro-IF serotype I) from both urethral and conjunctival material. They considered that it was probably significant that the positive specimens were obtained early in the course of disease, that is one month before the onset of arthritis. They had inoculated cell cultures with a further 54 specimens from 15 other patients with negative results.

Experimental infection of animals

Chlamydia isolated from a patient suffering from Reiter's disease has been used for the experimental inoculation of animals.

Ostler and others (1970) reported that some rabbits developed Chlamydia-positive arthritis after the inoculation of the eye with Chlamydia.

Smith and others (1973) produced arthritis by inoculation of the knees of macaque monkeys, and of New Zealand white rabbits. Monkeys developed an acute self-limited arthritis; re-inoculation produced a similar arthritis. Repeated intraurethral inoculations produced Chlamydia-positive urethritis in one of two monkeys. The arthritis resulting from the intra-articular inoculation of rabbits became chronic; the agent was re-isolated from joints as long as 107 days after inoculation. Two rabbits developed Chlamydia-positive eye disease after intra-articular inoculation with Chlamydia.

Gilbert and others (1973) showed that tetracycline and penicillin could prevent or reverse the development of arthritis following intra-articular inoculation of rabbits with Chlamydia. Eight untreated controls developed arthritis; three developed disease of the eye. Rabbits treated with tetracycline, started prior to inoculation, or on the day of inoculation (there is a discrepancy between the text and the relevant figure), apparently did not develop arthritis. The longer the delay in starting tetracycline, the longer the arthritis lasted. The initial arthritis was thought to be the result of the infectious process; after this a chronic inflammatory reaction developed that could continue in the absence of Chlamydia.

Conclusion. It seems likely that Chlamydia may be a cause of Reiter's disease, but this has not yet been established beyond doubt.

It is essential that the relationship of Chlamydia to Reiter's disease should be defined by further studies aimed at isolating the agent, as well as investigating serological and cellular immunity. Attention must be directed to subgroup B Chlamydia as well as to subgroup A and to the study of control groups.

The genital reservoir of chlamydial infection

Non-gonococcal urethritis (NGU) is becoming increasingly common in men in England and Wales. If the equivalent infections in women are considered it is likely that the incidence of non-gonococcal genital infection in men and women must be considerably greater than that of gonorrhoea. About 90 per cent of NGU in men is NSU. In a joint study carried out at the Whitechapel Clinic of The London Hospital and the Institute of Ophthalmology, eight cases of gonococcal ophthalmia neonatorum were seen during a period in which 44 cases of ophthalmia neonatorum due to TRIC agent were seen. Factors concerned in this ratio include: the incidence of each infection in the community; the relative clinical silence of genital infection due to TRIC agent (so that the infected parents tend to remain untreated), and the longer incubation of ophthalmia neonatorum due to TRIC agent, than that due to gonorrhoea.

That ophthalmia neonatorum due to TRIC agent can result in scarring like that of classical trachoma has been confirmed (Jones and others, 1965; Freedman and others, 1966; Watson and Gardner, 1968; Forster and others, 1970; Mordhorst and Dawson, 1971; Goscienski and Sexton, 1972). It is considered that prompt and effective treatment lessens the chances of such scarring developing (Mordhorst and Dawson, 1971; Goscienski and Sexton, 1972).

LGV can now be defined by the precise identification of the agent after isolation. This has yet to be done for many of the lesions that are said to be due to LGV such as Parinaud's conjunctivitis, arthritis and proctitis. It may well be that, in areas where LGV is common, the agent may also be found to cause urethritis and cervicitis analogous to proctitis. As Schachter and Meyer (1969) have stated, LGV is a clinical entity that may be due to different members of the Chlamydia genus, including subgroup B Chlamydia (see p. 279) although subgroup A is more usually found.

Isolates have been obtained in cell culture from lymph node material from patients suffering from LGV (Gordon and Quan, 1971; Treharne and others, 1971, 1972; Philip and others, 1971). An isolate was obtained in yolk sac from the urethra of a man suffering from LGV and from discomfort on micturition (Philip and others, 1971).

Summary and conclusions

It seems that a considerable proportion of 'non-specific' genital infection in the UK is related to Chlamydia. The new developments will enable us to begin to define how big this proportion is; to study control groups; to determine if any of the Chlamydia are non-pathogenic in the eye, genital tract or elsewhere; to study the relationship of cellular and serological immunity to disease and, in particular, to study further special forms of inflammatory disease such as Reiter's disease, abacterial pyuria, proctitis and salpingitis. There is evidence already that salpingitis commonly occurs in the mothers of babies suffering from ophthalmia neonatorum due to TRIC agent (Dunlop and others, 1967; Mordhorst and Dawson, 1971). The culture of specimens obtained at laparoscopy should show whether Chlamydia is present in the affected Fallopian tubes or not. Such studies will lay the foundations for effective assessment of treatment for disease due to Chlamydia.

Further studies should include assessments of intradermal tests using known serotypes of the agent.

Thygeson (1967) reported that when he examined a single conjunctival scraping in the cases of Navajo Indians affected by trachoma, he found inclusions in 30 per cent of cases. By repeating the scrapings, he could obtain positive findings in 70 per cent. It seems likely that repeated tests of genital material also should raise the percentage of positive findings.

Nevertheless it would be surprising if there were no agent other than Chlamydia concerned as a cause of NSU. Therefore it will be of particular interest to test for other agents those patients in whose cases efficient tests (cell culture and immunological studies) for Chlamydia have given negative results.

REFERENCES

ASHTON, N., DUNLOP, E. M. C. and DAROUGAR, S. (1974). In preparation.

BARWELL, C. F., DUNLOP, E. M. C. and RACE, J. W. (1967). *Amer. J. Ophthal.*, **63**, 1527.

BECKER, Y., LOKER, H., SAROV, I., ASHER, Y., GUTTER, B. and ZAKAY-RONES, Z. (1971). 'Trachoma and Related Disorders', ed. Roger L. Nichols, p. 13. Excerpta Medica.

CHIANG, W. T., ALEXANDER, E. R., WEI, P. V. and FRESH, J. W. (1968). *Amer. J. Obst. Gynec.*, **100**, 422.

COLLIER, L. H. (1960). *Rev. int. Trachome*, **37**, 585.

COLLIER, L. H., DUKE-ELDER, S. and JONES, B. R. (1958). *Brit. J. Ophthal.*, **42**, 705.

DAROUGAR, S. (1973). Personal communication.

DAROUGAR, S., CUBITT, S. and JONES, B. R. (1974). *Brit. J. vener. Dis.* In press.

DAROUGAR, S., DWYER, R. ST. C., TREHARNE, J. D., HARPER, I. A., GARLAND, J. A. and JONES, B. R. (1971a). 'Trachoma and Related Disorders', ed. Roger L. Nichols, p. 445. Excerpta Medica.

DAROUGAR, S., JONES, B. R., KINNISON, J. R., VAUGHAN-JACKSON, J. D. and DUNLOP, E. M. C. (1972). *Brit. J. vener. Dis.*, **48**, 416.

DAROUGAR, S., KINNISON, J. R. and JONES, B. R. (1971b). 'Trachoma and Related Disorders', ed. Roger L. Nichols, p. 63. Excerpta Medica.

DAROUGAR, S., KINNISON, J. R. and JONES, B. R. (1971c). Ibid., p. 501.

DAROUGAR, S., TREHARNE, J. D., DWYER, R. ST. C., KINNISON, J. R. and JONES, B. R. (1971d). *Brit. J. Ophthal.*, **55**, 591.

DAWSON, C. R. and SCHACHTER, J. (1967). *Amer. J. Ophthal.*, **63**, 1288.

DURHAM, J., ROCK, J. and BELT, E. (1947). *J. Urol. Baltimore*, **58**, 212.

DUNLOP, E. M. C. (1965). Section XIII, 257. Excerpta Medica.

DUNLOP, E. M. C., AL-HUSSAINI, M. K., FREEDMAN, A., GARLAND, J. A., HARPER, I. A., JONES, B. R., RACE, J. W., DU TOIT, M. S., TREHARNE, J. D. and WRIGHT, D. J. M. (1966). *Trans. ophthal. Soc. U.K.*, **86**, 321.

DUNLOP, E. M. C., AL-HUSSAINI, M. K., GARLAND, J. A., TREHARNE, J. D., HARPER, I. A. and JONES, B. R. (1965a). *Lancet*, **1**, 1125, 1286.

DUNLOP, E. M. C., FREEDMAN, A., GARLAND, J. A., HARPER, I. A., JONES, B. R., RACE, J. W., DU TOIT, M. S. and TREHARNE, J. D. (1967). *Amer. J. Ophthal.*, **63**, 1073.

DUNLOP, E. M. C., HARE, M. J., DAROUGAR, S. and DWYER, R. ST. C. (1973). *Brit. J. vener. Dis.*, **49**, 301.

DUNLOP, E. M. C., HARE, M. J., DAROUGAR, S. and JONES, B. R. (1971a). 'Trachoma and Related Disorders', ed. Roger L. Nichols, p. 494. Excerpta Medica.

DUNLOP, E. M. C., HARE, M. J., DAROUGAR, S. and JONES, B. R. (1971b) 'Trachoma and Related Disorders', ed. Roger L. Nichols, p. 507. Excerpta Medica.

DUNLOP, E. M. C., HARE, M. J., DAROUGAR, S., JONES, B. R. and RICE, N. S. C. (1969). *J. infect. Dis.*, **120**, 463.

DUNLOP, E. M. C., JONES, B. R. and AL-HUSSAINI, M. K. (1964). *Brit. J. vener. Dis.*, **40**, 33.

DUNLOP, E. M. C., JONES, B. R. and AL-HUSSAINI, M. K. (1965b). *Rev. int. Trachome*, **42**, 14.

DUNLOP, E. M. C., JONES, B. R., DAROUGAR, S. and TREHARNE, J. D. (1972a). *Brit. med. J.*, **2**, 575.

DUNLOP, E. M. C., VAUGHAN-JACKSON, J. D. and DAROUGAR, S. (1972c). *Brit. J. vener. Dis.*, **48**, 421.

DUNLOP, E. M. C., VAUGHAN-JACKSON, J. D., DAROUGAR, S. and JONES, B. R. (1972b). *Brit. J. vener. Dis.*, **48**, 425.

DWYER, R. ST. C., TREHARNE, J. D., JONES, B. R. and HERRING, J. (1972). *Brit. J. vener. Dis.*, **48**, 452.

EDITORIAL (1973). *Lancet*, **1**, 703.

FORD, D. K. (1968). *Canad. med. Ass. J.*, **99**, 900.

FORD, D. K. and McCANDLISH, L. (1971). *Brit. J. vener. Dis.*, **47**, 196.

FORSTER, R. K., DAWSON, C. R. and SCHACHTER, J. (1970). *Amer. J. Ophthal.*, **69**, 467.

FREEDMAN, A., AL-HUSSAINI, M. K., DUNLOP, E. M. C., EMARAH, M. H. M., GARLAND, J. A., HARPER, I. A., JONES, B. R., RACE, J. W., DU TOIT, M. S., TREHARNE, J. D. and WRIGHT, D. J. M. (1966). *Trans. ophthal. Soc. U.K.*, **86**, 313.

GEAR, J. H. S., GORDON, F. B., JONES, B. R. and BELL, S. D. (1963). *Nature, Lond.*, **197**, 26.

GERLOFF, R. K. and WATSON, R. O. (1967). *Amer. J. Ophthal.*, **63**, 1492.

GILBERT, R. J., SCHACHTER, J., ENGLEMAN, E. P. and MEYER, K. F. (1973). *Arthr. Rheum. N.Y.*, **16**, 30.

GORDON, F. B., DRESSLER, H. R. and QUAN, A. L. (1967). *Amer. J. Ophthal.*, **63**, 1044.

GORDON, F. B., HARPER, I. A., QUAN, A. L., TREHARNE, J. D., DWYER, R. ST. C. and GARLAND, J. A. (1969). *J. infect. Dis.*, **120**, 451.

GORDON, F. B. and QUAN, A. L. (1965). *J. infect. Dis.*, **115**, 186.

GORDON, F. B. and QUAN, A. L. (1971). 'Trachoma and Related Disorders', ed. Roger L. Nichols, p. 476. Excerpta Medica.

GORDON, F. N., QUAN, A. L., STEINMAN, T. E. and PHILIP, R. N. (1973). *Brit. J. vener. Dis.*, **49**, 376.

GOSCIENSKI, P. J. and SEXTON, R. R. (1972). *Amer. J. Dis. Child.*, **124**, 180.

HALBERSTAEDTER, L. and VON PROWAZEK, S. (1907). *Arb. Gesundh.Amt., Berl.*, **26**, 44.

HANNA, L., DAWSON, C. R., BRIONES, O., THYGESON, P. and JAWETZ, E. (1968). *J. Immunol.*, **101**, 43.

HANNA, L., ZICHOSCH, J., JAWETZ, E., VAUGHAN, D. G. JR. and THYGESON, P. (1960). *Science*, **132**, 1660.

HARE, M. J., DUNLOP, E. M. C. and TAYLOR-ROBINSON, D. (1969). *Brit. J. vener. Dis.*, **45**, 282.

HARKNESS, A. H. (1950). 'Non-gonococcal Urethritis'. E. & S. Livingstone Ltd., Edinburgh.

HARPER, I. A., DWYER, R. ST. C., GARLAND, J. A., JONES, B. R., TREHARNE, J. D., DUNLOP, E. M. C., FREEDMAN, A. and RACE, J. W. (1967). *Amer. J. Ophthal.*, **63**, 1064.

JAWETZ, E. (1969). 'Advances in Pharmacology and Chemotherapy', ed. S. Garrallini, A. Goldin, F. Hawking and I. J. Kopin, 7, 253. Academic Press, New York and London.

JAWETZ, E., HANNA, L., DAWSON, C., WOOD, R. and BRIONES, O. (1967). *Amer. J. Ophthal.*, **65**, 1413.

JONES, B. R. (1964). *Rev. int. Trachome*, **41**, 425.

JONES, B. R. (1972). *Brit. J. vener. Dis.*, **48**, 13.

JONES, B. R., AL-HUSSAINI, M. K. and DUNLOP, E. M. C. (1965). *Rev. int. Trachome*, **42**, 27.

JONES, B. R. and COLLIER, L. H. (1962). *Ann. N.Y. Acad. Sci.*, **98**, 212.

JONES, B. R., COLLIER, L. H. and SMITH, C. H. (1959). *Lancet*, **1**, 902.

JUCHAU, S. V., LINSCOTT, W. D., SCHACHTER, J. and JAWETZ, E. (1972). *J. Immunol.*, **108**, 1563.

KINSELLA, T. D., NORTON, W. L. and ZIFF, M. (1968). *Ann. rheum. Dis.*, **27**, 241.

MAGRUDER, G. B., GORDON, F. B., QUAN, A. L. and DRESSLER, H. R. (1963). *Arch. Ophthal.*, **69**, 300.

MCCALLUM, F. O. and FINDLAY, G. M. (1938). *Lancet*, **2**, 136.

MEYER, K. F. (1967). *Amer. J. Ophthal.*, **63**, 1225; 1425.

MITSUI, Y., KONISHI, K., NISHIMURA, A., KAJIMA, M., TAMURA, O. and ENDO, K. (1962). *Brit. J. Ophthal.*, **46**, 651.

MORDHORST, C. H. (1967). *Amer. J. Ophthal.*, **63**, 1283.

MORDHORST, C. H. and DAWSON, C. (1971). *Amer. J. Ophthal.*, **71**, 861.

MOULDER, J. W. (1964). 'The Psittacosis Group as Bacteria, Ciba Lectures in Microbial Biochemistry', p. 1. Wiley, New York.

MOULDER, J. W. (1966). *Ann. Rev. Microbiol.*, **20**, 107.

NEISSER, A. (1879). *Zbl. med. Wiss.*, **17**, 497.

ORIEL, J. D., REEVE, P., POWIS, P. MILLER, A. and NICOL, C. S. (1972). *Brit. J. vener. Dis.*, **48**, 429.

OSTLER, H. B., DAWSON, C. H., SCHACHTER, J. and ENGLEMAN, E. P. (1971). *Amer. J. Ophthal.*, **71**, 986.

OSTLER, H. B., SCHACHTER, J. and DAWSON, C. R. (1970). *Invest. Opthalmol.*, **9**, 256.

PAGE, L. A. (1966). *Int. J. system. Bact.*, **16**, 223.

PHILIP, R. N., HILL, D. A., GREAVES, A. B., GORDON, F. B., QUAN, A. L., GERLOFF, R. K. and THOMAS, L. A. (1971). *Brit. J. vener. Dis.*, **47**, 114.

PUKHNER, A. F. and KOZLOVA, V. I. (1965). *J. Gynaec.*, **6**, 47.

PUKHNER, A. F., PORUDOMINSKY, I. M., KOZLOVA, V. I. and NYUNIKOVA, O. I. (1966). *Urol. Nephrol.*, **4**, 42.

RICHMOND, S. J., HILTON, A. L. and CLARKE, S. K. R. (1972). *Brit. J. vener. Dis.*, **48**, 437.

RODIN, P. (1971). *Brit. J. vener. Dis.*, **47**, 452.

SCHACHTER, J. (1967a). *Amer. J. Ophthal.*, **63**, 1049.

SCHACHTER, J. (1967b). *Amer. J. Ophthal.*, **63**, 1082.

SCHACHTER, J. (1971). *Amer. J. Ophthal.*, **7**, 857.

SCHACHTER, J., BARNES, M. G., JONES, J. P. JR., ENGLEMAN, E. P. and MEYER, K. F. (1966). *Proc. Soc. exp. Biol. N.Y.*, **122**, 283.

SCHACHTER, J. and MEYER, K. F. (1969). *J. Bact.*, **99**, 636.

SCHACHTER, J., SMITH, D. E., DAWSON, C. R., ANDERSON, W. R., DELLER, J. JR., HOKE, A. W., SMARTT, W. H. and MEYER, K. F. (1969). *J. infect. Dis.*, **120**, 372.

SCOTT, J. G. (1968). *S. Afr. med. J.*, **42**, 928.

SHAABAN, M. M., SHOKEIR, A. A., WASFY, I. A. and AL-HUSSAINI, M. K. (1972). *J. Obstet. Gynaec. Brit. Commonw.*, **79**, 360.

SHIPLEY, A., BOWMAN, S. J. and O'CONNOR, J. J. (1968). *Med. J. Aust.*, **1**, 794.

SIBOULET, A. and GALISTIN, P. (1962). *Brit. J. vener. Dis.*, **38**, 209.

SMITH, D. E., JAMES, P. G., SCHACHTER, J., ENGLEMAN, E. P. and MEYER, K. F. (1973). *Arthr. Rheum. (N.Y.)*, **16**, 21.

STORZ, J. (1971). 'Chlamydia and Chlamydia-induced Diseases'. Charles C. Thomas, Illinois.

T'ANG, F.-F., CHANG, H.-L., HUANG, Y.-T. and WANG, K.-C. (1957). *Chin. med J.*, **75**, 429.

THYGESON, P. (1967). *Amer. J. Ophthal.*, **63**, 1426.

THYGESON, P. (1971). *Amer. J. Ophthal.*, **71**, 975.

TREHARNE, J. D., DAROUGAR, S. and JONES, B. R. (1973). *Brit. J. vener. Dis.*, **49**, 295.

TREHARNE, J. D., DAVEY, S. J., GRAY, S. J. and JONES, B. R. (1972). *Brit. J. vener. Dis.*, **48**, 18.

TREHARNE, J. D., KATZENELSON, E. DAVEY, S. J. and GREY, S. J. (1971). 'Trachoma and Related Disorders', ed. Roger L. Nichols, p. 289. Excerpta Medica.

VAUGHAN-JACKSON, J. D. (1974). In preparation.

VAUGHAN-JACKSON, J. D., DUNLOP, E. M. C., DAROUGAR, S., DWYER, R. ST. C. and JONES, B. R. (1972). *Brit. J. vener. Dis.* **48**, 445.

WANG, S.-P. (1971). 'Trachoma and Related Disorders', ed. Roger L. Nichols, p. 273. Excerpta Medica.

WANG, S.-P. and GRAYSTON, J. T. (1970). *Amer. J. Ophthal.*, **70**, 367.

WANG, S.-.P. and GRAYSTON, J. T. (1971). 'Trachoma and Related Disorders', ed. Roger L. Nichols, p. 305. Excerpta Medica.

WANG, S.-P., GRAYSTON, J. T. and GALE, J. L. (1973). *J. Immunol.*, **110**, 873.

WEISS, E. (1967). *Amer. J. Ophthal.*, **63**, 1098.

30 Therapeutic Aspects

R. S. Morton

Since the cause or causes of NSU is by definition unknown, treatment is largely empirical. There is, however, some indication, both *in vivo* and *in vitro*, that the tetracyclines have advantages over other anti-bacterials.

Trials with 5-iodo-2-deoxyuridine, by Hutfield (1964), and nalidixic acid (Negram), by Willcox (1965), were found of no value. Csonka (1965) reviewed trends in the investigation of NSU and the lines of thought used in treatment. He suggested that since aetiology is generally obscure every new drug offering a chance of success should be investigated and even negative results recorded.

Sulphonomides alone or in combination have been tried. Alergant (1964) compared two regimes: (a) 1 g of sulphamethoxydiazine combined with 0·5 g of streptomycin and (b) 1 g of sulphadimidine four times daily for 5 days combined with 0·5 g of streptomycin. Cure rates showed no statistical difference. Jelinek (1964) used streptomycin with a long-acting sulphonamide with disappointing results. Fernandes (1965) had a cure rate of 70 per cent with a 5 to 8 day course of a triple sulphonamide, supranol. Sulphonamides owe their activity to their ability to inhibit the conversion of paramino-benzoic acid to dihydro-folic acid in the metabolic pathway that leads, through purine synthesis, to DNA. A substance called trimethoprim which interferes with purine synthesis would therefore be expected to potentiate sulphona-mide activity. Carroll and Nicol (1970) reported a trial of these two drugs in combination. Each patient was given two tablets, each containing 80 mg trimethoprim and 400 mg sulphamethoxazole, twice daily for 4 days. Of the 14 treated, two defaulted immediately and eight failed to show any improvement. The trial was abandoned.

Cephaloridine was compared with other antibiotics in a randomly selected group of patients by Csonka and Murray (1967). Following 1·0 g of cephaloridine the cure rate lay between 36–41 per cent. Where 2·0 g was given for gonorrhoea, 15 per cent developed PGU as compared with 22 per cent after penicillin therapy, 13 per cent after kanamycin and 6 per cent after tetracycline. The authors note that these findings parallel the antibiotic sensitivity levels of the *M. hominis* and T-mycoplasma isolated from the their patients. Csonka (1967) reported on the use of a single 2·0 g dose given to each of 60 men with NSU. The results were compared with those following tetracycline 250 mg four times per day for 4 days. At the end of 1 month, kanamycin was found effective in 67 per cent of 54 patients and tetracycline in 89 per cent of 120. The authors conclude that tetracycline is still the most effective preparation available for the treatment of NSU.

A wide variety of tetracyclines have been tried. Limecycline (Tetralysal) was found to be as effective as conventional tetracycline by Willcox (1965). Methacycline (Rondomycin) was used in 49 patients in a dosage of 150 mg four times daily for 4 days by Morton and Wray (1966) with 79·6 per cent success. Statham and Morton (1968) reported on the use of roliotetracycline nitrate (Tetrex PMT). They treated 45 men with a single intramuscular injection of 350 mg daily for 4 days. Of 42 patients who completed the course, 37 (88 per cent) responded satisfactorily but 6 (16 per cent) required retreatment later. Ten men reported discomfort at the site of injection. Schofield and Masterton (1969) also tried this preparation, giving two injections only to 101 patients. Six failed to attend for the second injection while 23 others complained of discomfort at the site of injection. Of 83 treated and followed, 24 either failed or had a recurrence within 2 months. Wijetunga and Morton (1969) used tetracycline hydrochloride, acidified with sodium hexametaphosphate (Tetrex). The preparation was given orally in a dosage of 500 mg 12-hourly for 4 days. The regime was successful in 87 per cent but later recurrence, calling for retreatment, occurred in 17 per cent. Heinke (1967) claimed good results with tetracycline combined with oleandomycin (Sigmamycin). Wright (1969) found the results with methacycline much like those obtained with tetracycline. Promising results using rifampicin (Rimactate) were reported by Meyer Rohn (1969). Doxycycline (Vibramycin) was used by Lassus et al (1971). An initial dose of 200 mg was followed by 100 mg daily. Of the 99 men involved 60 per cent had T-mycoplasmas. Cures were claimed in 92 per cent of those with the organism and in 95 per cent of the culture negative patients. Although clinically cured, 26 per cent of the culture positive cases still yielded T-mycoplasma. Masterton and Schofield (1972) gave 134 men with NSU a single oral dose of doxycycline. Of 119 men followed-up, 6·7 per cent failed to respond. Holmes et al (1967) in one of a series of articles on NSU report a double blind trial comparing tetracycline hydrochloride with a placebo. The tetracycline was given in an initial dose of 1·5 g followed by 0·5 g 6-hourly for 4 or 7 days. The duration of follow-up varied from 5 to 25 days only. The failure rates with the tetracycline courses were 35 and 10 per cent respectively. With the placebo the failure rate was 86 per cent. This well-planned trial was conducted on an aircraft carrier where the possibility of reinfection was virtually eliminated.

Willcox (1968) tested erythromycin in 106 men with uncomplicated NSU. He used erythromycin stearate in a dosage of 6·25 g over 6 days. The retreatment rate in the 92 men followed up was 28·3 per cent at 3 months. There was no significant difference between these results and those of a similar trial conducted 12 years earlier. Willcox provides a table comparing his findings with those obtained using 23 other preparations. Tetracycline and oxytetracycline offer the lowest retreatment rates. Grimble (1968) in a similar trial had 28 failures in 95 patients treated with erythromycin as against 13 failures in an identical number treated with tetracycline. He postulated that the difference could be due to the presence of *M. hominis* which, unlike T-mycoplasma, is unaffected by erythromycin.

Shepard (1970) who isolated T-mycoplasma from 70–84 per cent of men with NSU, compared with 21–26 per cent from controls, found that 500 mg of tetracycline given 6-hourly for 7 days or erythromycin in like dosage for 10 days eliminated the organism. When the organism persisted, recurrence could be expected. He advised treatment of wives.

Morrison (1967) noted that patients apparently reinfected by the same consort usually responded to the same drug which had cleared the original infection. Where a new consort was involved a different drug was more likely to be required.

Csonka and Spitzer (1969) reported a trial of lincomycin in NSU. They prescribed 500 mg four times daily for 5 days. In 51 men the cure rate at 7 days was only 25·5 per cent; about the same as that found when using a placebo. Retreatment with tetracycline or erythromycin gave much more satisfactory results. The authors note that T-mycoplasma is resistant to lincomycin but not to tetracycline or erythromycin. They found T-mycoplasma in 63 per cent of the lincomycin treated group before treatment and in 71 per cent of those unsuccessfully treated with the drug. Csonka and Corse (1970) showed that lincomycin inhibits the growth of *M. hominis* but not that of T-mycoplasma. Lincomycin therefore provides a method of differentiating the mycoplasmas and of facilitating culture and recognition of T-mycoplasma.

Weström and Mårdh (1971) in a clinical assessment of the value of metacycline, lincomycin and chloramphenicol in genital infection with mycoplasmas in the female, noted that after the first two drugs, *M. hominis* were rarely isolated and this was associated with disappearance of signs and symptoms. Neither happened after chloramphenicol. Such findings correlate with sensitivity testing in the laboratory. Cultures for T-mycoplasma showed that these organisms could be recovered in about the same frequency before and after exhibition of the drugs mentioned. Similar findings were made by Markham et al (1972).

Fowler (1970) undertook a therapeutic trial of 600 men with NSU.

He used three regimes in double blind fashion:

(a) Tetracycline 250 mg four times daily for 4 days.
(b) One lactose tablet four times daily for 4 days.
(c) Streptomycin 1·0 g followed by sulphadimidine 1·0 g four times per day for 5 days.

Assessment about 3 weeks after starting treatment gave cure rates of 72, 37 and 53 per cent respectively. Re-assessment at 3 months showed that 16·7, 2·5 and 8·9 per cent respectively had had a recurrence necessitating retreatment. These findings together with return cases in later years lead Fowler to the conclusion 'Tetracycline benefited only 10 per cent more patients than . . . placebo treatment'.

The chemotherapy of chlamydial infections was reviewed by Jawetz (1969).

So far there has been no serious attempt to determine the presence or absence of Chlamydia before and after treatment of non-specific genital infections in sexual partnerships. Chlamydial infections are generally recognised as requiring more prolonged treatment, or repeated courses of treatment, than bacterial infections. The following reports may, in future, be seen as the shadows cast by coming scientific events.

In a useful contribution John (1971) questioned the 'common knowledge' that tetracyclines cure 70–80 per cent of men with NSU. From a review of the literature he decided to assess the value of larger dosage for a more prolonged time than has been customary. Three groups were studied:

(a) 132 men given oxytetracycline 500 mg three times daily for 5 days.
(b) 200 men given oxytetracycline 250 mg four times daily for 21 days.
(c) 169 men given oxytetracycline 500 mg four times daily for 10 days.

Cure rates at 3 months were 55·0, 87·5 and 72 per cent respectively.

Side effects were minimal and John recommends the 21-day course for general use.

Bhattacharyya and Morton (1973) used a triple tetracycline (Deteclo) offering adequate blood levels on a 12-hourly regime. They gave 300 mg bi-daily for 21 days. The recurrence rate at 3 months follow-up was 11·8 per cent. There were no recurrences in the first month after completion of treatment. The number of recurrences increased with time. After short courses of tetracyline, recurrences were highest in the first month and declined. These findings are discussed.

In summary, 'cure' of NSU continues to be written in inverted commas.

REFERENCES

ALERGANT, C. D. (1964). *Brit. J. vener. Dis.*, **40**, 196.
BHATTACHARYYA, M. N. and MORTON, R. S. (1973). *Brit. J. vener. Dis.*, **49**, 521.

CARROLL, B. R. T. and NICOL, C. S. (1970). *Brit. J. vener. Dis.*, **46**, 31.

CSONKA, G. W. (1965). *Brit. J. vener. Dis.*, **41**, 1.

CSONKA, G. W. and MURRAY, M. (1967). *Postgrad. med. J.*, **43**, 123.

CSONKA, G. W. (1967). *Postgrad. med. J.*, **43**, Suppl., 63.

CSONKA, G. W. and SPITZER, R. J. (1969). *Brit. J. vener. Dis.*, **45**, 52.

CSONKA, G. W. and CORSE, J. (1970). *Brit. J. vener. Dis.*, **46**, 203.

FERNANDES, G. (1965). *Indian J. Derm.*, **31**, 72.

FOWLER, W. (1970). *Brit. J. vener. Dis.*, **46**, 464.

GRIMBLE, A. S. (1968). *Brit. J. vener. Dis.*, **44**, 230.

HEINKE, E. (1967). *Med. Welt.*, **5**, 265.

HOLMES, K. K., JOHNSON, D. W., FLOYD, T. M. and KVALE, P. A. (1967). *J. Amer. med. Ass.*, **202**, 474.

HUTFIELD, D. C. (1964). *Brit. J. vener. Dis.*, **40**, 146.

JAWETZ, E. (1969). *Adv. Pharmacol.*, **7**, 253.

JELINEK, G. (1964). *Brit. J. vener. Dis.*, **40**, 268.

JOHN, J. (1971). *Brit. J. vener. Dis.*, **47**, 266.

LASSUS, A., PERKO, R. L. et al (1971). *Brit. J. vener. Dis.*, **47**, 126.

MARKHAM, N. P., MARKHAM, J. G. and SMITH, E. R. (1972). *Brit. J. vener. Dis.*, **48**, 200.

MASTERTON, G. and SCHOFIELD, C. B. S. (1972). *Brit. J. vener. Dis.*, **48**, 121.

MEYER ROHN, J. (1969). 'Symposium on Rimactane', Ciba, Basle, **72**, 6.

MORRISON, A. I. (1967). *Brit. J. vener. Dis.*, **43**, 170.

MORTON, R. S. and WRAY, P. M. (1966). *Brit. J. vener. Dis.*, **42**, 195.

SCHOFIELD, C. B. S. and MASTERTON, G. (1969). *Brit. J. vener. Dis.*, **45**, 47.

SHEPARD, M. C. (1970). *J. Amer. med. Ass.*, **211**, 1335.

STATHAM, R. and MORTON, R. S. (1968). *Brit. J. vener. Dis.*, **44**, 228.

WESTRÖM, L. and MÅRDH, P. (1971). *Acta obstet. gynaec. scand.*, **50**, 25.

WIJETUNGA, E. B. and MORTON, R. S. (1969). *Brit. J. vener. Dis.*, **45**, 50.

WILLCOX, R. R. (1965). *Clin. Trials J.*, **2**, 239.

WILLCOX, R. R. (1968). *Brit. J. vener. Dis.*, **44**, 157.

WRIGHT, D. J. M. (1969). *Brit. J. vener. Dis.*, **45**, 167.

Part 7
Reiter's Syndrome

31 Epidemiology

J. R. W. Harris

In patients attending venereology units in the United Kingdom the onset of Reiter's syndrome follows sexual intercourse. This disease appears to have a sexually transmitted origin in Great Britain, the United States (Nicol, 1966), Russia (Klinyshkova, 1972) and Papua and New Guinea (Maddocks, 1967). Outbreaks are also associated with various forms of dysentery and have been reported from many countries in Europe, North Africa and Asia. However, the reports of individual cases or series from different countries give little idea of the true incidence of the condition or indeed the geographical pattern related to the dysenteric and sexually transmitted types. There is little doubt that the dysenteric and sexually transmitted forms can co-exist in the same community (Davies et al, 1969), and many of the early studies described the syndrome as it presented in military populations, where both dysentery and sexually transmitted disease occur (Hahn and Masi, 1968).

In 1971 450 patients with the syndrome attended units for the treatment of sexually transmitted disease (Chief Medical Officer of Health Report, 1971). The incidence in males was 1·8 per 100 000 in that year. It would be unwise to assume that this is the true incidence of the disease in our community. The prevalence of any multisystem disease process presenting to various specialities will be underestimated if the statistics from only one medical speciality are considered (Harris, 1970).

REFERENCES

DAVIES, N. E., HAVERTY, J. R. and BOATWRIGHT, M. (1969). *Sth. med. J.*, **62**, 1011.
DEPARTMENT OF HEALTH AND SOCIAL SECURITY (1973). Report of the Chief Medical Officer of Health for Year 1971. *Brit. J. vener. Dis.*, **49**, 89.
HAHN, B. H. and MASI, A. T. (1968). *Johns Hopkins med. J.*, **122**, 387.
HARRIS, J. R. W. (1970). MSSVD Spring Meeting, Belfast.
KLINYSHKOVA, K. M. (1972). *Vestn. Derm. Vener.*, **11**, 31.
MADDOCKS, I. (1967). *Brit. J. vener. Dis.*, **43**, 280.
NICOL, C. S. (1966). In *Second Symposium on Advanced Medicine*, p. 187, Pitman, London.

32 Laboratory Aspects

J. R. W. Harris

Research during the last decade has attempted to ascertain why certain individuals seem prone to this syndrome, and to discover the initial infective agent involved in the disease process. Mowat and Nicol (1968) described the occurrence of Reiter's syndrome in two brothers and discussed the likelihood of a genetic basis for the disease. Csonka (1969), in his review of 332 consecutive cases, noted that the syndrome had occurred in two pairs of brothers. Lawrence (1974) studied the relatives of patients with Reiter's syndrome. During the study 110 relatives of 35 patients with Reiter's syndrome were examined clinically and radiologically. Comparison was made with relatives of patients with ankylosing spondylitis, psoriatic arthritis and Still's disease. Psoriasis was found to be nine times more common in male relatives of patients with Reiter's syndrome than in the population, and was almost as frequent as in psoriatic families. Ankylosing spondylitis was eight, and bilateral sacro-iliac involvement three times as frequent in the relatives of those with the syndrome as in the population. This was the same frequency as the spondylitic and Still's families. The conclusion was that there is a genetic association with both psoriatic and ankylosing spondylitis. As a result of their work, Dryll et al (1969) speculated that a genetic tendency to psoriasis could predispose to infection by an arthrogenic agent, thus producing Reiter's syndrome.

Recently there have been exciting reports of highly significant associations between HL-antigen 27 and ankylosing spondylitis (Caffrey and James, 1973; Schlosstein et al, 1973; *Lancet*, 1973; Brewerton et al, 1973a). Aho et al (1973) have identified this antigen in four out of five patients with Reiter's syndrome. It would appear that a susceptibility to reactive arthritis after certain infections is closely linked with the possession of HL-A27. The two large series of patients with the syndrome who have been tissue typed (Brewerton et al 1973b, Harris et al 1974) give similar results. Approximately 60 per cent of patients with the syndrome possess HL-A27, and a high proportion of these have the HL-A27/W10 combination. There is a close correlation between the occurrence of sacro-iliitis and iritis and the presence of HL-A27.

Dunlop has discussed in detail the work of the various investigators who were considering Chlamydia as being an aetiological factor in the development of Reiter's syndrome. The initial work of Mendlowski and Serge (1960) in Wisconsin demonstrated that sub-group B Chlamydia could be isolated from the joints of sheep with polyarthritis. Siboulet and Galistin (1962) described the isolation of Chlamydia from urethral and conjunctival material taken from patients with the syndrome. Schachter and her team from the Hooper Foundation and the University of California (Schachter et al, 1966; Schachter, 1967) noted that isolates from the joint, conjunctiva and urethra were sub-group B Chlamydia. Dunlop et al (1967) also noted that some of their isolates were sub-group B Chlamydia. (For further detail see section on N.S.U. by E. M. C. Dunlop.)

Mycoplasma are also firmly established as a cause of arthritis in animals (Decker and Ward, 1966) and there is still controversy over their potential role in initiating Reiter's syndrome. Ford and Rasmussen (1964) did not find any evidence implicating them with the syndrome but Bartholomew (1965) claimed to have isolated mycoplasma from patients with Reiter's. McCormack et al (1973) in an excellent review felt that consideration of the available data did not indicate a direct role for mycoplasma in Reiter's syndrome. There have been a few reports in the last decade of isolations of mycoplasma from the joint fluid of patients with the syndrome (Claus et al, 1964; Dunlop et al, 1969). None of these reported isolations has been consistently confirmed by other investigators (Sharp, 1970). Taylor-Robinson et al (1969) felt that there was no causal relationship between mycoplasma and Reiter's syndrome. Smith and Ward (1971) and Ford (1970) both felt that the relationship between mycoplasma and this syndrome should be investigated further. Infection by a fastidious mycoplasma, that cannot be isolated by currently available techniques, or infection at a distant site triggering immunopathologic mechanisms, have not yet been excluded.

Other possible mechanisms of the syndrome have been explored. Rats inoculated with complete Freund adjuvant (consisting of killed tubercle bacilli in an oil and water emulsion) develop a polyarthritis with associated ophthalmic, urethral and dermatological pathology (Pearson, 1963). This experiment was repeated with the same results in Athens (Katsimantis, 1966). Muirden and Peace (1969) carried out light and electron microscopic studies in carragheenin, adjuvant and tuberculin induced arthritis. They postulated that the initial inflammation releases a tissue antigen which then produces a local immune response. Stone (1968) believed that the form of hypersensitivity in Reiter's syndrome was an inability to inactivate the mediators of early cellular inflammation following initial infection. Solenn and Lassen (1971) compared the arthropathy following infection with Yersinia enterocolitica and Reiter's syndrome. They stated that on occasions Yersinia infection preceded Reiter's syndrome and speculated that the arthropathy following Yersinia infection had the same immunopathology as Reiter's syndrome.

Following detailed observations by Weinberger (1962) on cellular and glucose concentrations in synovial fluid, various workers have investigated the complement activity of this fluid. Fostiropoulos et al (1965) noted that total haemolytic complement activity is normal in patients with Reiter's syndrome and that this is another distinguishing feature from rheumatoid arthritis in which the haemolytic complement activity is reduced. Peltier et al (1966) reported that serum complement was increased in Reiter's syndrome and that the synovial complement activity was also increased. Peltier et al (1970) continued the investigation and found there was a significant correlation between complement levels and total protein and gammaglobulin in the synovial fluid. Pekin et al (1967) observed very high haemolytic complement activity in the synovial fluids from these patients and also noted the presence of macrophages containing polymorphonuclear leucocytes in this fluid. They found a correlation between the severity and duration of joint involvement and the degree of elevation of synovial fluid complement. They felt that the presence of the macrophages may represent an early response to the provocative factor responsible for the acute arthritis in the syndrome.

Highton and Raynes (1966) discussed the appearances of the synovium in Reiter's syndrome. They noted rod-like inclusion bodies in the cytoplasm of endothelial cells of synovial blood vessels in two out of six cases of Reiter's syndrome. The rods were randomly grouped and the groups occurred in random distribution. Preliminary observation after uranyl acetate staining suggested the presence of nucleic acid in the rods. Using radioactive tagging techniques, Sliwinski and Zvaifler (1970) studied two patients to determine if there was any local productions of IgG by the inflamed synovium. The results indicated that there was no such local production.

In the majority of patients with the syndrome a circulating antibody to a prostatic antigen can be detected using a haemagglutination test (Grimble and Lessof, 1965). However, the test is rather non-specific since positive results are also obtained in approximately one-third of patients with ankylosing spondylitis and one-fifth of patients who have psoriasis as their sole complaint.

REFERENCES

Aho, K., Ahvonen, P., Lassus, A., Sievers, K. and Tilikainen, A. (1973). *Lancet*, ii, 157.

Bartholomew, L. E. (1965). *Arthritis Rheum.*, **8**, 376.

Brewerton, D. A., Caffrey, M., Hart, F. D., James, D. C. O., Nicholls, A. and Sturrock, R. D. (1973). *Lancet*, i, 904.

Brewerton, D. A., Caffrey, M., Nicholls, A., Walters, D., Oates, J. K. and James, D. C. O. (1973). *Lancet*, ii, 996.

CAFFREY, M. and JAMES, D. C. O. (1973). *Nature, Lond.*, **242**, 121.
CLAUS, G., MCEWEN, C., BRUNNER, T. and TSAMPARLIS, G. (1964). *Brit. J. vener. Dis.*, **40**, 170.
CSONKA, G. (1969). *Brit. J. vener. Dis.*, **45**, 157.
DECKER, J. L. and WARD, J. R. (1966). *Bull. rheum. Dis.*, **16**, 412.
DRYLL, A., KAHN, M. F., SOLNICA, J. et al (1969). *Sem. Höp. Paris*, **45**, 499.
DUNLOP, E. M. C., FREEDMAN, A., GARLAND, J. A., HARPER, I. A., JONES, B. R., RACE, J. W., DU TOIT, M. S. and RENARNE, J. D. (1967). *Amer. J. Ophthal.*, **63**, Suppl., 1073.
DUNLOP, E. M. C., HARE, M. J., JONES, B. R. and TAYLOR-ROBINSON, D. (1969). *Brit. J. vener. Dis.*, **45**, 274.
FORD, D. K. and RASMUSSEN, G. (1964). *Arthritis Rheum.*, **7**, 220.
FORD, D. K. (1970). In *The Role of Mycoplasmas and L Forms of Bacteria in Disease*, p. 137. Charles C. Thomas, Springfield, Illinois.
FOSTIROPOULOS, G., AUSTEN, K. F. and BLOCH, K. J. (1965). *Arthritis Rheum.*, **8**, 219.
GRIMBLE, A. and LESSOF, M. H. (1965). *Brit. med. J.*, ii, 263.
HARRIS, J. R. W., GELSTHORPE K., DOUGHTY, R. W., LEE, D. and MORTON, R. S. (1974). *Acta derm.-venereol. Stockh.* (In press).
HIGHTON, T. C. and RAYNES, D. G. (1966). *Proc. Univ. Otago. med. Sch.*, **44**, 37.
KATSIMANTIS, D. M. (1966). *Rev. Rhum.*, **33**, 118.
Lancet (1973). i, 921.
LAWRENCE, J. (1974). *Brit. J. vener. Dis.*, **50**, 140.
MCCORMACK, W. M., BRAUN, P., LEE, Y.-H. KLEIN, J. O. and KASS, E. H. (1973). *New Engl. J. Med.*, **288**, 78.
MENDLOWSKI, B. and SERGE, D. (1960). *Amer. J. Vet. Res.*, **21**, 68.
MUIRDEN, K. D. and PEACE, G. (1969). *Ann. Rheum. Dis.*, **28**, 392.
MOWAT, A. G. and NICOL, C. S. (1968). *Brit. J. vener. Dis.*, **44**, 334.
PEARSON, C. M. (1963). *J. chron. Dis.*, **16**, 863.
PELTIER, A., COSTE, F. and DELBARRE, F. (1966). *Presse med.*, **74**, 1523.
PELTIER, A. P., VIAL, H. C., LEROY, C. and DE SEZE, S. (1970). *Path. Biol. (Paris)*, **18**, 969.
PEKIN, J. J. JR., MALININ, T. I. and ZUAIFLER, N. J. (1967). *Ann. intern. Med.*, **66**, 677.
SCHACHTER, J., BARNES, M. G., JONES, J. P. JR., ENGLEMAN, E. P. and MEYER, K. F. (1966). *Proc. Soc. exp. Biol. N.Y.*, **122**, 283.
SCHACHTER, J. (1967). *Amer. J. Ophthal.*, **63**, Suppl. 1082.
SCHLOSSTEIN, L., TERASAKI, P. I., BLUESTONE, R. and PEASSON, C. M. (1973). *New Engl. J. Med.*, **288**, 704.
SHARP, J. T. (1970). *Arthritis Rheum.*, **13**, 263.
SIBOULET, A. and GALISTIN, P. (1962). *Brit. J. vener. Dis.*, **38**, 209.
SLIWINSKI, A. J. and ZVAIFLER, N. J. (1970). *J. Lab. clin. Med.*, **76**, 304.
SMITH, C. B. and WARD, J. R. (1971). *J. infect. Dis.*, **123**, 313.
SOLENN, J. H. and LASSEN, J. (1971). *Scand. J. infect. Dis.*, **3**, 83.
STONE, O. J. (1968). *Derm. Int., (Philad).*, **7**, 137.
TAYLOR-ROBINSON, D., ADDEY, J. P., HARE, M. J. and DUNLOP, E. M. C. (1969). *Brit. J. vener. Dis.*, **45**, 265.
WEINBERGER, H. J. (1962). *Arthritis Rheum.*, **5**, 202.

33 Clinical Aspects

J. R. W. Harris

While the clinical manifestations of Reiter's syndrome had been well documented by the early sixties some observations made during the last decade are worthy of note.

Csonka (1966) in a study of 302 consecutive patients with Reiter's syndrome reported that 10 developed thrombophlebitis of the deep leg veins within a few days of the onset of arthritis. This phlebitis appeared to be associated with active arthritis in the adjacent knee joint. The thrombophlebitis settled quickly and was uncomplicated by pulmonary embolism. Csonka believed that this was part of the disease process and not a chance association. Most of the patients were ambulant at this time and had received no drug therapy. As they were healthy young males there was no predisposing cause for the thrombophlebitis. Lemke (1965) had noticed similar thrombophlebitis in two patients and discussed the possible relation between Reiter's syndrome and Behcet's disease in which thrombophlebitis is a common occurrence. Weese and McCarty (1969) described spontaneous rupture of the synovial capsule of the knee joint in a 64-year-old man with Reiter's syndrome. This occurred three days after admission to hospital. The knee had appeared normal the previous day and on examination there was a tense massive effusion related to the knee joint with associated pitting oedema of the lower part of the leg. The calf of the affected leg was 7 cm greater in circumference than that of the unaffected limb. An arthrogram demonstrated extravasation of the dye into the calf. The authors suggested that since neither arthrograms nor venograms were performed on the 10 patients in Csonka's series, some or all of them might have had undetected rupture of the knee joint. Garner and Mowat (1972) reported a similar case in a young man with relapsing Reiter's syndrome. He developed severe pain and tenderness in the calf which became markedly swollen some time after injection of the knee joint with hydrocortisone acetate. On examination he was found to have a cyst of the popliteal fossa which communicated with the knee joint. This cyst was excised and was lined with synovial tissue. Csonka (1973) reviewed his own cases and came to the conclusion that, while rupture of the joint capsule undoubtedly occurs in Reiter's syndrome, the patients he had reported had thrombophlebitis. Tait et al (1965) noted that following rupture of the joint capsule the effusion in the knee joint disappears concurrently with the appearance of a painful swelling in the calf. The symptoms clear up in a few days when treated. The treatment is aimed at reducing the production of synovial fluid by resting the patient, splinting the knee and by intra-articular injection of locally acting steroid.

Davies et al (1969) from Atlanta, Georgia, noted the difficulties associated with the diagnosis of the dysenteric type of Reiter's syndrome in countries where the venereal type is usually seen. Nicol (1966) in a symposium at the Royal College of Physicians of London had observed that the syndrome in the United States of America usually follows sexual intercourse. The three patients reported by Davies et al developed the post-dysenteric syndrome as a result of Shigella infection acquired while on vacation in Mexico. Verdaguer et al (1965) stressed the practical difficulty of making a biological diagnosis of recent shigellosis at the time when the syndrome initially occurs. They found that serological diagnosis, using an antigen prepared from freshly isolated strains was the only method of obtaining positive results in these patients. Warren (1970) noted that patients with arthritis following Salmonella infections can have conjunctivitis and reported two such cases. He wondered whether these cases could be related to Reiter's syndrome. The occurrence of pyogenic arthropathy following a dysenteric-like illness was documented by Vartiainen and Hurri (1964) and obviously the physician must exclude this possibility before diagnosing Reiter's syndrome.

Moss (1964) reviewed the literature on Reiter's syndrome in children and described a further case. He discussed 24 paediatric cases of whom 20 were preceded by dysentery and noted that iritis and keratitis were frequent and more severe than in adults. Lockie and Hunder (1971) outlined the development of the complete syndrome in a young boy whose initial symptoms began at the age of three and in whom the disease progressed during the next 10 years.

While Reiter's syndrome is not commonly diagnosed in females, Crocco and Formato (1964) described a 47-year-old woman whose presenting feature was haematuria associated with haemorrhagic cystitis. They felt that this type of case could be easily misdiagnosed and emphasised the importance of recognition of abacterial haemorrhagic cystitis as a manifestation of the syndrome. Reckless (1972) reported the association of parotitis in a 27-year-old woman. This was a non-tender, non-fluctuant swelling which enlarged and resolved at the same time as the conjunctivitis and arthritis. Klinyshkova (1972) from Omsk described in detail classical Reiter's syndrome in two women. Examination of urethral scrapings from the second patient revealed the

11

presence of the characteristic cytoplasmic inclusions of Chlamydiae. He also discussed the results obtained on examining the sexual contacts of both patients and referred to a further five female patients who were also under his care with the same disease. Reich (1966) noted that a 16-year-old girl with the syndrome had also generalised lymphadeno-pathy. He thought that this was a new component of the syndrome.

Ingram (1964) remarked that 2 per cent of the population suffer from psoriasis and the view has been proposed that the association between psoriasis and Reiter's syndrome is fortuitous. However, Wright and Reed (1964), Perry and Mayne (1965), Hammer and Graykowski (1964), and Maxwell et al (1966) all observed that keratoderma blenorrhagica was indistinguishable clinically and histopathologically from psoriasis. Kahn and Hall (1965) reported a series of seven adults with severe recurrent Reiter's syndrome, all of whom later exhibited the charac-teristic features of psoriatic arthropathy. Maxwell et al (1966) discussed similar cases.

Mason (1964) stated that in the radiological evaluation of patients with spondylitis, it was the character rather than the position of perio-stitis which seemed to be of importance in aiding the diagnosis of Reiter's syndrome. In this condition the new bone formation had an exuberant fluffy appearance when seen radiologically. He emphasised that diagnosis could not be made on radiological appearance alone. Sholkoff et al (1970) in their radiological review of 55 patients did not observe this exuberant fluffy periostitis of the calcaneum. They noted that the main toe involvement was the interphalangeal joint of the great toe. Good (1965) reported that 57 per cent of his series of 35 patients had sacroiliitis 2 or more years after the onset of the disease. Delbarre et al (1969) felt that the incidence and degree of spinal involvement increases with time to reach 75 per cent 5 years after the onset of the disease. Brousse et al (1966) compared the relative incidences of cal-caneal abnormalities in ankylosing spondylitis and Reiter's syndrome. They found a higher incidence in ankylosing spondylitis although the percentage of patients in each group with heel pain did not differ signifi-cantly. McEwen et al (1971) found that the spondylitis associated with Reiter's syndrome was indistinguishable from that found in psoriasis, but that they both could be separated radiologically from the spondylosis of ankylosing spondylitis by the radiographic appearance of the syndes-mophytes. This is contrary to the view expressed by Kahn and Hall (1965) that there is no radiological difference between the spondylosis of Reiter's syndrome and ankylosing spondylitis.

During the last decade there have been an increasing number of reports of both conduction defects and aortic valve disease as late manifestations of Reiter's syndrome. These were reviewed by Collins (1972). At that time there had been 20 reports in the literature of aortic incompetence occurring frequently in association with conduction defects. In the case that he reported himself there was evidence of active myocarditis shown by the elevated erythrocyte sedimentation rate and the changing electrocardiographic pattern from complete heart block through second degree block to first degree block with intermittent left bundle branch block. The interval of onset of aortic incompetence following the initial episode of Reiter's syndrome varied from 4 to 31 years. Cliff (1971) noted that two of the three patients in his series had been erroneously diagnosed as having subacute bacterial endocarditis, on the grounds of their having a febrile illness with elevated sedimentation rate and aortic incompetence. Rodnan et al (1964) described the pathological appearance of the meso-aortic disease with dilatation of the valve ring and rolling of the free margins of the semi-lunar cusps. Siquier et al (1970) considered the indications for valve replacement in such patients. Maddocks (1968) published the first recorded case from a developing country. Block (1972) reported the history of a patient who developed marked aortic incompetence within 1 month of a normal clinical and radiological examination. The patient had had recurrent attacks of the syndrome for 4 years. His electrocardiogram, 1 month prior to presentation with marked aortic incompetence, showed first degree heart block. This case demonstrates that acute aortic insufficiency may develop rapidly in Reiter's syndrome and suggests that patients should have careful cardiac examinations at frequent intervals. These patients can obviously benefit from recent advances in cardiac pacemakers and open-heart surgery if the conduction or valvular defect is diagnosed prior to permanent myocardial damage.

Catterall et al (1965) described the development of neuralgic amyotrophy in a patient with chronic relapsing Reiter's syndrome. This is a localised neuropathy affecting one or more nerves and leading to wasting and weakness of the muscles innervated by those nerves. Electro-myographical studies on the wasted muscles showed significant fibrillation activity at rest and a decreased jerking pattern of motor unit activity on voluntary contraction in the right infraspinatus and deltoid muscles. The condition responded to prednisone 30 mg daily. Bálint (1966) mentioned that two cases of peripheral paralysis developed during the course of Reiter's. Kitov and Stantchev (1971) discussed the presentation of Reiter's syndrome with an encephalomengitic picture. This improved as the patient was treated. Klempel (1970) related the development of a slowly progressive encephalitic process in a 47-year-old man to the Reiter's syndrome he had at the age of 26. Despite these reports neurological complications of the syndrome are very uncommon.

Sairanen et al (1969) reviewed 100 patients who had had the syndrome following the dysentery epidemic in Finland in the Karelian isthmus 20 years previously. The disease had resulted in permanent disability in 42 per cent of the patients. They were compared with a control group of 100 males matched for age and occupation. Examination of the prostate was carried out in each group and the authors felt, from results of the study, that the importance of prostatitis as a focus of infection in the disease was open to doubt. Tryapichnikov and his colleague Iliyn (1970) noted that the prognosis was guarded as only 54 per cent of their patients were able to resume their original occupation following the disease and the remainder were either disabled or dead. Death resulting from the side effects of treatment were reported by Denko and von Haam (1963) and Catterall (1968). Bleehen et al (1966) described the clinical history and post-mortem findings in a patient whose Reiter's syndrome was complicated by amyloidosis. The severe amyloid deposition in the colon caused a protein losing enteropathy necessitating total colectomy. The patient died in the post-operative period. The authors suggested that corticosteroid has an enhancing effect of the development of amyloidosis and that this had been a contributory factor in the case.

This multisystem disease can have many manifestations and complications. It can present with single system involvement separated by variable time intervals (Schimer and Böni, 1967) or with multiple system involvement with unusual clinical symptoms. At times all the physician concerned can do is make a provisional diagnosis and await further developments (Hammer and Graykowski, 1964).

REFERENCES

BÁLINT, G. (1966). *Rheumatol. Balneol. Allerg.*, **7**, 205.
BLEEHEN, S. S., EVERALL, J. D. and TIGHE, J. R. (1966). *Brit. J. vener. Dis.*, **42**, 88.
BLOCK, S. R. (1972). *Arthritis Rheum.*, **15**, 218.
BOYLE, J. A. and BUCHANAN, W. W. (1971). In *Clinical Rheumatology*, pp. 262–281. Blackwell, Oxford and Edinburgh.
BROUSSE, J. P., BRAUN, S. AMOR, B. and COSTE, F. (1966). *Sem. Hôp. Paris*, **42**, 795.
CATTERALL, R. D. (1965). *Brit. J. vener. Dis.*, **41**, 62.
CATTERALL, R. D. (1968). *Brit. J. vener, Dis.*, **44**, 151.
CLIFF, J. M. (1971). *Ann. rheum. Dis.*, **30**, 171.
COLLINS, P. (1972). *Brit. J. vener. Dis.*, **48**, 300.
CROCCO, J. A. and FORMATO, A. A. (1964). *J. Urol.*, **92**, 45.
CSONKA, G. (1966). *Brit. J. vener. Dis.*, **42**, 93.
CSONKA, G. (1973). Personal communication.
DAVIES, N. E., HAVERTY, J. R. and BOATWRIGHT, M. (1969). *Sth. med. J.*, **62**, 1011.
DELBARRE, F., AMOR, B. and PANAHI, F. (1969). *Sem. Hôp. Paris*, **45**, 563.
DENKO, C. W. and VON HAAM, E. (1963). *J. Amer. med. Ass.*, **186**, 632.
GARNER, R. W. and MOWAT, A. G. (1972). *Brit. J. Surg.*, **59**, 657.
GOOD, A. E. (1965). *Acta rheum. scand.*, **11**, 305.
HAMMER, J. E. and GRAYKOWSKI, E. A. (1964). *J. Amer. Dent. Ass.*, **69**, 560.
INGRAM, J. T. (1964). *Lancet*, i, 121.
KAHN, M. Y. and HALL, W. H. (1965). *Arch. intern. Med.*, **116**, 911.
KITOV, D. and STANTCHEV, T. (1971). *Med. Probl. (Plovdiv.)*, **23**, 105.
KLINYSHKOVA, V. M. (1972). *Vestn. Derm. Vener.*, **11**, 31.
LEMKE, L. (1965). *Munch. med. Wschr.*, **107**, 936.
KLEMPEL, K. (1970). *Schweiz. Arch. Neur. Neuroch. Psychiat.*, **106**, 283.
LOCKIE, G. N. and HUNDER, G. G. (1971). *Arthritis Rheum.*, **14**, 767.

McEwen, C. di Tata, D., Lingg, C., Porini, A., Good, A. and Rankin, T. (1971). *Arthritis Rheum.*, **14**, 291.

Maddocks, I. (1968). *Papua N. Guin. med. J.*, **11**, 33.

Maxwell, J. D., Greig, W. R., Boyle, J. A., Pasieczny, T. and Schofield, C. B. S. (1966). *Scot. med. J.*, **11**, 14.

Moss, I. S. (1964). *Brit. J. vener. Dis.*, **40**, 166.

Nicol, C. S. (1966). In *Second Symposium on Advanced Medicine*, p. 187. Pitman, London.

Reckless, J. P. D. (1972). *Brit. J. vener. Dis.*, **48**, 207.

Reich, H. (1966). *Hautarzt*, **17**, 406.

Rodnan, G. P., Benedek, T. G., Shaver, J. A. and Fennell, R. H. (1964). *J. Amer. med. Ass.*, **189**, 889.

Perry, H. O. and Mayne, J. G. (1965). *Arch. Derm.*, **92**, 129.

Sairanen, E., Paronen, I. and Mähonen, H. (1969). *Acta med. scand.*, **185**, 57.

Schimer, A. and Böni, A. (1967). *Z. Rheumaforsch.*, **26**, 142.

Sholkoff, S. D., Glickman, M. G. and Steinbach, H. L. (1970). *Radiology*, **97**, 497.

Siguier, F., Godeau, P., Herreman, C. et al (1970). *Coeur Med. Interne*, **9**, 457.

Tait, G. B. W., Bach, F. and Dixon, A. St. J. (1965). *Ann. rheum. Dis.*, **24**, 273.

Tryapichnikov, P. F. and Iliyn, I. I. (1970). *Soviet Med.*, **33**, 109.

Vartiainen, J. and Hurri, L. (1964). *Acta med. scand.*, **175**, 771.

Verdaguer, S., Gaubert, Y., Phelippon, M., Churet, J., Thiery, M., Legros, B. and Carteaud, M. (1965). *Presse Med.*, **73**, 961.

Warren, C. P. W. (1970). *Ann. rheum. Dis.*, **29**, 483.

Weese, W. C. and McCarty, D. J. (1969). *J. Amer. med. Ass.*, **208**, 825.

Wright, V. and Reed, W. B. (1964). *Ann. rheum. Dis.*, **23**, 12.

34 Therapy

J. R. W. Harris

There is a long-established relationship between rest and relief from pain. The broad principles of general management have altered little in the last decade. The reduction in physical activity, as a result of hospitalisation, frequently produces an appreciable improvement in symptoms. Local immobilisation of a joint produces the maximal rest in the joint. At the same time gentle non-weightbearing passive movements of the joint should be encouraged twice daily to prevent stiffness. There is still controversy as to the advisability of active non-weight bearing movement at an early stage of the inflammatory process. Some workers believe that exercise of the joint may milk foreign antigenic substances in the synovial fluid down to the deeper layers of the synovial membrane and so perpetuate the inflammatory process. Rest diminishes this process and facilitates a more speedy recovery (Ziff, 1965). Certainly vigorous exercise must be condemned as there is the possibility of causing further intra-articular damage and of tearing weakened ligaments.

Today there is a greater appreciation than ever before of the importance of correct posture during periods of bed rest (Boyle and Buchanan, 1971). The patient should be nursed on fracture boards or a firm mattress. A back rest should be provided and this should be removed at night. Despite the protestations of the patient the neck should not be allowed to flex and he should use one pillow at night. A bed cage will take the weight of the clothes off the feet and wrist- or foot-drop must be prevented at all costs with adequate supports. Nicol (1970) advocates aspiration of large joint effusions for rapid relief of pain. Boyle and Buchanan (1971) argue that as patients with Reiter's syndrome are often the largest producers of synovial fluid among those with arthritic diseases, the resultant joint distension is often a source of acute discomfort to the patient.

Numerous drug regimes have been advocated in the treatment of Reiter's syndrome indicating that no therapy is perfect. Acetylsalicyclic acid (aspirin) is the most popular analgesic in use today. Although it has an anti-inflammatory action (Boardman and Hart, 1967) it would usually be prescribed for its analgesic effect. The patient should be maintained on the lowest dosage which will relieve pain. This usually in the region of 3–6 g per day. To maintain adequate plasma levels of 15 mg per cent the drug should be administered 4-hourly. However, if enteric-coated aspirin is used, the longer half-life permits less frequent doses (Ansell, 1963). This preparation may be of use in those patients whose disease process takes a prolonged course and complain of early morning stiffness. As approximately one-quarter of patients complain of dyspepsia, buffered and soluble preparations have come into use. Aloxiprin (Palaprin), a polymeric condensation product of aspirin, enteric-coated aspirin and aluminium oxide may be tolerated better in those patients complaining of dyspepsia, but is a less effective analgesic as the blood levels attained are much lower (Cummings and Martin, 1964). Aspirin has been known to induce massive gastro-intestinal haemorrhage (Perry and Wood, 1967), and even death (Denko and von Haam, 1963). This complication must, however, be considered in the light of the massive aspirin consumption of the community as a whole and is undoubtedly uncommon. Nevertheless as there is evidence that aspirin ingestion is on occasions a factor in precipitating overt haemorrhage from acute or chronic peptic ulcers, its use should be avoided in patients with histories of such conditions (Valman et al, 1968). Chronic haemorrhage occurs in the absence of dyspepsia and there does not appear to be any relation between blood salicylate levels and faecal blood content. The amount lost seems to be the same whether the aspirin is plain, buffered or soluble. Aloxiprin and enteric-coated preparations diminish but do not abolish chronic blood loss (Wood, 1963). Patients with Reiter's syndrome will rarely require sufficiently long-term treatment with aspirin compounds to develop an iron deficiency anaemia. It is important not to confuse the normocytic or hypochromic anaemia which frequently occurs during an acute episode of Reiter's syndrome with a supposed iron deficiency anaemia caused by aspirin therapy. Croft (1963) reported that blood loss following salicylate therapy was the result of a local effect on the gastric mucosa and that soluble aspirin might cause exfoliation of the mucosal epithelial cells. Later he and his co-workers suggested that the rate of surface cell replacement might be the determinant factor in the ability of aspirin to cause bleeding from this site (Croft et al, 1966). Quick (1966) has noted that the prolongation of the bleeding time and a decrease in platelet stickiness caused by aspirin may also be an aetiological factor. The only other serious complication of aspirin therapy which has received attention in recent years is the recognition of the rare occurrence of aspirin allergy. This has a clinical spectrum ranging from cutaneous urticaria to life threatening laryngeal oedema. The anaphylactoid reaction is treated along the usual lines with subcutaneous adrenaline and intravenous hydrocortisone (Samter and Beers, 1968).

Phenylbutazone (Butazolidin) and oxyphenylbutazone (Tanderil) are pyrazalone derivatives. They have powerful analgesic and anti-inflammatory actions. Unfortunately these drugs have many unpleasant toxic side-effects (*Brit. med. J.*, 1965). Blood dyscrasias including thrombocytopenia, agranulocytosis and aplastic anaemia may occur. A peripheral blood picture suggestive of acute leukaemia has been observed (Chalmers and McCarthy, 1964). Fatal hepatic necrosis has been reported by Catterall (1968). Exfoliative dermatitis and other cutaneous rashes have been observed. Swelling of the salivary glands, peptic ulceration and gastro-intestinal haemorrhage have also been noted. Some patients have developed goitres. As many of the toxic effects are dose dependent it is unwise to use the drugs for any length of time. It is probably inadvisable to prescribe more than 300 mg per day of phenylbutazone and indeed the drug would be best retained for those patients who fail to obtain relief from either aspirin or indomethacin.

Indomethacin (Indocid) has a definite place in the treatment of Reiter's syndrome. Mullins et al (1966) found it highly effective in the management of the arthropathy in refractory cases of Reiter's syndrome. Dunlop (1973) has observed that the 100 mg suppository inserted last thing at night often relieves early morning stiffness. The drug has both analgesic and anti-inflammatory properties. It is prescribed in capsules or suppository form. The side-effects are dose related and it is apparently unwise to prescribe more than 150 mg per day as oral medication (Rothermich, 1966). This drug would appear to be of value in the treatment of Reiter's syndrome especially as its rapid action should provide optimum benefit to the patient in a very short time.

There has been controversy as to the place, if any, of chloroquine in the management of this condition. Pernod and Mémin (1963) advocate its use in patients who have relapsed or where the disease process is of long duration. Baker (1966) noted that it may severely exacerbate localised keratoderma blennorrhagica and reported a case where localised keratoderma blennorrhagica was converted to generalised exfoliative dermatitis under such therapy. Retinopathy occurs often enough with the drug to warrant careful consideration before embarking on its use. This retinopathy can be irreversible and lead to blindness (von Sallman and Bernstein, 1963).

Initially glucocorticosteroids were used in the treatment of severe cases of Reiter's syndrome (Ogryzlo and Graham, 1950). Nowadays there is no place for the use of such compounds as they have major mineralocorticoid effects compared with prednisolone or prednisone. Oral corticosteroid administration may impair the ability of the hypothalamic–pituitary–adrenal axis to increase circulating plasma corticosteroid levels in response to stress. Grant et al (1965) have shown that oral corticosteroid will not produce lasting suppression of this axis if given in daily morning dose for a short period of time. However, if the same dose is given at midnight complete suppression of the axis occurs for 24 hours. Although the side-effects of corticosteroid therapy are dose dependent some patients tend to show evidence of the side-effects earlier than others. Protein metabolism is affected and if the patient's appetite is poor a negative nitrogen balance may develop. Under these circumstances atrophy of muscles may be augmented. As corticosteroid drugs restrict the energy supply of the cells in inflamed tissue they can bring the inflammatory process to a halt (Boyle and Buchanan, 1971). This renders the patient liable to asymptomatic pyogenic infection especially as his immunity responses are also impaired. Pyogenic infections of already damaged joints have been reported in patients with rheumatoid arthritis under treatment with corticosteroids (Rimoin and Wennberg, 1966). Nordin (1960) observed that gastro-intestinal complications were the commonest causes of death associated with corticosteroid therapy. This is still relevant today. As the drugs either cause or exacerbate peptic ulceration they should be withheld from those patients who have a history of peptic ulceration, and the development of dyspepsia in a patient on corticosteroid therapy is thought by many to be an indication for withdrawal of the drug. The absolute indications for these drugs in Reiter's syndrome are posterior uveitis, and pericarditis. Intra-articular injection of corticosteroid has been advocated by Colson and Palus (1964) during the acute stage of the disease but this form of therapy is of value in joint diseases where there is obvious synovial hypertrophy and this is not the case in early Reiter's syndrome. Injection of long-acting steroid such as methyl prednisolone acetate 20–40 mg will reduce the quantity of synovial fluid produced (Nicol, 1970). The danger of producing a destructive Charcot-like arthropathy with repeated intra-articular corticosteroid injections must be remembered (Alarcón-Segovia and Ward, 1965). Corticotrophin (ACTH) has the disadvantage that it is given by injection. Also the patient's own cortisol has marked mineralocorticoid activity and many patients gain weight rapidly. As one hopes that steroid therapy will only be used for a short time in Reiter's syndrome there appears to be little advantage in using ACTH.

Folic acid antagonists have been used in the treatment of selected cases of Reiter's syndrome. Methotrexate and aminopterin were used by Mullins et al (1966) to control the cutaneous lesions in six severely affected patients. The arthropathy improved in two of the patients under this regime. Farber et al (1967) found that both the arthropathy and the cutaneous lesions responded satisfactorily to methotrexate. Hancock (1967) felt that there was insufficient evidence that folic acid antagonists could produce such striking improvements in the arthritis component of Reiter's syndrome to justify their use. He also pointed out that in the management of severe and prolonged Reiter's syndrome the successful control of the arthritis is far more important than the relief of symptoms due to keratoderma. However, Jetton and Duncan (1969) outlined what they believed to be the indications for the use of methotrexate in Reiter's syndrome. They felt that it should be used in persistent, active and disabling joint disease which has not been controlled by other methods of therapy in a patient with normal renal, hepatic and bone marrow reserve. After remission of active arthropathy the drug should be stopped. They then reported the use of this drug in two patients, one of whom had failed to respond to 40 mg prednisone daily given full trial, and the other who was very ill and had had a previous partial gastrectomy for peptic ulceration. They emphasised the importance of constant supervision during therapy and obtained a remission in both cases within 3 months. The highest weekly dosage of methotrexate used was 25 mg and the maximum time that this dosage was given was 12 weeks. Krebs et al (1971) reported a similar case of successful response to methotrexate following prednisone failure. Therapy with folic acid antagonists should be approached bearing in mind that all mitotic cells of the body are susceptible to inhibition of DNA synthesis; that therapeutic and toxic effects are inseparable and that renal and hepatic function of the patient must be adequate.

Popert et al (1964) carried out a prospective study to determine whether treatment with oxytetracycline 500 mg four times daily for 5 days was of any value in this condition. They were not able to find any evidence that treatment of the genito-urinary component had a beneficial influence on the course of the syndrome. Following the initial report by Mowat et al (1967) that lincomycin hydrochloride therapy over a 2-week period produced a remission in the condition, Whaley et al (1969) carried out a double-blind trial using this drug. Altogether 22 patients were included in the trial and the authors were unable to find any significant difference between lincomycin hydrochloride and a placebo.

Gold therapy was advocated in severe or protracted cases by Pernod and Mémin (1963) and by Colson and Palus (1964). Griseofulvin was used over a 6-month period by Nicolau et al (1967). Laird et al (1965) reported the results of stilboestrol therapy in 10 patients. Daily prostatic massage was not found to have any beneficial effect on the disease process (Popert et al, 1964) although Morton (1972) advocates its use three times per week in these patients who have prostatis.

REFERENCES

Alarcón-Segovia, D. and Ward, L. E. (1965). *J. Amer. med. Ass.*, **193**, 1052.
Ansell, B. M. (1963). *Salicyclates, an International Symposium*, p. 35. Churchill Ltd., London.
Baker, H. (1966). *Brit. J. Derm.*, **78**, 161.
Boardman, P. L. and Hart, F. D. (1967). *Brit. med. J.*, iv, 264.

BOYLE, J. A. and BUCHANAN, W. W. (1971). In *Clinical Rheumatology*, pp. 262–281. Blackwell, Oxford and Edinburgh.

Brit. med. J. (1965). ii, 773.

CATTERALL, R. D. (1968). *Brit. J. vener. Dis.*, **44**, 151.

CHALMERS, T. M. and McCARTHY, D. D. (1964). *Brit. med. J.*, i, 747.

COLSON, J. A. and PALUS, J. C. (1964). *Rev. Rhum.*, **31**, 129.

CROFT, D. N. (1963). *Salicylates, an International Symposium*, p. 204. Churchill Ltd, London.

CROFT, D. N., POLLOCK, D. J. and COGHILL, N. F. (1966). *Gut*, **7**, 333.

CUMMINGS, A. J. and MARTIN, B. K. (1964). *Biochem. Pharmac.*, **13**, 767.

DENKO, C. W. and VON HAAM, E. (1963). *J. Amer. med. Ass.*, **186**, 632.

DUNLOP, E. M. C. (1973). Personal Communication.

FARBER, G. A., FORSHNER, J. C. and O'QUINN, S. E. (1967). *J. Amer. med. Ass.*, **200**, 171.

GRANT, S. D., FORSHAM, P. H. and DI RAIMONDO, V. C. (1965). *New Engl. J. med.*, **273**, 1115.

HANCOCK, J. A. H. (1967). *Brit. J. vener. Dis.* **43** 146.

JETTON, R. L. and DUNCAN, W. C. (1969). *Ann. intern. Med.*, **70**, 349.

KREBS, A., KUNG, D. and HONNAT, A. (1971). *Bull. Soc. franc. Derm. Syph.*, **78**, 239.

LAIRD, S. M., GILL, A. J. and PITKEATHLY, D. A. (1965). *Brit. med. J.*, i, 970.

MORTON, R. S. (1972). *Practitioner*, **209**, 637.

MOWAT, A. G., CHALMERS, T. M., ALEXANDER, W. R. M. and DUTHIE, J. J. R. (1967). *Brit. med. J.*, i, 478.

MULLINS, J. F. MABERRY, J. D. and STONE, O. J. (1966). *Arch. Derm.*, **94** 335.

NICOL, C. S. (1970). In *Current Medical Treatment*, p. 787. Staples Press, London.

NICOLAU, S. G., NOAGHEA, G. and BUCUR, G. (1967). *Derm. Vener., Buc.*, **12**, 537.

NORDIN, B. E. C. (1960). *Brit. J. Derm.*, **72**, 40.

OGRYZLO, M. A. and GRAHAM, W. (1950). *J. Amer. med. Ass.*, **144**, 1239.

PERNOD, J. and MÉMIN, Y. (1963). *Vie Méd.*, **44**, 249.

PERRY, D. J. and WOOD, P. H. N. (1967). *Gut*, **8**, 301.

POPERT, A. J., GILL, A. J. and LAIRD, S. M. (1964). *Brit. J. vener. Dis.*, **40**, 160.

QUICK, A. J. (1966). *Amer. J. med. Sci.*, **252**, 265.

RIMOIN, D. L. and WENNBERG, J. E. (1966). *J. Amer. med. Ass.*, **196**, 617.

ROTHERMICH, N. O. (1966). *J. Amer. med. Ass.*, **195**, 531.

SAMTER, M. and BEERS, R. F. JR. (1968). *Ann. intern. Med.*, **68**, 975.

SALLMAN, L. VON and BERNSTEIN, H. N. (1963). *Bull. rheum. Dis.*, **14**, 327.

VALMAN, H. B., PARRY, D. J. and COGHILL, N. J. (1968). *Brit. med. J.*, ii, 661.

WHALEY, K., DOWNIE, W. W., DICK, W. C., NUKI, G., SCHOFIELD, C. B. S. and ANDERSON, J. (1969). *Brit. med. J.*, ii, 421.

WOOD, P. H. N. (1963). *Salicylates, an International Symposium*', p. 194. Churchill Ltd., London.

ZIFF, M. (1965). *Ann. rheum. Dis.*, **24**, 103.

Part 8
Other Sexually Transmissible Diseases

Preamble

The term 'venereal diseases' or 'V.D.' is applied worldwide to syphilis and gonorrhoea. Inclusion of other diseases under this head varies from one part of the world to another. In the U.K. for instance, 'V.D.' is legally defined and includes syphilis, gonorrhoea and chancroid.

In recent years, clinical and epidemiological observations, social awareness and laboratory work have combined to bring a growing realisation that there are at least a dozen diseases which may be passed from man to woman, woman to man or man to man during sexual activity. Hence the terms 'sexually transmitted diseases' and 'sexually transmissible diseases' or 'S.T.D.' have been increasingly used.

The diseases to be dealt with in this section are all sexually transmissible. This term does not preclude an appreciation that they may be disseminated by social as well as sexual contact; nor does it prevent understanding that the proportion of cases sexually and socially acquired varies from one disease to another, from one place to another and from time to time. Such proportions not only depend on the individual disease but on social dynamics. Furthermore, since the borderline between social and sexual intercourse is not clear in every case, and definitions may vary from one society to another, such facets call for recognition by those who would endeavour to effect epidemiological as well as clinical control.

Appreciation of these observations has far-reaching effects. There is, for example, now no place for the 'two diseases' venereologist and this calls for recognition by medical administrators. In practical terms the clinician can no longer escape concomitant responsibility for all diseases acquired sexually. Involvement of other specialists is also essential. Thus local or national programmes aimed at epidemiological control, for example of scabies, should ensure involvement and commitment of both dermatologists and venereologists.

Such a comprehensive approach to sexually transmitted and transmissible diseases has been increasingly adopted over the last 50 years in

323

the U.K. It accounts, in part, for such success in control and disability prevention as that sexually free society may claim. Similar approaches are being made in some other European countries and sporadically elsewhere. Doubtlessly all these countries would welcome a growing number of enlightened neighbours.

35 Herpes Genitalis

R. S. Morton

Introduction

Herpes genitalis is caused by *Herpes virus hominis* type II (see Figs. 23, 24). The condition is sexually transmissible. As with herpes facialis the primary infection may be severe with marked regional adenitis and systemic symptoms. Clinically more limited recurrences may be frequent and troublesome and interfere with a regular sex life.

The itchy blisters, which characterise the first stage of herpes genitalis, usually break down within 24 hours and present themselves to the clinician as a cluster of small, round, regularly edged, areolated and sloughy based, shallow ulcers. Differentiation from syphilis calls for both sound clinical judgment and repeated dark-ground examinations.

In recent times neonatal herpes infection has become widely recognised as a clinical entity. The recent association of herpes genitalis and cervical cancer is at the time of writing circumstantial rather than one of cause and effect.

EPIDEMIOLOGY AND SOCIAL ASPECTS

The morbidity rate of genital herpes infection is unknown. Nahmias et al (1969b) suggest that it is commoner than formerly, may well become commmer; and be found to parallel, at a low level, the trend in gonorrhoea.

Some idea of the incidence is reflected in a paper by Shelley (1967). He found one case in every 500 cervical cytology specimens. Intranuclear inclusions were used as the diagnostic criterion. Nahmias et al (1967) found 103 (0·016 per cent) such specimens in 60 000 cervical scrapings. Beilby et al (1968) grew the herpes virus from the cervix of eight (3·8 per cent) of 209 patients attending a venereal diseases clinic. Most of the 209 were named sex contacts of men with gonorrhoea. The virus's presumed predilection for the cervix is questioned by Cederqvist et al (1970) in Sweden. They found cytological changes due to herpes in

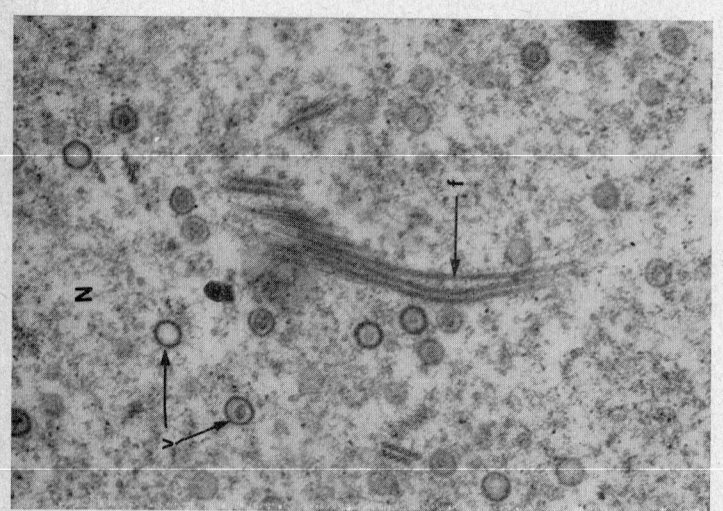

(b)

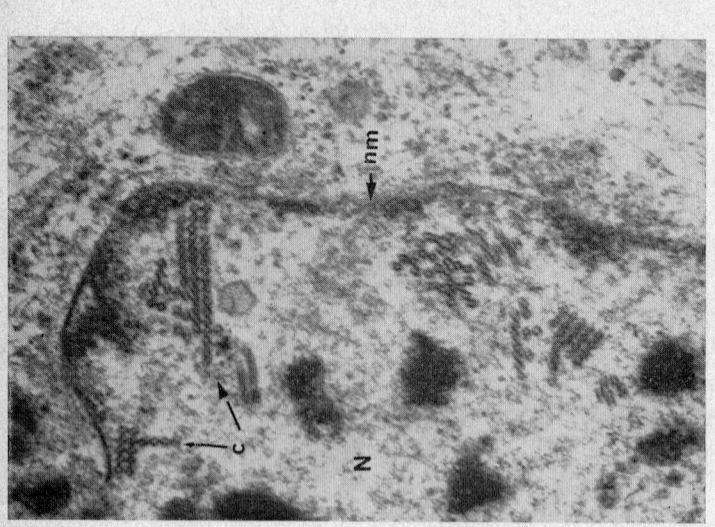

(a)

FIG. 23. Electron micrographs of BHK cells infected with Type 2 HVH. N = nucleus; nm = nuclear membrane; c = 'chain-mail' structures; v = virus particles; f = filaments. Lead citrate, uranyl acetate (a) = 60×000, (b) = 40×000. (From a paper by Isabel W. Smith and others (1973). *Brit. J. vener. Dis.*, **49**, 385. Reproduced by kind permission of the authors and the Editor of the *British Journal of Venereal Diseases*.)

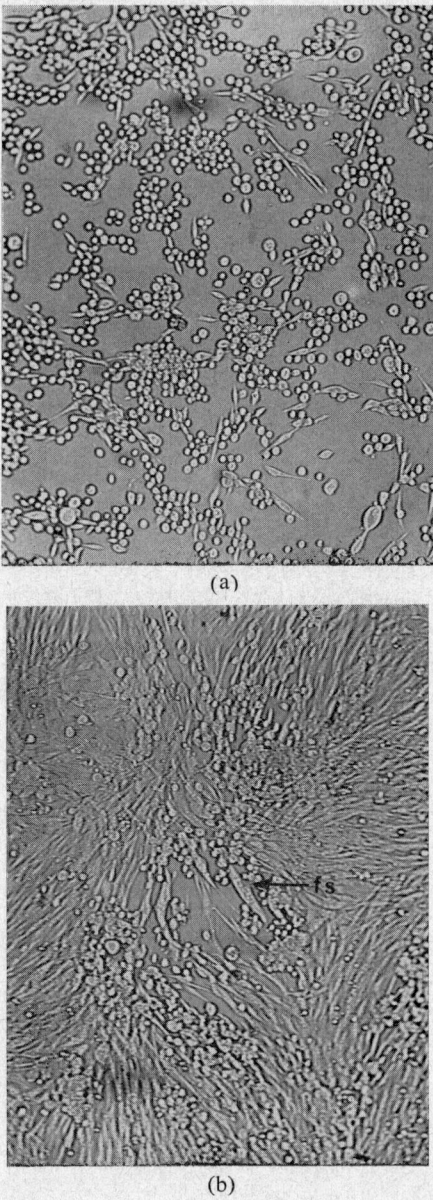

(a)

(b)

FIG. 24. Unstained light micrographs, showing the cytopathic effect produced by (a) HVH Type 1 and (b) HVH Type 2 in BHK cells. fs= fusiform syncytium. × 70. (From a paper by Isabel W. Smith and others (1973). *Brit. J. vener. Dis.*, **49**, 385. Reproduced by kind permission of the authors and the Editor of the *British Journal of Venereal Diseases*.)

0·04 per cent of 68 000 vaginal specimens. Ng et al (1970) described the intracellular manifestations of herpes as seen in primary and recurrent cases.

A measure of sexual transmissibility of genital herpes was given in a paper by Kleger et al (1968). They recovered the virus from 0·1 per cent of 1 899 women attending cervical cytology clinics but from 1·6 per cent of 494 promiscuous females attending a venereal diseases clinic. Four forms of culture media were used. Although the evidence presented supports the sexual transmission theory no data is presented to link the infection with cervical cancer.

There is other evidence of sexual transmission, Nahmias et al (1969a) found the type II *Herpes virus hominis* in seven of eight female contacts of seven men with herpetic penile lesions. Rawls et al (1971) examined 18 female contacts of men with genital herpes and grew the virus from 14 (78 per cent). Further support for genital transmission can be found in the papers of Amstey and Baluzzi (1970), Davies and Longson (1970), Jeansson and Molin (1970) and Hutfield (1970). Indirect support for genital herpes as a sexually transmissible infection comes from the work of Nahmias et al (1970a) who found type II virus antibodies only in persons over the age of 14 years.

Rawls et al (1971) studied genital herpes in two social groups. Amongst Caucasians of upper socio-economic class with symptomatic primary herpes 78 per cent lacked antibodies to either types I or II herpes virus. Amongst Negroes of lower socio-economic class the corresponding figure was only 29 per cent. Antibody response to *Herpes virus hominis* type II followed a similar pattern in both social groups.

Nahmias et al (1968) found genital herpetic lesions in six children aged 3–12 years. Type I virus was isolated in two and type II in four. On the basis of the evidence presented genital infection in children can be either sexually or non-sexually transmitted.

This takes us to consideration of the possibilities of neonatal or even intra-uterine infection. Wheeler and Huffines (1965) noted that infection in the baby may be widely disseminated over skin and oral mucus membranes with generalised lymphadenopathy and splenomegaly. In some of their cases the baby died. Infantile herpetic infections of varying severity have been described by Hudson and McFarland (1969), Torphy et al (1970) and Zavoral et al (1970). In one series by Nahmias et al (1969b) 25 of 28 cases of infantile infection were due to Type II herpes virus. The authors leave us in no doubt that they believe the babies were infected by their mothers. Some of the babies demonstrated elevation of IgM levels.

What are the chances of neonatal infection? This aspect has been examined by Nahmias and his co-workers. In 1967 they offered the belief (Nahmias et al, 1967) that the baby would be safe if the mother's infection had cleared at least 3 to 4 weeks prior to delivery. Infection presenting, occurring or recurring later they saw as a potential hazard. So very real did they consider the possibility that they recommended that in such cases Caesarian section should be considered. Pursuing this subject in more depth and detail they reported (Nahmias et al 1970a) on a series of 283 women with cytological evidence of genital herpes during pregnancy or immediately thereafter. They noted an abortion rate three times that of the general hospital population during the first 20 weeks of pregnancy. The premature birth rate was slightly higher than might be expected. The risk of neo-natal infection was 10 per cent if infection occurred after 32 weeks of pregnancy. The risk increased to 40 per cent if infection was present at confinement. Four babies in this last 'at risk' group were delivered by Caesarian section and none was infected. The authors are firm in their advice regarding isolation and barrier nursing for all babies born to mothers with herpes infection at time of delivery. Ng et al (1970) described 256 instances of herpes during pregnancy. They found no evidence that the infection increased foetal mortality.

Unlike another member of the herpes group of virus, the cytomegalic virus, *Herpes virus hominis* type II does not appear to create the formidable problem of intra-uterine infection. There is need for further observation. Goldman (1970) has reported herpes virus inclusions in endometrial cells and suggests that foetal infection must be considered a possibility if the placenta is formed from infected endometrium.

Josey et al (1972) reviewed the epidemiology of Type II (genital) herpes infection. A prostitute population was studied for evidence of herpes type II infection by Duenas et al (1972).

CLINICAL ASPECTS

According to Yen et al (1965) as many as 90 per cent of primary herpes genitalis infections are sub-clinical. This is said to be particularly true of infections in females say Rawls et al (1966) and Nahmias et al (1969a).

Parker and Banatvala (1967) noted that recurrences were common and that in men the condition was commonest in the uncircumcised.

Josey et al (1966) drew special attention to the clinical condition in in females and listed it as a cause of vaginal discharge and dysuria. Willcox (1968a, b), commenting on how much more frequently the condition is recognised in males, described six cases of acute primary herpes of cervix and vaginal vault. The commonest presenting sign was unusually severe cervicitis. The report is illustrated. Complement fixation tests originally negative became positive after 2 or 3 weeks. Hutfield (1968) also working at St. Mary's Hospital, London, noted that genital herpes was five to six times as common as primary syphilis. He noted also that 81 per cent of all patients attending the venereal diseases department were found to have neutralising antibodies. From this he concluded that probably four out of five cases of genital herpes are recurrences.

Minikin and Lynch (1968) in a letter to the editor of the *Journal of the American Medical Association* noted that genital herpes in servicemen returning from Vietnam was frequently classified as recurrent chancroid. Six cases were seen in a period of 4 weeks. A plea is made by the writers for greater awareness of herpes and other 'minor' sexually transmitted diseases. Juel-Jensen (1969) emphasises that active herpetic infections are highly infectious and illustrates why they should be handled with caution by doctors and nurses. He gives the incubation period as 2–7 days.

Recurrences may be precipitated by a wide variety of stimuli according to Fenner and White (1970). The same point it made by Logan et al (1971) who give special mention to trauma, consitutional disease, fever, genito-urinary infection and immunological defect.

Hutfield (1966) described the history of herpes and in particular reviewed the eighteenth and nineteenth century literature on the subject. Not surprisingly, French and German workers are widely represented. Jonathan Hutchinson was the only British contributor of note. An up-to-date clinical description of herpes genitalis is given by Young (1972). He deals very fully with the differential diagnosis and illustrates the article in black and white.

Recently 190 randomly selected males have been searched for type II virus. Specimens for culture were obtained from urethral swabs, prostatic fluid and testicular biopsy. No patient had a clinical history of genital herpes, but 41 carriers were identified (Centifanto et al, 1972).

Nahmias et al (1970b) reviewed 148 infections in the newborn. Incubation period varied but never exceeded 21 days. Between 80–95 per cent were due to herpes virus type II. In one-third of the cases lesions were localised and prognosis was fairly good. A few babies were asymptomatic. Two-thirds of cases however showed varying degrees of dissemination of infection. Any or many organs could be involved—skin, eyes, liver, adrenals, mouth, trachea, etc. Conjunctivitis, convulsions, jaundice, neurological involvement and evidence of a bleeding diathesis were common. The overall fatality rate was 71 per cent; it was 95 per cent of the disseminated cases. Of those recovering, 15 per cent had sequels, mostly C.N.S. defects. It is recommended that babies born of mothers with genital herpes should not only have a herpes C.F.T. done repeatedly but should also have IgM estimations.

Herpes virus type II has been isolated from brain tissue of the newborn by Juel-Jensen and MacCallum (1972), Craig and Nahmias (1973) and in two cases of meningitis, by Craig and Nahmias (1973). In a further three cases of proven type II genital herpes, meningitis occurred 5–10 days after the appearance of the genital vesicles. Terni et al (1971), who made this report, did not isolate the virus from the C.S.F. Skoldenberg et al (1973) believed that when type II affects the C.N.S. of young adults it causes meningitis in contrast to type I which causes encephalitis. They describe seven cases of type II meningitis and note that the ages of the patients correspond to the age distribution of patients attending a venereal diseases clinic with genital herpes.

Laboratory

Dowdle et al (1967) were amongst the first to demonstrate that the virus of genital herpes (type II) is distinct from that causing labial herpes (type I). They used a micro-neutralising technique. Herrman (1967) laid down a routine for laboratory isolation of type II. The virus, he showed, can be grown on human amnion, embryo cells and fibroblasts, rabbit kidney and a variety of cell lines. Parker and Banatvala (1967) grew the genital virus on the chorio-allantoic membrane of 11-day-old fertile hens' eggs in 23 of 60 suspected cases. Unlike the virus of herpes labialis the type II viruses were found to produce large necrotic lesions in the eggs. This point was taken up by others. Figueroa and Rawls (1969) noted that in chick embryo culture herpes virus type II forms obvious plaques and that these are absent in type I cultures. Kleger and Prier (1969) found that eight strains of the herpes labialis virus produced multi-nucleated giant cells in cultures of human embryoid kidney cells as against nine genital herpes strains which did not. The authors note that the two virus types have previously been noted to produce differences in cultures of HeLa cells and chorio-allantoic membranes of eggs.

Plummer et al (1970) summarised the biological differences between the two types of herpes virus. More simplified methods of differentiating *Herpes virus hominis* types I and II have been sought.

Hutfield (1967) described cultural isolation of the virus. In 100 consecutive cases he found complement fixing antibodies against non-specific herpes viruses were present in 49 per cent as against neutralising antibodies against the genital strain in 81 per cent. There were other attempts to improve diagnosis. Gardner et al (1968) found that diagnosis by use of immunofluorescent antibody testing correlated well with virus culture results and a neutralisation test. Exploration of this method of diagnosis resulted in Geder and Skinner (1971) evolving a simpler and rapid immunofluorescent means of typing strains. The technique is given in detail. Using eight freshly isolated virus strains they found that cell membrane immunofluorescence with absorbed sera gave clear-cut results. Culture of the clinically suspected virus is still the favoured diagnostic method principally because, in contrast to culture of some viruses, it is a relatively rapid and conclusive method. Dealing with genital lesions, Nahmias et al (1969a) found that 63 of 64 isolates from males and 155 of 165 isolates from females were genital (type II) strains. The remainder were type I. In contrast, Kaufman and Rawls (1972) described cases of extragenital type II herpes virus infection. Terni and Roizman (1970) recorded cases where both types of virus affected the same patient at different sites.

Roizman et al (1970) described the glyco-protein structure and classification of herpes viruses.

Nahmias et al (1970a) claimed that the use of a micro-neutralisation test clearly differentiated the circulating antibodies of types I and II viruses. Type II antibodies were found only in patients aged 14 years and over. In a series of 122 patients they were able to demonstrate that the presence of type I antibodies does not preclude infection with type II virus.

Rodin et al (1971) came forward with the useful observation that Stuart's transport medium was satisfactory for the transport of the herpes virus. They compared the findings with those by the standard method, using a plain swab and a virus transport medium. Men with genital lesions were used in this study.

Treatment

It is generally agreed that there is no specific treatment for herpes. Simple hygiene and the avoidance of steroids, which may precipitate systemic spread, form the principles of present-day care. In men, only circumcision appears to offer hope of diminishing the frequency and number of recurrent attacks in some. A number of experimental treatment methods have been reported in recent years.

Schofield (1964) treated 50 cases of genital herpes (with 54 episodes of infection) with topical applications of an ointment containing 0·5 per cent 5-iodo-2-deoxyuridine (5-IDU). It was claimed that the clinical duration of the herpes was cut by half, and without side-effects. 5-IDU acts by blocking thymidine, an essential for the formation of virus DNA. Hutfield (1964) compared the results of treating 20 patients with 5-IDU, with 20 treated with penotrane and 20 treated with a placebo. The first two both appeared to shorten the duration of lesions by a few days, probably by promoting healing. In this respect 5-IDU was marginally better.

Joosting (1971) on the basis of laboratory experience of cultural inhibition of viruses by metronidazole tried the drug in the clinical condition in children and reported favourably on the trial.

MacCallum and Partridge (1968) and Partridge and Millis (1968) discuss the systemic use of 5-IDU in generalised neonatal herpes.

Söltz-Szöts (1971) using a herpes simplex antigen, vaccinated 532 patients with histories of recurrent herpes including genital herpes. The procedure was repeated at 3–6 monthly intervals. Three-quarters of the patients ceased to have recurrences. The author also reported his findings with other treatment measures. Five-IDU he described as 'disappointing'. Stimulating interferon production by vaccination with inactivated influenza virus is said to reduce the duration of herpes zoster.

An old method has recently been revived. The relationship—presumed to be immunological—between the herpes and smallpox viruses has long been the basis for smallpox vaccination as a means of trying to prevent recurrence of genital herpes. Kern and Schif (1968) recommend weekly vaccination for 6 weeks.

Many experienced dermatologists and venereologists might see more hope in the suggestions of Felber (1971). He attempted photodynamic inactivation of the herpes viruses and claimed some degrees of success. The routine is as follows. Firstly, the lesions are photosensitised by application of 0·1 per cent aqueous solution of netural red. Alternatively, proflavine dye can be used. Thereafter, and repeatedly, the affected area is exposed to a cool white 15-watt fluorescent bulb. Similar methods and claims had been used and made by Wallis et al (1969). The latest report on the method comes from Friedrich (1972) who in a series of 30 patients claimed that 24 obtained marked relief within 36 hours.

GENITAL HERPES AND CERVICAL CANCER

The opinion that herpes virus type II is a likely candidate as a cervical carcinogen has gained ground since the publications of Rawls et al (1968) and Josey et al (1968). The first paper reported finding the virus in four of 23 cervical biopsy specimens showing either dysplasia or carcinoma in situ. The second paper reviews all the evidence and finds that the association of Type II virus with cervical cancer is circumstantial only. The authors are in no doubt that the findings justify the prolonged follow-up of all women diagnosed as having genital herpes. In recent years a great deal has been written about the association, for example by Naib et al (1969) and Goodheart (1970), who showed that antibodies in women without carcinoma of the cervix increased with age and that higher titres are more usual in the lower socio-economic classes. It has been shown in a series of papers by Rawls et al (1969, 1970, 1971) that the kind of people who develop carcinoma of the cervix have the same kind of social background and life style as those with genital herpes. Similar work has been reported by Willbanks and Campbell (1972).

Aurelian et al (1971) identified herpes type II virus in cervical cancer cells undergoing degeneration in tissue culture. These electron-microscopy findings strengthen further the association of the two conditions. Serological tests have also been employed to explore the associations. Aurelian et al (1972) in a further study have shown that *in vivo* cervical tumour cells only reveal type II antigens when exposed to high pH induced by glandular secretions. The presence or absence of antigen in 29 patients was determined by immuno-fluorescent tests. The absence of virus particles in exfoliated cervical cells is thought to be due to faulty virus assembly.

The sera of 335 women with normal and abnormal cervical cytology were tested for neutralising antibodies to types I and II herpes virus by Skinner et al (1971). High type I antibody titres were equally distributed in the two groups. With type II tests, higher titres, and more of them, were found in the women with histological evidence of cervical changes than in controls. The differences were independent of age and socio-economic states. Furthermore, preliminary evidence is presented to show that cone biopsy of the cervix in cases of carcinoma *in situ* is followed by a fall in the titre of neutralising type II antibody.

In sexually free societies where the attitudes and behaviour of young women currently show marked change, the question of the association of genital herpes and carcinoma of the cervix has need of urgent attention. The resolution of this problem must be seen as the paramount need in future research into herpes genitalis.

REFERENCES

AMSTEY, M. S. and BALUZZI, P. C. (1970). *Amer. J. Obstet. Gynec.*, **106**, 188.
AURELIAN, L., STRANDBERG, J. D. et al (1971). *Science, N.Y.*, **174**, 704.
AURELIAN, L., STRANSBERG, J. D. and DAVIS, H. J. (1972). *Proc. Soc. exp. Biol. (N.Y.)*, **140**, 404.
BEILBY, J. O. and CAMERON, C. H. (1968). *Lancet*, **1**, 1065.
CRAIG, C. P. and NAHMIAS, A. J. (1973). *J. infect. Dis.*, **127**, 365.
CENTIFANTO, Y. M. and DRYLIE, D. M. (1972). *Science, N.Y.*, **178**, 318.
CEDERQVIST, L. and ELASSON, B. (1970). *Acta obstet. gynec. scand.*, **49**, 13.
DAVIES, R. M. and LONGSON, M. (1970). *Oral Surg.* **30**, 41.
DOWDLE, W. R. and NAHMIAS, A. J. (1967). *J. Immunol.*, **99**, 974.
DUENAS, A. and ADAM, E. (1972). *Amer. J. Epidem.*, **95**, 483.
FELBER, T. D. (1971). *J. Amer. med. Ass.*, **217**, 307.
FENNER, F. and WHITE, D. D. (1970). *Medical Virology*. Academic Press, New York, 232 pp.
FIGUEROA, M. E. and RAWLS, W. E. (1969). *J. gen. Virol.*, **4**, 259.
FRIEDRICH, E. G. (1973). *J. Obstet. Gynaec.*, **41**, 74.
GARDNER, P. S. and McQUILLAN, J. (1968). *Brit. med. J.*, **4**, 89.
GEDER, L. and SKINNER, G. R. B. (1971). *J. gen. Virol.*, **12**, 179.
GOLDMAN, R. L. (1970). *Obstet. Gynec.*, **36**, 603.
GOODHEART, C. R. (1970). *J. Amer. med. Ass.*, **211**, 91.
HERRMAN, E. C. (1967). *Mayo Clin. Proc.*, **42**, 744.
HUTFIELD, D. C. (1964). *Brit. J. vener. Dis.*, **40**, 210.
HUTFIELD, D. C. (1966). *Brit. J. vener. Dis.*, **42**, 263.
HUTFIELD, D. C. (1967). *Brit. J. vener. Dis.*, **43**, 48.
HUTFIELD, D. C. (1968). *Brit. J. vener. Dis.*, **44**, 241.
HUTFIELD, D. C. (1970). *Brit. J. Hosp. Med.*, **3**, 881.
HUDSON, A. W. and McFARLAND, C. (1969). *J. Amer. med. Ass.*, **208**, 859.

JEANSSON, S. and MOLIN, L. (1970). *Lancet*, **1**, 1064.
JOOSTING, A. C. C. (1971). *S. Afr. med. J.*, **45**, 486.
JOSEY, W. E. et al (1966). *Amer. J. Obstet. Gynec.*, **96**, 493.
JOSEY, W. E.,NAHMIAS, A. J. and NAIB, Z. M. (1968). *Amer. J. Obstet. Gynec.*, **101**, 718.
JOSEY, W. E., NAHMIAS, A. J. and NAIB, Z. M. (1972). *Obstet. Gynec. Ser.*, **27**, 295.
JUEL-JENSEN, B. E. (1969). *Brit. J. Hosp. Med.*, **2**, 1687.
JUEL-JENSEN, B. E. and MACCALLUM, F. O. (1972). *Herpes Simplex, Varicella and Zoster*, Heinemann, London.
KAUFMAN, R. H. and RAWLS, W. H. (1972). *Amer. J. Obstet. Gynec.*, **112**, 866.
KERN, A. B. and SCHIF, B. L. (1966). *Arch. Derm.*, **89**, 844.
KLEGER, B. and PRIER, J. E. (1968). *Amer. J. Obstet. Gynec.*, **102**, 745.
KLEGER, B. and PRIER, J. E. (1969). *J. infect. Dis.*, **120**, 376.
LOGAN, W. S., TINDALL, J. P. & ELSTOM, M. L. (1971). *Arch. Derm.* **103**, 606.
MINKIN, W. and LYNCH, P. J. (1968). *J. Amer. med., Ass.*, **203**, 526.
MACCALLUM, F. O. and PARTRIDGE, J. W. (1968). *Arch. Dis. Childh.*, **43**, 265.
NAHMIAS, A. J. and ZUHER, M. N. (1967). *Obstet. Gynec.*, **29**, 395.
NAHMIAS, A. J. and DOWDLE, W. R. (1968). *Pediatrics*, **42**, 659.
NAHMIAS, A. J. and DOWDLE, W. R. (1969a). *Brit. J. vener. Dis.*, **45**, 294.
NAHMIAS, A. J. and DOWDLE, W. R. (1969b). *J. Pediat.*, **75**, 1194.
NAHMIAS, A. J. and JOSEY, W. E. (1970a). *Amer. J. Epidem.*, **91**, 539 and 547.
NAHMIAS, A. J., ALFORD, C. A. and SHELDON, B. K. (1970b). *Adv. Pediat.*, **17**, 185.
NAIB, Z. M. and NAHMIAS, A. J. (1969). *Corcv.*, **23**, 940.
NG, A. B. P., REAGAN, J. W. and YEN, S. S. C. (1970). *Obstet. Gynec.*, **36**, 645.
PARKER, J. D. J. and BANATVALA, J. E. (1967). *Brit. J. vener. Dis.*, **43**, 212.
PARTRIDGE, J. W. and MILLIS, R. R. (1968). *Arch. Dis. Childh.*, **43**, 377.
PLUMMER, G. and WANER, J. L. (1970). *J. Virol.*, **5**, 51.
RAWLS, W. E. and TOMPKINS, W. A. F. (1966). *Science, N.Y.*, **161**, 1255.
RAWLS, W. E. and LAUREL, D. (1968). *Amer. J. Epidem.*, **87**, 647.
RAWLS, W. E., TOMPKINS, W. A. F. and MELNICK, J. L. (1969). *Amer. J. Epidem.*, **89**, 547.
RAWLS, W. E., GARDNER, H. L. and KAUFMAN, R. L. (1970). *Amer. J. Obstet. Gynec.*, **107**, 710.
RAWLS, W. E. and GARDNER, H. L. (1971). *Amer. J. Obstet. Gynec.*, **110**, 682.
RODIN, P. and HARE, M. J. (1971). *Brit. J. vener. Dis.*, **47**, 198.
ROIZMAN, B., KELER, J. M. and SPEAR, P. G. (1970). *Nature, Lond.*, **225**, 1253.
SCHOFIELD, C. B. S. (1964). *Brit. J. Derm.*, **76**, 465.
SHELLEY, W. B. (1967). *J. Amer. med. Ass.*, **201**, 153.
SKINNER, G. R. B., THOULESS, M. E. and JORDAN, J. A. (1971). *J. Obstet. Gynaec. Brit. Commonw.*, **78**, 103.
SKOLDENBERG, B., JEANSSON, S. and WOLONTIS, S. (1973). *Brit. med. J.*, **2**, 611.
SÖLTZ-SZÖTS, J. (1971). *Z. Haut-u-Geschl.-Kr.*, **46**, 755.
TERNI, M. and ROIZMAN, B. (1970). *J. infect. Dis.*, **121**, 212.
TERNI, M., CACCIALANZA, P., CASSAI, E. and KIEFF, E. (1971). *New Engl. J. Med.*, **285**, 503.
TORPHY, D. E. and RAY, C. G. et al. (1970). *J. Pediat.*, **76**, 405.
WALLIS, C., TRULOCK, S. and MELNICK, J. L. (1969). *J. gen. Virol.*, **5**, 53.
WHEELER, C. E. and HUFFINES, W. D. (1965). *J. Amer. med. Ass.*, **191**, 455.
WILLBANKS, L. D. and CAMPBELL, J. A. (1972). *Amer. J. Obstet. Gynec.*, **112**, 924.
WILLCOX, R. R. (1968a). *Brit. med. J.*, **1**, 610.
WILLCOX, R. R. (1968b). *Br. J. clin. Pract.*, **22**, 358.
YEN, S. S. C., KEGAN, J. W. and ROSENTHAL, M. S. (1965). *Obstet. Gynec.*, **25**, 479.
YOUNG, A W. JR. (1972). Clinicis of North America, *Venereal Diseases*, **56**, 1175.
ZAVORAL, J. H. and RAY, W. L. (1970). *J. Amer. med. Ass.*, **213**, 1492.

36 Molluscum Contagiosum

R. S. Morton

This condition is a viral infection, well recognised as being contracted through close body contact. The virus is the largest of the pox group of viruses. Marital and family contacts have long been recognised. Traditionally, infection is said to originate in swimming and Turkish baths. The incubation period varies from 3 weeks to 3 months. The cells lining the small, waxy and umbilicated papules show ballooned cells with inclusions. Treatment consists of emptying the papules and applying phenol.

Overfield and Brody (1966) described an epidemic of the infection amongst close living children in Alaska. Blattner (1967) found work with the virus difficult as its growth could not be sustained by repeated subculture.

Ayres et al (1964) described and discussed molluscum contagiosum of the penis. Lynch and Minkin (1968) suggested that venereal contact probably accounted for many cases. They recorded 55 instances in 7 months in servicemen returning from Vietnam and Korea. Lesions were primarily sited on the penis, pubis and inner aspects of the thighs. The men were aged 18–27 years and all but two admitted pre- or extra-marital intercourse. Non-venereal transmission is discussed as are the difficulties of treatment.

Jacobs (1970) described 14 cases following coitus. Lesions in individual patients numbered from one to 63. Effective treatment was by liquid paraffin.

Cobbold and MacDonald (1970) question the current relevance of standard textbook descriptions that molluscum contagiosum is a disease of children, and adults who attend Turkish bath-houses. Working at St. Mary's Hospital, London, they found that the average annual number of cases attending the department of dermatology was 14 with 50 per cent of them children. This contrasted sharply with 23 cases, in 3 months, attending the department of venereology. The average age of these patients was 24 years and all had genital lesions. Twenty of these patients had other forms of sexually transmitted disease. The authors claim that the need today is to re-classify molluscum contagiosum as a sexually transmissible disease.

Further work in this condition will no doubt revolve around improved handling of the virus in the laboratory and development of serological methods of diagnosis.

REFERENCES

AYRES, S. JR. and MIHAW, R. (1964). *Arch. Derm., Chicago*, **89**, 465.
BLATTNER, R. J. (1967). *J. Pediat.*, **70**, 997.
COBBOLD, R. J. C. and MACDONALD, A. (1970). *Practitioner*, **204**, 416.
JACOBS, P. H. (1970). *Aerospace Med.*, **41**, 1196.
LYNCH, P. J. and MINKIN, W. (1968). *Arch. Derm., Chicago*, **98**, 141.
OVERFIELD, J. M. and BRODY, J. A. (1966). *J. Pediat.*, **69**, 640.

37 Genital Warts

R. S. Morton

Condylomata accuminata are caused by a papilloma virus. There is no morphological difference between the virus of ordinary skin warts and that causing genital warts. There may be antigenic differences. Warmth and moisture appear to encourage the growth of genital warts. Rapid development is associated with conditions, for example, trichomoniasis and thrush, pregnancy and a long prepuce. In cases of peri-anal spread a thorough search for the gonococcus is generally indicated. The recent cult in both sexes of wearing tight, supporting, stretch nylon, if persisted with, does not accelerate response to treatment. The presence of genital warts should be seen as an indication to look for other forms of sexually transmissible disease. The incubation period is generally less than 3 months but may be more than twice that.

A wide variety of treatment is available. Local applications of CO_2 snow, trichloracetic acid or podophyllin 25 per cent in spirit are amongst the favoured. The tendency for podophyllin to cause severe local reaction may be countered by night and morning application of hydrocortisone lotion 1 per cent. This can be done without interference to the anti-mitotic activity of podophyllin. Curettage of various kinds may be used either under local or general anaesthetic. Circumcision and cautery is indicated in men with extensive growths. Trimming and cauterisation is frequently indicated in women.

When listing tumours of the vulva, Gardner et al (1965) listed genital warts. Theokharov (1966) of Omsk studied 428 cases over 15 years, He found that 69·5 per cent of their sexual contacts either had or developed genital warts. The longest incubation period was 8 months. The author insists that it is sound epidemiology to see all sex contacts of persons with genital warts and to keep the apparently unaffected under observation for 6 months. Writing again on the same subject Theokharov (1969) says the epidemiological and clinical evidence accumulated by him leads him to believe that genital 'condylomatosis' is probably independent of ordinary skin warts and certainly sexually transmissible. He notes that 20 per cent of affected women have concomitant vaginitis.

That the subject was beginning to demand growing attention in the late 1960s is reflected in the papers during these years. Bafverstedt (1967) reviewed past and present knowledge. Bieniak and Pietraszun (1967) described cancerous changes in a case of penile warts.

Inevitably the growing incidence of the condition has led to greater depth of study. Oriel and Almeida (1970) confirmed the work of Dunn and Ogilvie (1968). Using the electron microscope and negative staining they identified intranuclear virus particles in thin sections of genital warts in 13 of 25 patients (see Figs. 25, 26, 27). These two pieces of work put the viral origin of genital warts beyond any doubt. Ogilvie (1970) reported further on the virus. He found it prompted IgM antibodies in rabbits but not in humans. Almeida et al (1969) using complement

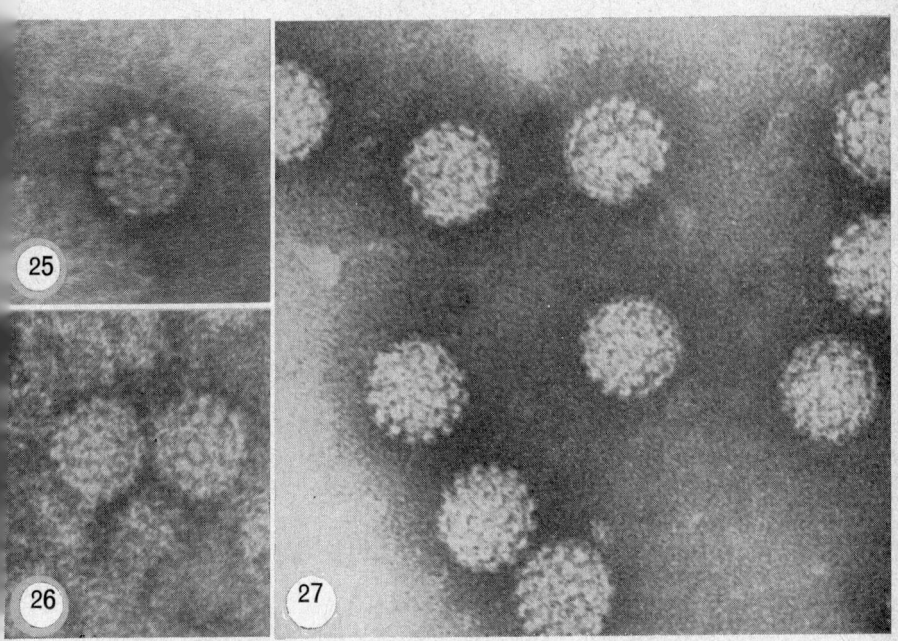

FIG. 25. Over 50 per cent of lesions examined by the negative-staining technique revealed small numbers of undoubted virus particles. One such particle, from a penile wart, is illustrated here. × 300, 000.

FIG. 26. Example of result obtained when genital warts were only very lightly disrupted. More numerous particles were present and could be easily identified against the rather greater amount of background material. × 300, 000.

FIG. 27. Group of particles from a common skin wart for comparison with Figs. 25 and 26. × 300, 000. (Figs. 25, 26, and 27. From an article by J. D. Oriel and June D. Almeida (1970). *Brit. J. vener. Dis.*, **46**, 37. Reproduced by kind permission of the authors and the Editor of the *British Journal of Venereal Diseases*.)

fixation methods found one-way cross-reactivity between genital and skin wart antibodies. These findings bear some relationship to clinical observations that genital warts are not capable of auto-inoculation on to the general skin surface. In other words the immunology studies support this 'one-way' phenomenon. (*Brit. med. J.*, 1972).

Oriel (1971a) studied 191 men and 141 women with genital warts. He concluded that the infection is sexually transmissible, that the age of onset parallels that of gonorrhoea and that the infected commonly have associated sexually transmitted diseases. Oriel noted also that ordinary skin warts are no more common in those with genital warts than in controls although skin warts of the penis could appear in patients with warts elsewhere. He noted that 64 per cent of sex contacts developed genital warts and that not infrequently the incubation was over 2 years. The author classifies genital warts and illustrates his findings in black and white.

Oriel (1971b) described 72 men and eight women with peri-anal warts. Sixty (83 per cent) of the men and five of the women admitted anal intercourse. There was, however, no conclusive evidence of sexual transmission from this study although contact tracing was admittedly limited. A retrospective study of 500 homosexual males showed anal warts to be seven times commoner than penile warts. The author considers that there are other reasons besides sexual contact which may account for the peri-anal wart findings.

Treatment was discussed by Rowe (1970). Powell et al (1970) used an autogenous vaccine while Halverstadt and Parry (1969) drew attention to intrameatal warts as a frequent source of recurrence.

Patel and Groff (1972) report the case of an 18 month old child with massive peri-anal warts. The infant's mother was known to have had condylomata accuminata during pregnancy and delivery. Treatment of the child consisted of ligation and excision, podophyllin and 5 per cent ammoniated mercury ointment.

Chamberlain et al (1972) report severe peripheral neuropathy and stillbirth in a primegravida treated for vulvar warts under general anaesthesia with 7·5 ml of 25 per cent solution of podophyllin resin in compound tincture of benzoin. Recovery took more than 3 months. Whether podophyllin should be used at all during pregnancy is questioned by some. Because of its anti-mitotic effect it should certainly not be used in the early months.

Shah and Jertz (1972) describe two women with extensive condylomata accuminata of the ano-rectum (Bashke–Lowenstein tumour). Fistulae were present and recurrence followed a variety of treatments. In spite of extensive surgery one patient died. Massive warts of the ano-rectum are not common. Another case was reported by Judge (1969). Other sites are commoner, particularly the penis. Such cases are described by Davies (1964), Powley (1964), Litvak et al (1966), Gilbert

(1966), Becker et al (1969), Evans and Dische (1969), Alfthan et al (1970) and Oriel and Whimster (1971).

The chromosomes of condylomata accuminata and other genital lesions were studied by Katayama et al (1972), and wart virus antibodies by Pyrhonen and Penttinen (1972). They found 57 per cent of 182 patients had measurable antibodies. The longer the duration and the more extensive the condition the lower the titre. Anibodies of IgG type were associated with a good chance of recovery. A micro-diffusion method was used. Complement fixation antibodies of the IgG type were domonstrable only in 12 per cent.

Recently, Rogerson (1972), has drawn attention to the increasing number of students complaining of vulvar warts. She notes the frequent association with trichomoniasis; and that recurrence of both conditions simultaneously is not uncommon. Her study is based on 31 patients.

Future work in this field will no doubt concentrate on treatment methods, both preventative and curative; better handling of the virus in the laboratory; improved differentiation of genital and skin warts by immunological studies and greater awareness of the high degree of infectivity of the disease.

REFERENCES

ALFTHAN, O., RAPOLA, J., RIMTALN, R. et al (1970). *Scand. J. Urol. Nephrol.*, **4**, 71.
ALMEIDA, J. D., ORIEL, J. D. and STANNARD, L. M. (1969). *Microbios.*, **3**, 225.
BAFVERSTEDT, B. O. (1967). *Acta derm.-venereol. Stockh.*, **47**, 376.
BECKER, F. T., WALDER, H. J. and LARSEN, D. M. (1969). *Arch. Derm.*, **100**, 184.
BIENIAK, B. and PIETRASZUN, R. (1967). *Przgel. Derm.*, **54**, 383.
Brit. med. J. (1972). **2**, 179.
CHAMBERLAIN, M. J., REYNOLDS, A. L. and YEOMAN, W. B. (1972). *Brit. med. J.*, **2**, 391.
DAVIES, S. W. (1964). *J. Bact.*, **88**, 111.
DUNN, A. E. G. and OGILVIE, M. M. (1968). *J. Ultrastruct. Res.*, **22**, 282.
EVANS, R. L. and DISCHE, F. E. (1969). *J. Obstet. Gynec. Brit. Commonw.*, **76**, 757.
GARDNER, H. L. (1965). *Clin. Obstet. Gynec.*, **8**, 938.
GILBERT, C. F. (1966). *Arch. Derm.*, **93**, 714.
HALVERSTADT, D. B. and PARRY, W. L. (1969). *J. Urol.*, **101**, 729.
JUDGE, J. R. (1969). *Arch. Path.*, **88**, 46.
KATAYAMA, K. P. and WOODRUFF, J. D. (1972). *Obstet. Gynec.*, **39**, 346.
LITVAK, A. S. et al (1966). *J. med. Soc., New Jersey*, **63**, 165.
OGILVIE, M. M. (1970). *J. Hyg., Camb.*, **68**, 479.
ORIEL, J. D. and ALMEIDA, J. D. (1970). *Brit. J. vener. Dis.*, **46**, 37.
ORIEL, J. D. (1971a). *Brit. J. vener. Dis.*, **47**, 1.
ORIEL, J. D. (1971b). *Brit. J. vener. Dis.*, **47**, 373.
ORIEL, J. D. and WHIMSTER, C. W. (1971). *Brit. J. Derm.*, **84**, 71.
PATEL, R. and GROFF, D. B. (1972). *Pediatrics*, **50**, 152.
POWELL, L. C. JR., POLLARD, M. and JINKINS, J. L. (1970). *Sth. med. J.*, **63**, 202.
POWLEY, J. M. (1964). *Brit. J. Surg.*, **51**, 76.
PYRHONEN, S. and PENTTINEN, K. (1972). *Lancet*, **2**, 1330.
ROGERSON, E. B. (1972). *Amer. J. Obstet. Gynec.*, **40**, 327.
ROWE, R. J. (1970). *Post-grad. med. J.*, **47**, 229.
SHAH, I. C. and JERTZ, R. E. (1972). *Dis. Colon. Rect.*, **15**, 207.
THEOKAROV, B. A. (1966). *Akush. Ginek.*, **42**, 41.
THEOKAROV, B. A. (1969). *Brit. J. vener. Dis.*, **45**, 334.

38 *Phthiris Pubis* Infestation

R. S. Morton

'Crab' lice are not uncommonly found from the level of the umbilicus to the knees. Chest and axillary hair may be affected on occasion. The eyebrows of babies and adults are known to be involved but rarely. Dicophane emulsion (D.D.T.) or gamma benzone hexachloride are the favoured forms of treatment.

Valasquez (1968) claimed to be the first to report *Phthiris pubis* on the eyelashes of Filipino women. The crab louse is widely believed to be almost exclusively confined to Caucasians.

Altchek (1970) writing from the U.S.A. suggested that checking for the presence of *Phthiris pubis* and gonorrhoea may well become an essential part of the routine examination in gynaecology departments. Both of these conditions have to date been seen together infrequently but often separately in such departments. Now both are common amongst young adults and the finding of one should lead to a search for the other. A high and rising index of suspicion is called for. The author emphasises that specific therapy is available for both conditions.

This was underlined in the U.K. by Fisher and Morton (1970) working in a major city V.D. department. They showed that infestation with crab lice was increasing year by year with gonorrhoea. In 1964, of 1 642 new patients 18 (1·1 per cent) were found to be infested. Increasing incidence was real and steady and amounted to 69 (3·2 per cent) of 2 110 new patients in 1968. In terms of age, sex, marital status the infested were found to match very closely the patients found with gonorrhoea. The only exception was the relative absence of coloured immigrants amongst those with pubic lice. In the 225 infested patients seen over the 5 year study period there were another 105 forms of sexually transmitted disease. D.D.T. emulsion was the only treatment used. One application well rubbed in was advised. The hair absorbs sufficient and fixes it for long enough to deal with any emerging young. No evidence of D.D.T. resistance was noted. Kinmont (1972) in a discussion on an alleged case of resistance to treatment agrees with this last point.

Wright and Pal (1965) reported the results of insecticide resistance in body lice gathered from 22 countries and made estimations of LC50 values. This work was followed up by Busvine (1967) who studied the inheritance of laboratory-induced resistance. He was able to show inheritance in hybrids. His work confirms the earlier suggestion that 5 per cent D.D.T. dust is suitable for testing for resistance.

Further observations will no doubt concern themselves with the possible emergence of strains of Phthiris pubis showing resistance to D.D.T.

REFERENCES

ALTCHEK, A. (1970). *Obstet. Gynec.*, **35**, 638.
BUSVINE, J. R. (1967). *Bull. Wld Hlth Org.*, **36**, 431.
FISHER, I. and MORTON, R. S. (1970). *Brit. J. vener. Dis.*, **46**, 326
KINMONT, P. D. C. (1972). *Practitioner*, **209**, 342.
VALASQUEZ, C. C. (1968). *J. Parasit.*, **54**, 1140.
WRIGHT, J. W. and PAL, R. (1965). *Bull Wld Hlth Org.*, **33**, 485.

39 Scabies

R. S. Morton

Introduction

The typical burrows of scabies are formed by the ovigerous female *Sarcoptes scabiei* bent on egg-laying. Burrows may exist at any of the usual sites for some weeks before the onset of symptoms. This second stage is usually associated with papules on the belly wall, the flanks, thighs and forearms. Broken burrows may surmount excoriated papules on the penis, scrotum and axillary folds. Secondary infection is usually a late manifestation.

Diagnosis is placed beyond doubt by demonstration of the mite from burrows or in scales from excoriated papules, treated with potassium hydroxide.

Scabies is a disease of social contact and infected contacts within the family, at school, at work or within long-stay hospitals between staff and patients, are to be expected. The most intimate form of social contact occurs when a bed is shared or during sexual intercourse and so, particularly amongst young people, scabies may be accompanied by other sexually transmissible diseases.

Benzyl benzoate (25 per cent) emulsion, gamma benzene hexa-chloride (1 per cent) cream or lotion and crotamiton (Eurax) as a 10 per cent cream or lotion are the favoured drugs used in treatment.

Apart from departmental reports few figures are available. In recent years the Chief Medical Officer to the Department of Health and Social Security in England has reported the number of cases in the 200 or so clinics for the sexually infested, as follows:

	1971	1972
1st Quarter	903	753
2nd Quarter	713	662
3rd Quarter	830	695
4th Quarter	816	661
	3 262	2 771

EPIDEMIOLOGICAL AND SOCIAL ASPECTS

Russell (1964) in a general review of scabies emphasised that it was a disease needing greater recognition as a 'disease of bedfellows'.

Mites are common in most animals. Such parasites are morphologically indistinguishable from the *Sarcoptes scabiei* of humans. Physiologically, however, they are distinct and cannot live for any length of time on humans. Madison (1965) reported two cases of dog scabies in humans.

Scabies has long been recognised as less common in the New World than in Europe. This appears to continue today. Epstein (1966) in the U.S.A. found only 1 per cent of his private dermatological practice patients with the disease. He blamed therapeutic resistance for recently increased incidence. At about the time of this report Grant and Keczkes (1964) in Glasgow were finding that 7 per cent of dermatological hospital outpatients had scabies.

In the mid-1960s several writers mention a rising incidence and some talk of epidemics. Shrank and Alexander (1967) working in London found an increase in scabies in their dermatological department from 0·9 per cent of new patients to 2·4 per cent in a period of 3 years. The greatest increase was in those aged 16–29 years. On the basis of this last observation and a study of past epidemics and the interval between them, Shrank and Alexander present the hypothesis of 'herd hypersensitivity'. According to this, a generation builds up 'herd immunity'. This, together with a high index of suspicion amongst doctors and early diagnosis and treatment of patients and their contacts, brings a period of control which lasts for some 15 years, before a new generation of susceptibles again suffer. Danby et al (1967) subscribe to this theory. Some 45 per cent of their scabetics were aged 10–19 years. Hellier (1966) who supports the hypothesis believes there is another potent factor in the resurgence. He believes many younger doctors have never seen scabies and fail to recognise it or its variants until the epidemic is widespread. He predicted that the U.K. trend would be repeated in the U.S.A. An editorial in the *British Medical Journal* (1967) under the title 'The Scabies Epidemic' reviews the reasons for the resurgence. The herd immunity/hypersensitivity hypothesis is accepted. Attention is also drawn to the upward trends in other sexually transmissible diseases and increasing promiscuity is suggested as a factor.

Hellier's forecast has become fact. Pace and Puress (1970) report a ten-fold increase in scabies in Ontario in a 6 months' period. They see Canada as joining the growing number of countries reporting epidemic levels of incidence. From the U.S.A., Haydon and Caplan (1971) report three associated epidemics. The originating patient in each was a mongol with Norweigan scabies. Nationwide epidemic levels are predicted. The writers, subscribing to the hypersensitivity idea, believe the incubation period, that is, to onset of symptoms should be shorter in those not previously infested, ie the younger generations.

Orkin (1971) decided it was time to take a worldwide view. He sent a questionnaire to 94 American and 120 foreign dermatologists and received 86 and 73 replies. It was generally agreed by the respondents that scabies was uncommon in the 1950s and that increases date from around 1963. There had been a progressively deteriorating situation since and in some areas and countries the disease was epidemic. This was not yet so in the U.S.A. or Canada except amongst some groups of hippies. Incidence in the U.S.A. was variously reported as 1 to 8 per cent of dermatological patients. Orkin illustrates his report with maps. He says the reasons for the worldwide resurgence of scabies are not clear. He lists the following: poverty and poor hygiene, sexual promiscuity, mis-diagnosis, migration, increased travel and tourism and loss of herd immunity. Broad agreement comes from Maleville and Heid (1972). They point out that scabies, like syphilis, is traditionally a disease with wartime peaks. The peak incidences of both infections have coincided for 400 years. They agree that presently occurring high levels in the incidence of scabies are therefore unusual. The most potent currently operating factors they see as population movement and promiscuity. These they consider as far outweighing loss of herd immunity. The emergence of hypersensitivity they see manifest in earlier onset of symptoms, more lesions than the number of mites warrant, esinophilia and post-treatment pruritis.

Jelliffe (1972) points to the part played in the spread of scabies in some areas by poor nutrition, falling resistance due to secondary infection, poor hygiene and inadequate water supplies. Richardson (1972) gives emphasis to these. He points out that in South Africa the incidence of scabies is just as high in rural as in urban areas. The common factors in both are overcrowding and poor standards of personal hygiene.

CLINICAL ASPECTS

Although the *Sarcoptes scabiei* attacks many areas of the body it never attacks the face. According to Madsen (1965) this is due to the high follicle density. It is probably as much as 16 times greater on the face than on the extremities. Follicles are seen as obstructing the passage of the mites. This theory is supported by the claim that the sites commonly attacked are those with the lowest follicle density. Madsen (1970) follows this up by observing that ovigerous mites do not burrow into the head skin of infants but do burrow into crusts and that these are worthy of microscopy, using potash in difficult cases.

Norwegian scabies is the name given to the disease when its chief manifestations are many crusted lesions and exfoliative dermatitis.

Logan et al (1966) reported such a case in which leukaemia was diagnosed a few months after successful treatment. The authors suggest that leukaemia lowers resistance to the mite. The patient was one of 50 treated during an outbreak of scabies in an old people's home. This association of leukaemia and scabies is the third in the literature.

Apart from secondary infection there are few complications of scabies. Persistent pruritic nodules were described in five patients by Berg and Krook (1967). The lesions, all on parts of the skin exposed to daylight, measured an average of 12 mm in diameter. They had been present for 9–18 months. No parasites were found in the lesions. Biopsy showed histiocytes, lymphocytes and esinophils all involved in peri-vascular cuffing. The authors offer no wholly acceptable explanation for the complication.

Hersch (1967) described acute glomerular nephritis as associated with secondarily infected scabies in non-white South Africans. The subject was looked at in two ways. Of 75 consecutive cases of acute glomerular nephritis, 44 had infected scabies, 12 had other skin infections and 19 had no skin disease. In 155 pediatric patients with acute glomerular nephritis the corresponding figures were 45, 31 and 79. As a corollary, evidence of acute glomerular nephritis was found in 8 per cent of patients with scabies and this in a department seeing more than 5 000 cases annually. The authors recommend that all patients with scabies should have their urine tested for albumen. Three further reports of the association appeared in 1972. Gordon (1972) also writing from South Africa stated that in spite of evidence of epidemics of scabies there had been no recent increased incidence of nephritis. Allen (1972) reported a case of scabies with acute nephritis from Edinburgh. Lastly, there was an outstanding study from Trinidad by Svartman et al (1972). Monthly admissions of cases of acute glomerular nephritis increased from 10 to 30 in the 7 months September 1970 to March 1971. The outbreak corresponded with a scabies epidemic. The 139 patients with nephritis showed an increasing incidence of scabies from 32 per cent at the start of the outbreak to 80 per cent in the last month. β-haemolytic streptococci were found to be present in the scabetics and in the members of their families. Secondarily infected scabies with β-haemolytic streptococci was found in local dogs.

LABORATORY ASPECTS

Alexander et al (1967) described atypical cases of scabies. He pointed out that in the absence of burrows it is sometimes useful to examine potash scrapings from scaly papules. Lyell (1967) in an excellent review of the subject says a high index of suspicion about scabies is needed in all cases of persistent generalised itch. Demonstration of the *Sarcoptes scabiei* puts the diagnosis beyond doubt.

TREATMENT ASPECTS

Erskine (1967) in reviewing treatment methods emphasises strict attention to detail in the routine to be followed. Epidemiological treatment of contacts, including the asymptomatic is seen as essential. Ramsay (1969) noted that in cases of reinfection, symptoms appear earlier. This he sees as in keeping with the hypersensitivity theory. Alexander (1969) agrees with this and says the hypersensitivity state persists for at least 6 months. He reviews scabies in children and states, 'Neglect of detail more than any other factor contributes to the perpetuation of scabies'.

Maleville and Heid (1972) recommend epidemiological treatment with benzyl benzoate of all domestic and sexual contacts. This view is based on their belief that population movement and promiscuity are the most potent factors at work in promoting the present problems.

James (1972) writing from Bengal, where the numbers presently infected are enormous, and 10 per cent are secondarily infected, treated all patients with one application of 1 per cent gamma benzene hexachloride. James was able to see 15 per cent of his patients for follow-up examination. All were cured. Long-term follow-up, however, revealed many late recurrences due to reinfections by untreated family contacts.

MacMillan (1972) warned against the use of steroids in scabies. The point had previously been made in a *British Medical Journal* editorial (1967) which pointed out that steroids may well suppress symptoms and delay treatment.

Alexander (1968) gave a brief review of the history of scabies.

Coda

Implementation of present knowledge could control scabies at some low irreducible minimum. Nevertheless epidemics are common and often become advanced before action is taken. Action is often sadly inadequate. Campaigns of eradication frequently disappear before the disease does. This area calls for study with a view to improved public and professional education not least about the value of the employment of permanent contact-tracers. Much demographic data associated with recent outbreaks calls for exploration. Immunological studies are also needed.

REFERENCES

ALEXANDER, J. O. (1967). *Brit. med. J.*, **2**, 766.
ALEXANDER, J. O. (1968). *Practitioner*, **200**, 632.
ALEXANDER, J. O. (1969). *Clin. Pediat.*, **8**, 73.
ALLEN, B. R. (1972). *Lancet*, **1**, 434.
BERG, T. and KROOK, G. (1967). *Acta derm.-venereal., Stockh.*, **47**, 20.

Brit. med. J. (1967). **2**, 193.

DANBY, P. R., CHURCH, R. E. and SNEDDON, I. B. (1967). *Brit. med. J.*, **1**, 496.

EPSTEIN, E. (1966). *Arch. Derm.*, **93**, 60.

ERSKINE, D. (1967). *Lancet*, **1**, 54.

GORDON, W. (1972). *Lancet*, **1**, 794.

GRANT, P. W. and KECZKES, K. (1964). *Arch. Derm.*, **89**, 239.

HAYDON, J. R. and CAPLAN, R. M. (1971). *Arch. Dermat.*, **103**, 168.

HELLIER, F. F. (1966). *Arch. Derm.*, **93**, 634.

HERSCH, C. (1967). *S. Afr. med. J.*, **2**, 766.

JAMES, B. H. (1972). *Brit. med. J.*, **1**, 178.

JELLIFFE, D. B. (1972). *Lancet*, **2**, 49.

LYELL, A. (1967). *Brit. med. J.*, **2**, 223.

LOGAN, J. C., GRANT, P. W. and KECZKES, K. (1966). *Brit. J. Derm.*, **79**, 303.

MACMILLAN, A. L. (1972). *Brit. J. Derm.*, **87**, 496.

MADISON, J. F. (1965). *J. Maine med. Ass.*, **56**, 131.

MADSEN, A. (1965). *Acta derm.-venereol., Stockh.*, **45**, 167.

MADSEN, A. (1970). *Acta derm.-venereol., Stockh.*, **50**, 391.

MALEVILLE, J. and HEID, E. (1972). *Munch. med. Wschr.*, **1**, 27.

ORKIN, M. (1971). *J. Amer. med. Ass.*, **217**, 593.

PACE, W. B. and PURESS, J. (1970). *Canad. med. Ass. J.*, **104**, 719.

RAMSAY, C. (1969). *Postgrad. med. J.*, **45**, 258.

RICHARDSON, B. D. (1972). *Lancet.*, **1**, 839.

RUSSELL, B. (1964). *Practitioner*, **192**, 621.

SHRANK, A. B. and ALEXANDER, S. L. (1967). *Brit. med. J.*, **1**, 669.

SVARTMAN, M. and POTTER, E. V. (1972). *Lancet*, **1**, 249.

40 Viral Hepatitis B

J. R. W. Harris

For many years serum hepatitis was believed to be transferred solely by parenteral means. The discovery of Australia antigen (HBAg) (Blumberg et al, 1965) and its association with viral hepatitis type B (Prince, 1968); Giles et al, 1969), has meant that the occurrence of sporadic cases of this disease, with no history of parenteral exposure, were observed. The nomenclature of viral hepatitis has had to be altered on the basis of these observations and the name 'serum hepatitis' has now been abandoned. Krugman et al (1967) and Giles et al (1969) indicated the importance of oral transmission while Almeida et al (1971) has implicated airborne transmission of HBAg hepatitis. Blumberg and his co-workers in 1968 felt that homosexual practice might well be responsible for the predominance of males among those affected by type B hepatitis. Vahrman (1970) endorsed this hypothesis. Prince et al (1970) found that 55 per cent of adult patients with hepatitis, who were HBAg positive, gave no history of parenteral exposure. Fulford et al (1973) commented in their publication that in the London area most patients were young adults and two-thirds were men. There were very few cases in children. Such a distribution would not be incompatible with the hypothesis that hepatitis type B is commonly a sexually transmitted disease. Hersh et al (1972), while being unable to establish the mechanism of transmission, presented evidence that hepatitis type B may spread between sexual partners by non-parenteral routes.

In 1973 several studies from London were published investigating the relationship between sexual practice and infection with hepatitis antigen (HBAg). Fulford et al (1973) described a retrospective study in which serum samples from 974 patients attending a clinic for sexually transmitted diseases were tested for HBAg and its antibody HBAb. Information from the clinical notes were then correlated with these results. They found that a high frequency of Australia antigen and its antibody occurred among these patients. This was established by comparison with the general population, represented by blood donors attending the North London Blood Transfusion Centre for the first time. The analysis of the case reports indicated that the patients belonged to two distinct groups. The antigen was found predominantly in non-promiscuous men of Mediterranean origin, who were thought to be chronic carriers. The antibody was commonly found among male homosexual and promiscuous patients of British origin. A highly significant correlation was found for the HBAb group, with a history of both syphilis and gonorrhoea. The HBAb group also had a significant distribution for sexual orientation and contact history. The immuno-diffusion test which was used for the detection of HBAb in this study is relatively insensitive compared with the haemagglutination test (Vyas and Schulman 1970). Because of this the authors feel that it will only detect antibody in rather less than a quarter of those who can be shown to have antibody by the haemagglutination test. Therefore if the more sensitive test had been used it is probable that over 80 per cent of the patients who admitted homosexual contact would have been HBAb positive.

In the discussion on the possible mechanisms of transmission no evidence was found to indict lice or scabies mites, and the frequency of drug abuse among patients attending the clinic was so low that paren-teral transmission was deemed to have little influence on the results.

Jefferies et al (1973) from St. Mary's Hospital, London, examined serological specimens for the presence of HBAg from 1 650 patients attending the unit of sexually transmitted diseases. The incidence was found to be more than 10 times the rate noted in blood donor popula-tion. Again the great majority of patients who were HBAg positive were either male homosexuals or non-European heterosexuals. 3·8 per cent of all male homsexuals studied had HBAg on testing by the techniques of immunoelectro-osmophoresis (Pesendorfer et al 1970) and gel diffusion. The authors speculate that transmission may well occur through the skin and mucous membrane lesions which are commonly found as a result of homosexual practice. They are also of the opinion that serious consideration must be given to the possibility of oral spread of HBAg by blood and serous exudates (Krugman and Giles, 1970).

The results of a survey of 67 patients admitted to two London hospitals with acute type B hepatitis were described by Heathcote and Sherlock (1973). The aim of the survey was to establish the source of infection with the hepatitis-B antigen HBAg. After the diagnosis of hepatitis had been made each patient was interviewed to establish whether they had been exposed to possible parenteral infection during the previous 6 months. Thus they were questioned regarding trans-fusions, injections with non-disposable or shared needles and tattoos. Possible contact with a jaundiced person either directly or by working in a hospital during the previous 6 months was also ascertained. Discreet inquiries were then made into the patient's sexual activities.

Whenever possible the household and other close social contacts of the patient were traced and they were asked the same questions.

As a result of the epidemiological study 16 patients were assumed to have been infected by the parenteral route. A further 13 (two were male homosexuals) were judged to have been infected as a result of sexual contact with individuals who were either HBAg positive or were jaundiced. Twelve patients (four were male homosexuals) had non-sexual contact with individuals who were either jaundiced or HBAg positive. Two further patients had sexual contact with a person from West Africa and Greece where the incidence of HBAg positivity is higher than in the United Kingdom. No definite source of infection was identified in the remaining 24 patients but nine of them were either homosexual or bisexual.

Of the whole group, sexual or domestic contact was the definite or most likely source of infection in 27 patients (40 per cent). Fifteen of the 43 males in the survey admitted homosexual or bisexual orientation, *ie* 34·9 per cent.

Vahrman (1973) reviewed the patients with viral hepatitis whom he had seen from January 1970 until June 1971. He observed that 72 of the 110 patients (65 per cent) were male and that 45 per cent of these were HBAg positive. Of the 32 male patients who were HBAg positive 20 were homosexual. He found the correlation between homosexuality and the recognition of viral hepatitis to be highly significant.

On the basis of the studies above investigating the relationship between sexual practice and infection with the hepatitis B virus, it would appear that the most important factor in the spread of active type B hepatitis in an urban cosmopolitan community is contact with jaundiced or HBAg carriers. The contact needs to be close. There is a growing body of evidence that transmission is most likely to occur among sexual partners. Male patients with homosexual orientation are particularly prone to the disease. In certain contexts hepatitis B virus behaves as a sexually transmitted disease.

REFERENCES

ALMEIDA, J. D., CHISHOLM, G. D., KULATILAKE, A. E., MACGREGOR, A. B., MACKAY, D. H., O'DONOGHUE, E. P. N., SHACKMAN, R. and WATERSON, A. P. (1971). *Lancet*, ii, 849.

BLUMBERG, B. S., ALTER, H. J. and VISNICH, S. (1965). *J. Amer. med. Ass.*, **191**, 541.

BLUMBERG, B. S., SUTNICK, A. I. and LONDON, W. T. (1968). *Bull. N.Y. Acad. Med.*, **44**, 1566.

FULFORD, K. W. M., DANE, D. S., CATTERALL, R. D., WOOF, R. and DENNING, J.V. (1973). *Lancet*, i, 1470.

GILES, J., McCOLLUM, R. W., BERNDSTON, L. W. and KRUGMAN, S. (1969). *New Engl. J. Med.*, **281**, 119.

HEATHCOTE, J. and SHERLOCK, S. (1973). *Lancet*, i, 1468.

HERSH, T., MELNICK, J. L., GOYAL, R. K. and HOLLINGER, F. B. (1972). *New Engl. J. Med.*, **285**, 1363.

JEFFERIES, D. J., JAMES, W. H., JEFFERISS, F. J. G., MACLEOD, K. G. and WILLCOX, R. R. (1973). *Brit. med. J.*, ii, 455.

KRUGMAN, S., GILES, J. and HAMMOND, J. (1967). *J. Amer. med. Ass.*, **200**, 365.

KRUGMAN, S. and GILES, J. P. (1970). *J. Amer. med. Ass.*, **212**, 1019.

PESENDORFER, F., KRASSNITZKY, O. and WEWALKA, F. (1970). *Klin. W.schr*, **48**, 58.

PRINCE, A. M. (1968). *Proc. natn. Acad. Sci. U.S.A.*, **60**, 814.

PRINCE, A. M., HARGROVE, R. L., SZMUNESS, W., CHERUBIN, C. E., FONTANA, V. J. and JEFFRIES, G. H. (1970). *New Engl. J. Med.*, **282**, 987.

VAHRMAN, J. (1970). *Lancet*, ii, 774.

VAHRMAN, J. (1973). *Lancet*, ii, 157.

VYAS, G. N. and SCHULMAN, N. R. (1970). *Science, N.Y.*, **170**, 332.

41 *Corynebacterium Vaginale* Infection

J. R. W. Harris

Leopold in 1953 reported 'a heretofore undescribed organism isolated from the genito-urinary system'. He believed this organism was closely related to the Haemophilus species. The bacillus had been recovered from the urethras of men with prostatitis (with or without urethritis), and from the cervices of women with clinical evidence of cervicitis. He did not find any relationship between the presence of the organism and vaginitis or excessive vaginal discharge. Lutz and Wurch in 1954 observed small Gram-negative bacilli in vaginal discharge and in 1956, Lutz, Grotten and Wurch named the organism *Haemophilus vaginalis hemolyticus*. At the same time an independent clinical and laboratory study, with essentially the same findings, had been published by Gardner and Dukes (1955). They called the agent *Haemophilus vaginalis*.

In their study in 1955 Gardner and Dukes cultured the organism on blood agar with accessory growth factors. They found it to be a minute, rod-shaped, Gram-negative bacillus which was non-motile, non-encapsulated and did not form endospores. However, Zinnerman and Turner (1963) reported that the organism was Gram-positive when grown on impissated serum slopes; they recommended classification as *Corynebacterium vaginale*. The growth requirements were determined by Dunkelberg and McVeigh (1969). There is no necessity for blood, serum, hemin, DNA or other definable co-enzyme-like substances. The bacillus does have considerable vitamin B and nucleic acid base requirements.

Since the discovery of *C. vaginale* there has been controversy regarding its pathogenicity and the mode of transmission. Döll (1958) doubted that the organism had any pathogenicity at all, as he was unable to grow it either from patients with vaginitis or from the control group. Heltai and Taleghany (1959) and Lapage (1961) were able to demonstrate the bacillus in association with vaginitis but unable to prove any pathogenic role. Frampton and Lee (1964) found no statistical difference in the recovery rates of *C. vaginale* from patients with or without vaginitis.

Gardner and Dukes (1955) inoculated disease-free vaginas with material from the vaginas of patients who exhibited what they regarded as *C. vaginale* infection. The inoculated patients were considered to have vaginal pH levels within normal limits. The donor material yielded five cultures of *C. vaginale*. Of the 15 normal patients inoculated 11 had the classical disease within 7 to 14 days. *C. vaginale* was the predominant bacterium in the vaginal material from all 11. Criswell et al (1969) inoculated nine volunteers intravaginally with 2×10^{10} organisms of *C. vaginale* type strain 594 which had been cultured for 12 hours. Vaginitis developed in five subjects. They inoculated 20 other volunteers with 24-hour-old cultures of several *C. vaginale* strains and only two of the women developed vaginitis. Thus it would appear that the organism has a low degree of virulence.

Many workers corroborated the reports by Gardner and Dukes in 1955; Ray and Maughan (1956), Rico (1959), Bergman et al (1961) and Lewis et al (1971) all found significant differences in the incidence of *C. vaginale* cultures from patients with vaginitis and symptomatic vaginal discharge compared with control groups. The bulk of evidence would apparently indicate that *C. vaginalis* has some degree of pathogenicity and a low degree of virulence in the vagina.

There have been reports of the association of the organism with non-gonococcal urethritis. Leopold (1953) isolated the organism from patients showing signs of 'moderate prostatitis'. Dunkelberg and Woolvin (1963) found *C. vaginale* to be the predominant bacterial organism in the urethral discharges of five men with non-gonococcal urethritis. Mehta et al (1967) believed that some of the patients they saw had non-gonococcal urethritis due to *C. vaginale*. Furness et al (1971) reported that 47 per cent of the patients with non-gonococcal urethritis, when examined, had Corynebacterium species. This followed the earlier work of Furness and Csonka (1966) on isolation of Corynebacterium species from patients with non-gonococcal urethritis. Despite these isolated reports the consensus of opinion suggests that *C. vaginale* is not a significant aetiological factor in non-gonococcal urethritis. This is not surprising since Edmunds (1962) recognised that the main source of energy for the bacterium is the glycogen of the vaginal and urethral epithelium. The glycogen content of male urethral epithelium is much less than that of vaginal epithelium, as demonstrated by staining fixed smears.

The discoverer of the bacillus, Leopold (1953), found it especially significant that husbands of infected wives showed a high incidence of positive urines on culture. De la Fuente et al (1960) found *C. vaginale* in the urethras of 37 of 44 men whose wives had *C. vaginale* vaginitis. Gardner and Dukes (1959) found that *C. vaginale* was the predominant organism in the urethra of 91 of 101 men whose wives had vaginitis due to the bacillus. Teokharov (1967) found *C. vaginale* in the urethras of males who were sexual contacts of patients with *C. vaginale*.

While many workers would be hesitant to accept '*H. vaginalis* transmission occurs in almost all cases via sexual intercourse' (Gardner and Kaufman, 1969), most would agree with Dunkelberg et al (1970a) that '*C. vaginale* seems to qualify as a sexually transmitted disorder'.

The reported incidence of this organism among women varies from 6–52 per cent. Factors thought to be directly responsible for variations in incidence are racial composition, socio-economic status, sexual habits and criteria for identification of the bacillus. In Scandanavia, Renkonen et al (1970) found an incidence of 30·5 per cent. In the U.S.A. Dunkelberg et al (1962) found a prevalence of 24·4 per cent in asymptomatic married Negro women and 9·5 per cent in asymptomatic married white women. Desai et al (1966), from India, studied 183 women attending an obstetric and gynaecological clinic and found 14·2 per cent had *C. vaginale*. In the United Kingdom, Frampton and Lee (1964) found 21 per cent of asymptomatic females had *C. vaginale*. In Vietnam, Dunkelberg and Scherman (1969) found an incidence of 7 per cent in married Vietnamese women. The most probable explanation for the enormous variation in incidence of infection with this organism is the diverse diagnostic criteria used. Many workers used blood agars which precluded microscopic examination of colonial morphology by transmitted light. The results in some series were based on the finding of 'clue cells' alone, while others diagnosed on the presence of 'clue cells' and cultivation of Gram-negative and Gram-variable bacilli on blood agar. Certain workers utilised microscopic examination in transmitted light for colony morphology and others depended on sugar fermentation reactions. It is obvious that such series and incidences are not suitable for comparison.

Perhaps the most reliable information on the incidence of *C. vaginale* is gained from the two groups who have most experience with the organism. Dunkelberg et al (1970a), while investigating 200 females attending the Fulton County Health Department in Atlanta, Georgia, found 62 had *C. vaginale* and the *Trichomonas vaginalis* : *C. vaginale* ratio was 113 : 62. Gardner and Kaufman (1969) found the *T. vaginalis* : *C. vaginale* ratio in private practice in Houston, Texas, was 4 : 1.

Dunkelberg et al (1970a) found that infection with *C. vaginale* was less common than infection with either gonorrhoea or trichomonas species. They postulated that this was the result of the low virulence of the corynebacterium and prior alteration in the vaginal pH. Women who maintain a normal vaginal pH are unlikely to become hosts of *C. vaginale* unless they are infected when the vagina is more alkaline. This occurs during menstruation or prior infection with trichomonads. This conjecture is based on the work reported by Gardner and Dukes (1959) which showed that the pH of the vagina infected with *C. vaginale* was between 5·0 and 5·5.

C. vaginale is the most benign of the common infections of the vagina. Despite the paucity of symptoms it is a well-defined vaginitis (Lewis et al, 1971). The majority of patients do not have any complaints; others are conscious of symptoms from the onset of the infection. The most common symptom is leucorrhoea or excessive discharge. Less than 25 per cent of patients with *C. vaginale* vaginitis mention this problem (Gardner and Kaufman, 1969). Malodour is frequently the most distressing symptom and pruritis and burning occurs in only a minority. The incidence of vaginitis varies in reported series from 13 per cent (Gardner and Dukes, 1959) to 32 per cent (Gardner and Dukes, 1955).

Certain workers believe that leucorrhoea is the most common sign of the disease. Brewer et al (1957) described the discharge as white or grey in almost 90 per cent of cases. Occasionally the discharge is frothy. Gross changes in the vulva and vagina are observed in less than 10 per cent of patients with the infection (Ray and Maughan, 1956). The odour of the discharge is characteristic according to Teokharov (1969).

While *C. vaginale* infection is usually benign there have been reports of serious illness, and death from disseminated infection with this organism. Edmunds (1959) indicts it as a cause of puerperal pyrexia. Rotherham and Schick (1969) believe that *C. vaginale* is frequently the agent responsible for septic abortions. Carney (1973) describes two mothers with septic abortions who were found to have *C. vaginale* septicaemia. Platt (1971) presents two cases and reviews a further seven of maternal/neonatal infection. As a result of such infections, in his series, there was a stillbirth, three neonatal deaths and two septic abortions. Several of the reported infants who survived had discharging scalp lesions from which *C. vaginale* was cultured. Hence in certain circumstances the organism is a pathogen.

Microscopic examination of Gram-stained preparations of vaginal exudate containing *C. vaginale* show a profusion of small Gram-negative or Gram-variable rods associated with epithelial cells. Unless there is some other clinical abnormality or infective agent present there is noticeable absence of pus cells. In wet mounts, many vaginal specimens display the so called 'clue cells' (Gardner and Dukes, 1955); these are squamous epithelial cells whose surfaces are covered by great numbers of the bacilli. The epithelial cells described present a distinctly granular appearance when viewed on wet film. There is considerable controversy about the diagnostic reliability of these 'clue cells' (Davidson and Layton, 1968), and even those who believe that they are a valuable clinical indicator (Dunkelberg and McVeigh, 1969) are not prepared to diagnose solely on their presence.

The organism was originally cultured on blood agar and classified as *Haemophilus vaginalis* (Leopold, 1953; Gardner and Dukes, 1955). True Haemophilus species require hemin (x factor), nicotinamide, adenine, dinucleotide (v factor) or other definable co-enzymes. This organism was successfully cultured in a medium containing only carbohydrates, nucleic acid bases, salts, vitamins, casein hydrolysate and trace metals, hence it cannot be Haemophilus species. While cultivation does not require x or v factors, the organism needs extensive vitamin B and purine-pyrimidine which can be obtained from proteose-peptone. Proteose Peptone No. 3 (Difco) is a satisfactory medium developed for the organism containing the nitrogen, vitamin and nucleic acid base requirements. Thus *C. vaginale* species can be isolated (Dunkelberg and McVeigh, 1969).

A suitable transport medium is Difco Porteose Peptone No. 3, 1·5 per cent in distilled water. The broth pH is maintained at 6·8. The isolation medium is Peptone-starch-dextrose (P.S.D) medium developed by Dunkelberg and McVeigh in 1969. The maintenance medium is the same as the isolation medium except that a lower concentration of agar is used. The fermentation media contain bromocresol purple as an indicator in the absence of buffers (Dunkelberg et al, 1970b).

The isolation medium plates are incubated for 48 hours at 35–37°C in candle extinction jars. After incubation the colonies are examined using a stereoscopic microscope with a total magnification of $40 \times$ and a substage light source. Suspect *C. vaginale* colonies are transferred to fresh PSD agar plates and re-incubated for 48 hours. The plates are then examined for colonial and cellular morphology. Reaction to H_2O_2, catalase reaction and sugar fermentation tests substantiate the diagnosis (Dunkelberg et al, 1970a). All *C. vaginale* isolates display a large zone of inhibition on PSD agar plates centrally spotted with 3 per cent H_2O_2 (Zinnermann and Turner, 1963).

Redmond and Kotcher (1963) reported the presence of a specific common antigen in *C. vaginale* which indicates that sero-identification might be feasible but no reliable serological test has appeared. Immuno-fluorescent diagnostic techniques have been applied to *C. vaginale* by Redmond and Kotcher (1963) but have not come into general use. McFadyen and Eykyn (1968) utilised cultures of aseptically aspirated urine to diagnose the presence of *C. vaginale*.

Treatment

In the experience of Davidson and Layton (1968) and Gardner and Kaufman (1969) the organism is insensitive to sulphonamides both *in vivo* and *in vitro*. Vaginal pessaries containing chloramphenicol were used by Davidson and Layton (1968) with success. The disadvantage of this treatment was the overgrowth of Candida which almost invariably followed the removal of Corynebacterium. Gardner (1973) recommends oxytetracycline vaginal pessaries and advised that the patient should be carefully observed for the onset of vulvovaginal candidiasis. Other workers have found oral oxytetracyclines effective. Gardner and

Kaufman (1969) believe that male sexual contacts should be treated at the same time since more than 90 per cent of them are infected. They prescribe oral ampicillin or tetracycline. Teokharov (1967) advocates urethral irrigations with a solution of mercury oxycyanide (1 : 6 000).

REFERENCES

BERGMAN, S., LUNDGREN, K. M. and LUNDSTROM, P. (1965). *Acta obstet. gynec. scand.*, **44**, 8.

CARNEY. F. E. (1973). *Obstet. Gynec.* **41**, 78.

CRISWELL, B. S., LADWIG, C. L., GARDNER, H. L. and DUKES, C. D. (1969). *Obstet. Gynec.*, **33**, 195.

DAVIDSON, A. J. L. and LAYTON, K. B. (1968). *Med. J. Aust.*, i, 757.

DESAI, Z. D., VAISHNAV, V. P. and ANKLESHWARIA, S. B. (1966). *J. Postgrad. Med., Bombay*, **12**, 91.

DÖLL, W. (1958). *Zentbl. Bakt.*, **171**, 372.

DUNKELBERG, W. E. and MCVEIGH, I. (1969). *Antonie van Leeuwenhock J. Microbiol. Serol.*, **35**, 129.

DUNKELBERG, W. E. and WOOLVIN, S. C. (1963). *Milit. Med.*, **128**, 1098.

DUNKELBERG, W. E., SKAGGS, R., KELLOG, D. S. and DOMESCIK, G. K. (1970a). *Brit. J. vener. Dis.*, **46**, 187.

DUNKELBERG, W. E., HEFNER, J. D., PATOW, W. E., WYMAN, F. J. and ORUP, H. I. (1962). *Obstet. Gynec.*, **20**, 629.

DUNKELBERG, W. E. and SCHERMAN, B. M. (1969). U.S. Medical Research Team (WRAIR) Vietnam: Annual Progress Report (Washington).

DUNKELBERG, W. E., SKAGGS, R. and KELLOGG, D. S. (1970b). *J. appl. Microbiol.*, **19**, 47.

EDMUNDS, P. N. (1962). *J. Path. Bact.*, **79**, 273.

EDMUNDS, P. N. (1959). *J. Obstet. Gynaec. Brit. Commonw.*, **66**, 917.

FUENTE, F. DE LA and SALCEDO, J. (1960). *Rev. Esp. Obstet. Gynec.*, **19**, 22.

FURNESS, G., KAMAT, M. H., KAMINSKI, Z. and SEEBODE, J. J. (1971). *J. Urol.*, **106**, 557.

FURNESS, G. and CSONKA, G. W. (1966). *Brit. J. vener. Dis.*, **42**, 185.

FRAMPTON, J. and LEE, Y. (1964). *J. Obstet. Gynaec. Brit. Commonw.*, **71**, 436.

GARDNER, H. L. and DUKES, C. D. (1955). *Amer. J. Obstet. Gynec.*, **69**, 962.

GARDNER, H. L. and DUKES, C. D. (1959). *Ann. N.Y. Acad. Sci.*, **83**, 280.

GARDNER, H. L. and KAUFAMN, R. H. (1969). In: *Benign Diseases of the Vulva and Vagina*, 1st ed., p. 191. C. V. Mosby, St. Louis.

GARDNER, H. L. (1973). Personal communication.

HELTAI, A. and TALEGHANY, P. (1959). *Amer. J. Obstet. Gynec.*, **77**, 144.

LAPAGE, S. P. (1961). *Acta path. microbiol. scand.*, **52**, 34.

LEOPOLD, S. (1953). *U.S. Armed Forces med. J.*, **4**, 263.

LEWIS, J. F., O'BRIEN, S. M., URAL, U. M. and BURKE, T. (1971). *Amer. J. clin. Path.*, **56**, 580.

LUTZ, A. and WURCH, T. (1954). *Bull. Féd. Soc. Gynec. Obstet. franç.*, **6**, 115.

LUTZ, A., WURCH, T. and GROTTEN, O. (1956). *Gynec. Obstet.*, **55**, 75.

MCFADYEN, I. R. and EYKYN, S. G. (1968). *Lancet*, i, 1112.

MEHTA, U. S., RANA, C. S. and VAISHMAN, V. P. (1967). *Indian J. Path. Bact.*, **10**, 170.

PLATT, M. S. (1971). *Clin. Ped.*, **10**, 513.

RAY, J. L. and MAUGHAN, G. M. (1956). *Western J. Surg.*, **64**, 581.

REDMOND, D. L. and KOTCHER, E. (1963). *J. gen. Microbiol.*, **33**, 77.

RENKONEN, O. V., WIDHOLM, O. and VARTIAINEN, E. (1970). *Acta obstet. gynec. scand.*, **49**, Suppl. 2, 3.

RICO, R. J. (1959). *Bol. Soc. Ginec. Espan.*, **9**, 17.

ROTHERHAM, E. B. and SCHICK, S. F. (1969). *Amer. J. Med.*, **46**, 80.

TEOKHAROV, B. A. (1967). *Vestn. Derm. Vener.*, **41**, 63.

TEOKHAROV, B. A. (1969). *Brit. J. vener. Dis.*, **45**, 334.

ZINNERMANN, K. and TURNER, G. C. (1963). *J. Path. Bact.*, **85**, 213.

42 Cytomegalovirus Infection

J. R. W. Harris

While the characteristic cytomegalic cells found in affected tissues have been recognised for many years, the virus itself was not isolated until 1956. Since then its epidemiology and pathogenesis have been widely studied.

As cytomegalovirus is a member of the Herpes virus group, it causes persistent latent infection. This has hampered epidemiological studies for some time. The advent of fluorescent antibody techniques utilising C.M.V. antibody IgM has improved the situation (Hanshaw et al, 1968).

The methods of spread of C.M.V. infection are still poorly understood (Stern 1972). In patients with active infection virus is excreted into the throat and urine, on to the cervix in women and in the pregnant female even in milk (Diosi et al, 1967; Alexander, 1967). The virus has a well-recognised lability outside the body. Infection is widespread but occurs predominantly in infancy and early adult life. There appears to be distinct differences in the distribution of the virus between populations in developed and developing countries. In London 10 per cent of infants have acquired C.M.V. complement-fixing antibodies by 2 years of age (Stern and Elek, 1965). There is then a slow rise in the incidence of antibodies with age, so that 20 per cent of the 15-year-old population have antibodies. After 15 years of age there is again a rapid increase in antibody incidence to a maximum of 50–60 per cent by 25–30 years of age. However, the prevalence of infection is higher among those living in crowded and unhygienic conditions. Thus in Puerto Rico, 25–35 per cent of children have antibodies as have 70–80 per cent of adults (Mendez-Cashion et al, 1963); while in Tanzania women have 100 per cent sero-conversion rate by the time they reach child-bearing age (Kresh et al, 1971).

From the surveys above one could postulate that in children and indeed in adults spread can occur by the urine–hands–oral route. This hypothesis would explain the increased incidence of infection among individuals living in unhygienic overcrowded conditions (Mendez-

Cashion et al, 1963). It could also explain the disparity between the 50–80 per cent rate of infection among children in boarding schools and orphanages, compared with 15–20 per cent in children of the same age attending day schools in this country (Stern and Elek, 1965).

Spread of C.M.V. infection can also be caused by blood transfusion (Kaariainen et al, 1966). The virus can be isolated from the white blood cells of neonates with cytomegalic inclusion disease and adults with cytomegalovirus mononucleosis (Stulberg et al, 1966; Harnden et al, 1967). However, spread of infection by parenteral routes can only explain a small fraction of the total number of adult primary infection in a developed country.

Stern (1972) suggested that C.M.V. is essentially a 'kissing disease', as virus is excreted into the throat and efficient cross-infection requires close contact. The prevalence of infection in adolescents and young adults suggests some such method of transmission (Harris, 1973). Montgomery et al (1972), during their discussion of the probable epidemiology of this virus, suggested that it might be acquired and transmitted during sexual intercourse. As the virus is excreted in the urine and on to the cervix this appeared a possibility. However, the virus had not been isolated from the male genital tract and this point was emphasised by Stern et al (1972) as an argument against transmission in this manner. Then Lang and Kummer (1972) from Duke University, N. Carolina, reported that in a young adult male convalescing from cytomegalovirus mononucleosis, C.M.V. was replicating in his uro-genital tract. A high titre of this virus persisted in the semen of the asymptomatic host for at least 11 weeks. They maintained that the persistence of high titres of C.M.V. for weeks in this patient's semen, in the presence of circulating antibody, indicated that in the male reproductive tract the virus seems to evade humoral defences and can remain a protracted hazard.

The greater frequency of congenital C.M.V. infection in babies of young unmarried mothers when compared with the incidence in babies of married women is evidence for the importance of sexual contact (Walker and Tobin, 1970; Starr et al, 1970); the former are likely to have a higher promiscuity index than married women and would thus be exposed to a greater risk of infection. The work of Dr. Helene Mair in Leicester was quoted by Tobin (1973) during a discussion on the isolation of C.M.V. from the cervix in different groups of women. Mair found that 3·2 per cent of patients attending a V.D. clinic had C.M.V. on the cervix. This was identical to the figure of 3·2 per cent among patients at a remand home in Manchester, compared with 0·7 per cent of patients attending antenatal clinics in Manchester.

Frequently the acquired disease in young adults is asymptomatic. When a clinical syndrome does occur it is most commonly atypical glandular fever. The patient complains of malaise and pharangitis, and is found to have generalised lymphadenopathy with associated spleno-megaly. The peripheral blood picture shows the presence of atypical mononuclear cells and the Paul Bunnell is negative (Stern, 1972). C.M.V. infection in adults was also found by Walker and Tobin (1970) to be associated with hepatitis and polyneuritis on occasions. Another factor which has caused confusion is the ability of the latent C.M.V. to become reactivated. There is little evidence that this occurs the general population (Stern, 1972) but this undoubtably occurs in pregnancy. Approximately half of those women excreting C.M.V. during pregnancy already have antibody before the onset of pregnancy and show no significant rise in titre subsequently (Stern, 1971).

In a recent study in a department for the treatment of sexually transmitted diseases (Harris et al, 1974), 220 consecutive patients were screened, using the C.M.V. complement fixation test, for evidence of cytomegalovirus infection. A total of 9·1 per cent of the patients had elevated titre levels. Eight of these patients were in three sexual 'kindreds'. Thirteen of the 20 patients had paired sera estimations and in seven there was some evidence of recent infection. Not all the contacts of patients with the infection developed it. One man had two extra-marital sexual contacts as well as his wife. Of these four patients the only one who escaped infection with C.M.V. was the man's wife. Two of the patients with active infection had the pseudo infectious mononucleosis syndrome, but the remainder were asymptomatic. Further research is proceeding.

Cytomegalovirus which was largely unknown to most clinicians until recently is a widely distributed agent. Its clinical spectrum is largely undetermined and the adult infection appears to have an epidemiological pattern of transmission, requiring either close social or sexual contact. Its importance as being the commonest infectious agent to reach the foetus (Hanshaw et al, 1971) is shown by the birth of 400 infants with severe brain damage in England and Wales each year (Stern and Tucker, 1973). The mode of transmission in adult life deserves more intensive study.

REFERENCES

ALEXANDER, E. E. (1967). *Pediat. Res.*, **1**, 210.
DIOSI, P., BABUSCEAC, L., NEVINGLOVSCHI, O. and KUN-STOICU, G. (1967). *Lancet*, ii, 1063.
HANSHAW, J. B., STEINFELD, H. J. and WHITE, C. J. (1968). *New Engl. J. Med.*, **279**, 566.
HANSHAW, J. B., SCHULTZ, F. W., MELISH, M. M. and DUDGEON, J. A. (1973). *Intrauterine Infections*, p. 23, Ciba Foundation Symposium 10.
HARINDEN, D. G., ELSDALE, T, R., YOUNG, D. E. and ROSS, A. (1967). *Blood*, **30**, 120.
HARRIS, J. R. W. and MORTON, R. S. (1974). *Brit. J. vener. Dis.*, in press.
HARRIS, J. R. W. (1973). Paper read at M.S.S.V.D. meeting in Brussels, May 1973.
KÄÄRIÄINEN, L., KLEMOLA, E. and PALOHEIMO, J. (1966). *Brit. med. J.*, i, 1270.

KRESH, U., JUNG, M. and JUNG, F. (1971). *Cytomegalovirus Infections in Men.* Karger, Basle.

LANG, D. J. and KUMMER, J. F. (1972). *New Engl. J. Med.,* **287,** 756.

MENDEZ-CASHION, D., VALCARCEL, M. I., RAMIREZ DE ARELLANO, R. and ROWE, W. P. (1963). *Biol. Assoc. Med. P. Rico,* **55,** 447.

MONTGOMERY, R., YOUNGBLOOD, L. and MEDEARIS, D. N. (1972). *Pediatrics,* **49,** 524.

STARR, J. G., BART, R. D. and GOLD, E. (1970). *New Engl. J. Med.,* **282,** 1075.

STERN, H. (1972). *J. clin. Path.* **25,** Suppl. (Roy. Coll. Path.), **6,** 34.

STERN, H. and ELEK, S. D. (1965). *J. Hyg. Lond.,* **63,** 79.

STERN, H. (1972). *Brit. med. Bull.,* **28,** 180.

STERN, H. (1971). *Proceedings of the XII International Congress of Pediatrics,* Vienna, **6,** 301.

STERN, H. and TUCKER, S. M. (1973). *Brit. med. J.,* ii, 268.

STULBERG, C. S., ZUELZER, W. W., PAGE, R. H., TAYLOR, P. E. and BROUGH, A. J. (1966). *Proc. Soc. exp. Biol., N.Y.,* **123,** 976.

TOBIN, J. O'H. (1973). *Intrauterine Infections,* p. 59, Ciba Foundation 10.

WALKER, G. H. and TOBIN, J. O'H. (1970). *Archs Dis. Childh.,* **45,** 513.

43 Sexually Transmitted Protozoa and Helminths

J. R. W. Harris

In 1962, Mylius and Ten Seldam reported sexual transmission of *E. histolytica* between a married couple. Apparently the wife, suffering from a longstanding amoebic vaginitis, infected her husband causing cutaneous amoebiasis of the prepuce and glans penis. Munguia et al (1966) described genital amoebiasis in a female patient who practised anal, as well as vaginal, intercourse. Cohen (1973) reviewed the whole question of genital amoebiasis and came to the conclusion that venereal transmission did not appear to be very important. Nevertheless she does admit that urethritis due to *E. histolytica* has been reported following rectal intercourse with patients who have *E. histolytica* in their rectum (Sayed and Amin, 1962).

Shookhoff (1972) stated that repeated parasite infections were not uncommon among the male homosexuals seen by his colleagues and himself in the department of health clinics in New York. Lynch (1972) felt that ano-rectal contact or a combination of fellatio and rectal intercourse were transmission factors in certain parasitic infections among homosexual patients. Waugh (1972) observed infection with *Enterobius vermicularis* in homosexual patients with established sexually transmitted diseases attending the West London unit. During the last year he has treated another 12 homosexual patients for *Enterobius vermicularis* infection (Waugh 1973). Harris and Morton (1973) observed that sexual transmission of these infections would be found more frequently among patients who indulged in genito-oral contact, particularly homosexuals.

The organisms involved will be those parasites which do not require an intermediate host or do not have a time interval during the life cycle outside the host. Also the stage of organism excreted must be able to survive immediate ingestion and should usually depend on the anus–hand–mouth transmission route. The following protozoa have been implicated; *Dientamoeba fragilis* (Shookhoff, 1972), *Entamoeba histolytica* (as noted above), *Giardia lambia* (Abraham, 1972), *Endolimax nana* (Abraham, 1972) and *Iodamoeba buetschlii* (Abraham, 1972). The importance of helminths such as *Enterobius vermicularis* has already been mentioned and from the life cycle of *Hymenolepsis nana* (Edington and Gilles, 1969) one would expect it to be of equal significance in tropical and sub-tropical countries.

REFERENCES

ABRAHAM, P. M. (1972). *J. Amer. med. Ass.*, **221**, 917.

COHEN, C. (1973). *J. Obstet. Gynaec. Brit. Commonw.*, **80**, 476.

EDINGTON, G. M. and GILLES, H. M. (1969). *Pathology in the Tropics*, 1st ed., p. 188. Arnold, London.

HARRIS, J. R. W. and MORTON, R. S. (1973). *Brit. J. vener. Dis.*, **49**, 393.

LYNCH, V. DE P. (1972). *J. Amer. med. Ass.*, **222**, 1311.

MUNGUIA, H., FRANCO, E. and VALENZUELA, P. (1966). *Amer. J. Obstet. Gynec.*, **94**, 181.

MYLIUS, R. E. and TEN SELDAM, R. E. J. (1962). *Trop. Geog. Med.*, **14**, 20.

SAYED, B. A. and AMIN, S. P. (1962). *Brit. med. J.*, i, 157.

SHOOKHOFF, H. B. (1972). *J. Amer. med. Ass.*, **222**, 1310.

WAUGH, M. A. (1972). *Trans. St. John Hosp. Derm. Soc.*, **58**, 224.

WAUGH M. A. (1973). Personal communication.

Part 9
Control

Introduction

The tendency in recent years has been to view venereal disease as a by-product of society's structure and function rather than in the crude terms of war and poverty or relative peace and affluence. The first two have undoubtedly played a part recently in Vietnam and Bangladesh, and the last two increasingly in many Western countries, but what has proved more intriguing is how these factors operate, especially relative peace and prosperity. It is how the social changes interact with individuals, and individuals with society, to produce alterations of attitudes and changing behavioural patterns, which exercises a growing number of demographers and epidemiologists.

It has been said: 'It is for the venereologist on the spot to synthesise consciously the medico-social factors operating locally and, following an evaluation of this evidence, to formulate a rational programme aimed at control. If the programme is to be fully effective it will require to be progressive, expanding and in all ways dynamic' (Morton, 1971).

All the measures currently available for the control of venereal and other sexually transmissible infections can be seen as falling under one of three headings:

(a) Provision of an adequate network of clinics offering prompt, scientific diagnosis and treatment.
(b) Education of the public and the health professions about venereal diseases.
(c) The tracing and treating of the contacts of all infected persons.

It is under these headings that control will be reviewed. But first, with a minimum of repetition of work summarised elsewhere, a brief review of the size and nature of the problem as delineated in recent years.

369

44 Size and Nature of the Problem

R. S. Morton

The World Health Organisation (1964) reported that 74·4 per cent of 105 countries had shown a rise in early syphilis. This report complemented the W.H.O. Report (1963) showing that 47·7 per cent of 111 countries and areas were reporting persistent rises in gonorrhoea. Loss of control has continued.

Bent (1965) considered the outstanding problems requiring urgent attention to be the apparent increase in moral laxity, inadequate reporting of cases and contacts, inadequate legislation, deficient reporting of positive laboratory findings, lack of awareness of the possibility of infections in homosexuals and teenagers, population mobility, growing antibiotic resistance in the gonococcus, inadequate public education, poor standards of follow-up and the role of alcohol and narcotics in facilitating the dissemination of infection.

The worldwide figures comparing the start of the rise in 1955 with the deteriorating position between 1960–67 were published by W.H.O. (1969).

By 1968 the whole question as to whether syphilis can be controlled by treatment and epidemiological methods is seriously questioned by Donohue (1968). With the annual global incidence of gonorrhoea increased from 60 million cases to 160 million, failure to control the disease was admitted by King (1970).

The environmental changes determining the continuing trends were discussed by Guthe et al (1969) and again by Guthe and Willcox (1971). Both these papers emphasise the changing attitudinal and behavioural patterns, in developed and developing countries, and how the changes increase the risk of acquiring infection. The authors see the inherent dynamics of a multiplicity of factors as facilitating the spread of infections and so placing control beyond the endeavours of physicians. This state of affairs the authors see as likely to continue for some time in the future.

The degree to which individual factors operate to produce growing prevalence of infection varies regionally, *eg* Schaller (1968) found, in

371

Ethiopia, that between 30–50 per cent of the young had syphilis and among prostitutes the figure approached 80 per cent. Acquiring venereal disease was regarded as a sign of maturity. Kibukamusoke (1965) attributed rising infection rates to population movement into urban areas by unattached males seeking work. Tribal ethics were found to be breaking down. Amongst the Masai tribe of Tanzania, Mann et al (1966) found the highest incidence of syphilis amongst the prosperous men, in their thirties. They had easiest access to the prostitutes of neighbouring tribes. Maffre et al (1965) showed how socio-economic changes in West Africa had led to increased infection rates. Cirera and Lefeuvre-Witier (1967) found significantly higher levels of positive syphilis serology in Sahara nomads (8·2 per cent) as compared with sedentary workers (4·5 per cent) and semi-nomads (1·85 per cent).

The dramatic effect of movement by a third of the population of Bangladesh away from home and back again in the space of less than 2 years was noted by Morton (1973) as being mainly responsible for a doubling of the incidence of both syphilis and gonorrhoea.

In Mexico, Campos-Salas (1964) indicated that syphilis incidence was apparently growing whilst that of gonorrhoea was declining. He considered the latter was due to growing self-treatment and non-reporting.

In European countries there have been several efforts to delineate the problem. Bijkerk (1970) produced an excellently detailed monograph relating to Holland. Similar details were presented on behalf of Sweden (Liden, 1969), Switzerland (Wagner, 1969), and the U.S.S.R. (Nikitina, 1970). Such baseline studies are essential not only to delineate a country's V.D. problem but as a measure against which to plan, pursue and consider the success or otherwise of infection-control endeavours.

So much for the size of the problem. Its nature revolves round learning something of the age, sex and marital status of the infected; the geography, seasonality and import/export of infection and, above all, the identification of 'at risk' groups of individuals. Some of these factors will be briefly considered.

Young People

Since World War II the proportion of young people, teenagers and adolescents in most nations has risen rapidly. This, together with the fact that the young are the most sexually active, most prone to experiment and most likely to indulge in partner change has made them feature prominently in the demography of venereal diseases. Infection rates in young people have risen more rapidly than in populations as a whole (Rosenblatt and Kabasakalian, 1966). It has also been noted in the U.S.A. by Fiumara and Briley (1969) that pre-pubertal infections are increasingly common. The status of young people and venereal disease has been widely studied, *eg* in England by King (1965); in New Zealand by Platts (1965); and in South America by Sieff (1966). Arya and Bennet (1967) noted that in Uganda venereal disease accounted for 23 per cent of all student attendances at the student health service. A student stood a 1 in 4 chance of being infected. Juhlin (1968) in Sweden showed how changing sex behaviour patterns have altered the age structure of V.D. clinic populations and determined a growing preponderance of young people.

Sanders (1971) noted that in the U.S.A., gonorrhoea amongst adolescents and young adults accounted for more than half of that country's epidemic problem. In England the Chief Medical Officer's Annual Report for 1971 shows gonorrhoea morbidity rates for teenagers (female) to be highest in those aged 18–19 at 558·8 per 100 000. It was 281·22 in 1967. Morbidity rates in males were highest in those aged 20–24 years at 683·29 per 100 000 in 1971 as against 549·41 in 1967 (Department of Health and Social Security, 1972).

Homosexuals

Homosexuality in relation to venereal diseases in Holland, one of Europe's most liberal countries in this respect, was discussed by Hermans and De Cock (1965). Its background and nature was dealt with by Holeman and Winokur (1965). In England, Jefferiss (1966) showed that the percentage of late syphilitic males who were homosexual varied between 14 and 79 per cent in four large clinics in London. Fluker (1966), reporting from one of London's largest venereal disease departments, gave percentages of homosexuals as follows:

Early syphilis cases	38 per cent
Gonorrhoea, males	15·4 per cent
Other conditions in males	4·9 per cent

Homosexuals and bisexuals and the part played by them in the epidemiology of syphilis in the U.S.A. was discussed by Neser and Parrish (1969). Philip (1968) gave a similar account of the situation in New Zealand. Elste et al (1968) outlined the situation in East Germany and stressed how the worldwide tendency of homosexuals to make frequent partner changes was associated with a high incidence of infection and reinfection in them. Racz (1969) demonstrated how dramatically the situation had changed in Budapest. No case of infectious syphilis in a homosexual was reported in 1963 or 1964. The incidence in 1967 and 1968, however, was 32 and 27 per cent of all early infections in men. Vilotte (1970), reporting from France, found 5 per cent of early syphilis and 3 per cent of gonorrhoea to be homosexually acquired.

13

Immigrants

Immigrants, usually unattached males, appear high on the list of 'at risk' people all over the world. Their numbers in Europe alone must now exceed 4 million. As a rule they do not import infection, but acquire it from the indigenous population of the country of adoption. Beveridge (1964) has shown how childhood conditioning determines differences in sexual behaviour patterns between West Indians, Pakistanis and Adenese, and U.K.-born men. Willcox (1966) showed that West Indians in London had a gonorrhoea morbidity rate 19 times that of the indigenous population. Hossain (1970a) studied the Pakistani immigrant in the U.K. In further papers he dealt with their socio-economic status (1970b); their living conditions (1971a) and sexual behaviour (1971b).

Idsøe and Guthe (1967) have shown quite dramatically the growth of tourism and brought factual data to show how tourists, who may be viewed as temporary immigrants, come to import infections into their own country. In some countries in Northern Europe tourists import 20–25 per cent of the total early syphilis.

Seafarers and Servicemen

Schofield (1965) showed that of all patients attending two port clinics in North-east England, 53·6 per cent were mariners. They largely accounted for the imported infections which amounted to 44·5 per cent of the total number of cases. Guthe and Idsøe (1964) judged that seamen have a 15–20 times greater chance of infection than landlubbers. From Poland, Tomaszonas (1967) reported that 137 of 1 000 seamen were known to be infected in 1960 while in 1963–66 the rate was 194 per 1 000 per annum. Most of the infections were contracted in foreign ports. The author believes these rates to be higher than in Dutch seamen but lower than in Swedish seamen. Ratnatunga (1968) dealt with the problem of seamen visiting Ceylon, while Idsøe and Guthe (1967), taking a global view, dealt with the contribution to infection rates made by increased merchant shipping tonnage with its increase in personnel.

There are papers from several countries concerning venereal infection in armies and navies in the mid- and late-1960s. Scarpari and Zamberlin (1965) noted a syphilis rate of 0·56 per cent in 28 705 recruits. By the time of their discharge from service their rate was 4·48 per cent. According to Erber et al (1969), Italian law requires that all conscripts have a blood test for syphilis before entering and again before leaving the services. The number so far found positive on discharge is almost double the entry rate. White and Bloont (1967) reporting from a large military establishment in the U.S.A claimed to see 6·7 per cent of all the early syphilis in the total military population, although the establishment houses only 1 per cent of the total number of service personnel. Ongom (1970) examined 712 Ugandan soldiers. Twenty had infectious venereal disease and 9·3 per cent a positive Reiter Protein Complement Fixation Test.

Prostitutes

Ostaja and Storlazzi (1964) drew attention to the rising infection rates following the closing of brothels under Italy's Merlin law. Prophylactic measures for Parisian prostitutes were outlined by Garnier et al (1965). Traditional prostitution in India and its relationship to the spread of venereal diseases was discussed by Hossain (1966). The need to examine American women in detention for such infections was endorsed by the *Bulletin of the New York Academy of Medicine*. De Amorin (1966) examined 202 Brazilian prostitutes and found 55·9 per cent with gonorrhoea, 22·7 per cent with syphilis and 4·0 per cent with chancroid. Wren (1967), in Australia, examined 100 consecutive women entering a State reformatory. Many of them were prostitutes—44 had gonorrhoea and two had syphilis. More than half were aged under 21 years. The contribution which these women made to the rising infection rate was believed to be considerable. In France, Sepetjian et al (1967) blamed the de-registration of prostitutes for their increasing contribution to the rise in the venereal disease rates.

Johnson et al (1969) working in the Philippines examined a random selection of 702 prostitutes. Using cervical cultures, they found, initially, 8·5 per cent infected with gonorrhoea. Regular testing at weekly intervals is claimed to have raised detection rates to 19·7 per cent. Identical techniques in 163 named contacts gave figures of 22 and 44·6 per cent respectively. Matsuda (1969) argued a case for the abolition of 'red light' districts in Japan.

In Western countries, with their growing degrees of sexual freedom, prostitutes as a source of infection are declining. Dunlop (1971) in London, England, has shown that whereas in 1961 about 31 per cent of heterosexually infected men were infected by a paid source, the figure in 1969 was only 14 per cent. The corresponding figures for 'girl friends' were 27 and 49 per cent.

Behavioural Aspects

Wheldon (1964) administered a lengthy questionnaire to the crew of a British cruiser in the Far East and concluded, amongst other things, that venereal disease now carries no stigma; fear of infection is no deterrent and that chastity has no recognisable merit. Singh et al (1966) described the typical Indian venereal disease clinic patient as young;

single; a member of a large family; poorly educated, both generally and sexually, and whose religious faith is ill-founded.

Bird (1965) considered the emotional problems of patients attending a special clinic and Seale (1966), dealing with the same subject, mentions the suicide of a named contact. The sexual behaviour of the expectant father was studied by Hartman and Nicolai (1966); and of medical students by Sheppe and Hain (1966). The social and behavioural background of the 'repeater' was discussed by Glass (1967). He concluded that half his patients with gonorrhoea sooner or later had at least one more attack. Kite (1971) found 20 per cent of clinic patients with emotional disturbance due to morbid fear of infection, although all were of previously sound personality.

As regards associated social phenomena, Linken (1968), writing from London, found that 18·2 per cent of 252 patients under 30 years of age were currently using drugs: 25 used an amphetamine, 32 cannabis, six L.S.D., one heroin. Nearly 25 per cent used these drugs with a fair degree of regularity. A similar picture was found in San Francisco by Smith and Rose (1968).

Linken and Weiner (1970) found that 15 of 63 single females attending their clinic had previously been pregnant on at least one occasion and that at least 1 in 5 of 89 females used no contraceptives of any kind.

Morton (1971) explored in detail the background of social change and the changes themselves as they have occurred in the U.K. He sees socioeconomic change, technical and scientific innovation and the extension of general and sexual freedom as a single process inevitably leading to altered attitudes and behaviour. High infection rates he sees as being one of the many growing manifestations of the social pathology which has resulted (Morton, 1973).

Historical Aspects

Mason (1964) listed the known facts about the history of syphilis. Weisman (1966), following an examination of pre-Columbian sculpture in the U.S.A., concluded that syphilis did not exist there in the explorer's time. Chesterman (1964), reviewing the epidemic of the European morbus gallicus in the sixteenth and seventeenth centuries, stated that one in every five Frenchmen was infected. The situation in Elizabethan England was only marginally better. He makes the interesting point that the widespread existence of such fevers as malaria, typhus, typhoid and smallpox probably accounted for the relative infrequency of general paralysis of the insane. Wilcocks (1967) credits Paracelsus with the introduction of mercury for the treatment of morbus gallicus. Hutfield (1966) believes that the Romans were acquainted with genital herpes and that the first classical description was given by Astruc in 1736.

The fiftieth anniversary of the establishment of the British venereal diseases service was celebrated by articles in the *British Medical Journal* (1966) and the *British Journal of Venereal Diseases* (1966). The report of the Royal Commission of 1916, which led to the beginnings of the present, nationwide network of over 200 clinics for some 50 million population, gave it as its view that before and during the World War I some 10 per cent of Londoners were syphilitics (Willcox, 1967).

Hudson (1968) brought further evidence to support the Unitarian origin of syphilis in Europe. Morton (1968) put forward the theory that the morbus gallicus was two diseases, a non-venereal treponematosis from Africa and venereal syphilis from the New World. He explains the decline in the epidemic and the changing clinical nature of the infection in its first 100 years in Europe as due to a decline in the non-venereal element. This he sees as a giving way to the spread of Renaissance influence, the use of washing, *etc*, and shows how non-venereal forms lingered only on the periphery of the continent, with different names in different countries, even until recent times. Another approach to the subject was made by Boneff (1968).

The *Journal of the American Medical Association* (1968) presented a short biography of August von Wassermann. Fifty years of research at the Secherov Institute in Moscow was reviewed by Rachmanov (1967). Dr. Samuel Johnson's biographer, Boswell, had his many attacks of urethritis reviewed by Ober (1969). The historical aspects of general paralysis of the insane in four great men, and in Australia, are dealt with by Heine et al (1969) and Stoller and Emerson (1969).

From Poland come two articles concerning recent history. In the first, Lablotniak (1970) describes anti-venereal endeavours between the wars while in the second, Capińska (1970) deals with the situation in Cracow during World War II. Venereology in India since the end of British rule was described by Desai (1970).

Waugh (1971) reviewed the care of the venereally sick in London during the eighteenth and nineteenth centuries, while Wyke (1973) reviewed in some detail the nineteenth century hospital facilities available to the venereally infected in England as a whole. A short biography of Franz Richard Schaudin was presented by Thorburn (1971).

Morton (1971) points out that the present era of sexual freedom is the third in British history. The previous two were followed by times of restraint. He gives the impression that history will repeat itself but that man will drift into improved social health rather than plan it.

REFERENCES

ARYA, O. P. and BENNET, F. J. (1967). *Brit. J. vener. Dis.*, **43**, 275.
BENT, W. I. (1965). *Canad. J. Publ. Hlth*, **56**, 137.
BEVERIDGE, M. M. (1964). *Publ. Hlth*, **78**, 268.
BIJKERK, H. (1970). *Brit. J. vener. Dis.*, **46**, 247.
BIRD, M. S. (1965). *Brit. J. vener. Dis.*, **41**, 217.

Brit. med. J. (1966). Editorial, **2**, 1344.

Brit. J. vener. Dis., (1966). **42**, 223.

BONEFF, A. (1968). *Amer. J. Derm. Syph.*, **95**, 529.

CAMPOS-SALAS, A. (1964). *Bol. Oficina. Sanataria. Pan. am.*, **57**, 517.

CIRERA, P. and LEFEUVRE-WITIER, P. (1967). *Bull. Soc. Path. Exot.*, **60**, 33.

CHESTERMAN, C. C. (1964). *Trans. Hunterian Soc.*, **22**, 77.

CAPIŃSKA, K. (1970). *Przegl. Derm. Suppl.*, **85**, 91.

DE AMORIN, P. J. (1966). *Hospital, Rio do Janeiro*, **70**, 1739.

DEPARTMENT OF HEALTH AND SOCIAL SECURITY (1973). Chief Medical Officer's Report for 1971. *Brit. J. vener. Dis.*, **49**, 89.

DESAI, S. C. (1970). *J. Ass. Physicians, India*, **18**, 135.

DONOHUE, J. F. (1968). *Rer. Agrup. Odont. Argent.*, **20**, 1201.

DUNLOP, E. M. C., LAMB, A. M. and KING, D. M. (1971). *Brit. J. vener. Dis.*, **47**, 192.

ELSTE, G., JOST, W. and KRELL, L. (1968). *Derm. Wschr.*, **154**, 985.

ERBER, B. and FASULO, V. (1969). *Giov. Batt. Virol. Immunol.*, **62**, 3.

FIUMARA, M. J. and BRILEY, J. M. (1969). *Brit. J. vener.*, *Dis.*, **45**, 254.

FLUKER, J. L. (1966). *Brit. J. vener. Dis.*, **42**, 48.

GARNIER, G., SERRES, J. and BEVZELIN, J. P. (1965). *Prophyl. Sanit. Morde*, **37**, 12.

GLASS, L. H. (1967). *Brit. J. vener. Dis.*, **43**, 128.

GUTHE, T., IDSØE, O. and DANBOLT, N. (1969). *Tidsskr. norske Laegeforen.*, **89**, 1784.

GUTHE, T. and WILLCOX, R. R. (1971). *Roy. Soc. Hlth J.*, **91**, 122.

GUTHE, T. and IDSØE, O. (1964). *Tidsskr. norske Laegeforen*, **84**, 1262.

HARTMAN, A. A. and NICOLAI, R. C. (1966). *J. Abnorm. Soc. Psychol.*, **71**, 232.

HEINE, H., GONCOURT, J. DE and DAUDET, A. (1969), *Proc. Roy. Soc. Med.*, **62**, 669.

HERMANS, E. H. and DE COCK, P. (1965). *Acta Leidensia*, **33**, 107.

HOLEMAN, R. W. and WINOKUR, G. (1965). *Amer. J. Orthopsychiat.*, **35**, 48.

HOSSAIN, A. S. M. T. (1966). *Indian J. Derm. Venereol.*, **32**, 56.

HOSSAIN, A. S. M. T. (1970a). *Indian Pract.*, **23**, 753.

HOSSAIN, A. S. M. T. (1970b). *Pakistan med. Rev.*, **5**, 471.

HOSSAIN, A. S. M. T. (1971a). *Publ. Hlth*, **85**, 123.

HOSSAIN, A. S. M. T. (1971b). *Social Sci. Med. J.*, **5**, 227.

HUDSON, E. H. (1968). *Acta Trop.*, **25**, 1.

HUTFIELD, D. C. (1966). *Brit. J. vener. Dis.*, **42**, 263.

IDSØE, O. and GUTHE, T. (1967). *Brit. J. vener. Dis.*, **43**, 227.

J. Amer. med. Ass. (1968). Editorial, **204**, 655.

JEFFERISS, F. J. G. (1966). *Brit. J. vener. Dis.*, **42**, 46.

JOHNSON, D. W., HOLMES, K. K. et al (1969). *Amer. J. Epiderm.*, **90**, 438.

JUHLIN, L. (1968). *Acta derm.-venereol., Stockh.*, **48**, 75.

KIBUKAMUSOKE, J. W. (1965). *Trop. Med. Hyg.*, **59**, 642.

KING, A. J. (1970). *Brit. med. J.*, **21**, 45.

KING, A. J. (1965). *W.H.O. Chronicle*, **19**, 144.

KITE, E. DE C. (1971). *Brit. J. vener. Dis.*, **47**, 135.

LABLOTNIAK, R. (1970). *Prezgl. Derm.*, **57**, 785.

LINKEN, A. (1968). *Brit. J. vener. Dis.*, **44**, 337.

LINKEN, A. and WEINER, R. S. P. (1970). *Brit. J. vener. Dis.*, **46**, 243.

LIDEN, S. (1969). *Lakertidninegen*, **66**, 907.

MAFFRE, E., BA, H. et al (1965). *Bull. Soc. Méd. Afr. Noire. Lang. Fr.*, **10**, 603.

MANN, G. V., SCHAFFER, R. D. et al (1966). *Publ. Hlth Rep.*, **81**, 513.

MASON, W. A. (1964). *J. nat. med. Ass.*, **56**, 148.

MATSUDA, T. (1969). *Jap. J. Nurs. Art.*, **8**, 122.

MORTON, R. S. (1968). *Brit. J. vener. Dis.*, **44**, 174.

MORTON, R. S. (1971). *Sexual Freedom and Venereal Disease*. Peter Owen, London.

MORTON, R. S. (1973). W.H.O./SEARO Assignment Report—VD Control, Bangladesh.

MORTON, R. S. (1973). *Brit. J. vener. Dis.*, **49**, 155.

NESER, W. B. and PARRISH, H. M. (1969). *Sth. med. J.*, **62**, 177.
NIKITINA, N. V. (1970). *Vestn. Derm. vener.*, **41**, 3.
OBER, W. B. (1969). *Bull. N.Y. Acad. Med.*, **45**, 587.
ONGOM, V. L. (1970). *E. Afr. med. J.*, **47**, 479.
OSTAJA, A. and STORLAZZI, O. (1964). *Minerva Med.*, **55**, 2467.
PHILIP, E. (1968). *N.Z. med. J.*, **67**, 397.
PLATTS, W. M. (1965). *N.Z. med. J.*, **64**, Suppl., 14.
RACHMANOV, V. A. (1967). *Cesk. Derm.*, **42**, 361.
RACZ, E. (1969). *Orv. Hetil.*, **110**, 2146.
RATNATUNGA, C. S. (1968). *Indian J. Derm. Venereol.*, **34**, 93.
ROSENBLATT, D. and KABASAKALIAN, L. (1966). *Amer. J. Publ. Hlth*, **56**, 1104.
SANDERS, S. (1971). *J. Tenn. med. Ass.*, **64**, 1052.
SCHALLER, K. F. (1968). *Abstr. Hyg.* (1968), Abstr. 4642.
SCHOFIELD, C. B. S. (1965). *Brit. J. vener. Dis.*, **41**, 51.
SEALE, J. R. (1966). *Brit. J. vener. Dis.*, **42**, 31.
SEPETJIAN, M., AVON, P., BONDET, P. and THIVOLET, J. (1967). *Revue Hyg. Méd. Soc.*, **15**, 541.
SHEPPE, W. M. and HAIN, J. D. (1966). *J. med. Educ.*, **41**, 457.
SCARPARI, S. and ZAMBERLIN, P. (1965). *Am. Sclavo*, **7**, 430.
SIEFF, B. (1966). *Med. Proc.*, **12**, 224.
SINGH, K., MAHOMED, E. and SUKHIJA, C. L. (1966). *J. Indian med. Ass.*, **46**, 270.
SMITH, D. E. and ROSE, A. J. (1968). *Clin. Pediat.*, **7**, 313.
STOLLER, A. and EMERSON, R. (1969). *Med. J. Aust.*, **20**, 706.
THORBURN, A. L. (1971). *Brit. J. vener. Dis.*, **47**, 459.
TOMASZONAS, S. (1967). *Bull. Inst. Mar. Med., Gdansk*, **18**, 67.
VILOTTE, M. J. (1970). *Arch. Fr. Mal. Appar. Dis.*, Suppl. **59**, 3.
WAGNER, G. (1969). *Ther. Umsch.*, **26**, 60.
WAUGH, M. A. (1971). *Brit. J. vener. Dis.*, **47**, 146.
WEISMAN, A. I. (1966). *Bull. N.Y. Acad. Med.*, **42**, 284.
WHELDON, G. R. (1964). *J. roy. Mor. Serv.*, **50**, 109.
WHITE, P. C. J. and BLOONT, J. H. (1967). *Milit. Med.*, **132**, 252.
W.H.O. (1963). Technical Report Series, No. 262.
W.H.O. (1964). *Chronicle*, **18**, 45.
W.H.O. (1969). *Wld Hlth Statist. Rep.*, **22**, 309.
WILCOCKS, C. (1967). *Bull. Inst. Tech. Venereol.*, **7**, 105.
WILLCOX, R. R. (1966). *Brit. J. vener. Dis.*, **42**, 225.
WILLCOX, R. R. (1967). *Brit. J. vener. Dis.*, **43**, 1.
WREN, B. G. (1967). *Med. J. Aust.*, **1**, 847.
WYKE, T. J. (1973). *Brit. J. vener. Dis.*, **49**, 78.

45 Clinical Services

R. S. Morton

Introduction

Countries in Northern Europe were amongst the first to recognise that venereal diseases constituted a social as well as a medical problem. They saw the venereal diseases as too extensive, distressing, devastating and costly to be left to the care of quacks, pharmacists or even private practitioners. Increasingly, it has become apparent that the essential basis of control is a well-organised network of clinics, manned by trained staff, offering early diagnosis, prompt treatment and epidemiological follow-up.

Imitators have been all too few. Amongst the latest is Thailand which in recent years has expanded its clinics from nine to 69. Few nations have expanded their services even to meet the recent population explosion with its growing preponderance of young, sexually active peoples. There is no doubt that medical administrators and politicians could be more helpful.

Such evidence as there is, shows that adequate services do contribute to prevention, cure without complications and the avoidance of costly and permanent disability. It is only when the great majority of a nation's sexually infected seek care in a widespread network of clinics offering humane, dignified and scientific care, that control can begin and be developed effectively.

Since services and reporting methods vary from one country to another, comparison of the success of V.D. control measures is not easy. Disparity of morbidity rates, however, are sometimes striking and the availability and quality of clinic services presumably play some part. The United Kingdom has more than 200 clinics to serve its population of over 50 million. Probably more than 80 per cent of all the venereal infections which occur are treated in public service clinics. The U.K. is one of the diminishing number of countries still controlling syphilis. Furthermore, its gonorrhoea morbidity rate compares favourably with other nations, even those with similar social structure and with public clinics. For example, the U.K. gonorrhoea morbidity rate is about half that of Denmark, a third that of Sweden and a fifth that of the U.S.A. Unlike the countries mentioned, and many others, doctors manning the U.K. public service generally specialise exclusively in the care of the sexually infected and they are supported by trained nursing, technical and social work staff.

The problems and ways and means of resolving them

Rangiah (1964) discussed emergency situations in venereology. The anaphylactoid reaction to penicillin calls for installation and maintenance of emergency equipment in all public clinics.

The need for venereologists to initiate and involve doctors in other disciplines in detection of syphilitics by mass survey techniques was described by Kail and Steppert (1964) and Lietchi (1964). The effectiveness of the complementary technique of pre-marital testing in the U.S.A. was dealt with by Porter (1964) and the role of the laboratory in case finding by Dandoy and McKenna (1964). In 1963 these writers 'netted' some 8 000 syphilitics, more than a third of them in an infectious state. An approach to case finding through mass surveys in midwifery departments was presented by Gourlay (1966).

Mendl and Lund (1964) discussed the legal aspects of clinical care of the infected individual while Hagen (1965) gave consideration to secrecy of treatment in juveniles. The legal aspects of V.D. control in the U.S.A., with particular attention to pre-marital and antenatal preventive methods, were outlined by Hall (1966a, b). The law and professional secrecy in the care of the venereally infected in the U.K. was given detailed reviewing by Bernfeld (1967).

Allison (1965) and Gillespie (1965) made a plea for epidemiological treatment of all contacts of infectious syphilis cases seen in clinics. Both saw this method of aborting possible infection as essential to a policy of control to eradication. Brown (1966) saw a single injection of 2·4 mega units of the long-acting benzathine penicillin as adequate for the purpose. As an illustration of the use of this control technique Smith (1965) presented a paper concerning an epidemic consisting of 66 cases of primary syphilis, 14 secondary cases and two cases of early latency in a prison population of 1 076. These cases were found following interview of six original patients. A further 209 sex contacts, apparently not infected, were treated epidemiologically with 2·4 mega units of benzathine penicillin, as were 785 social contacts.

Prather (1967) on the other hand, sees the only hope of control as lying in a more thorough epidemiological approach, with treatment based on sound diagnosis. This is one of the first papers from the U.S.A. to show an awakening to the realisation that only a nationwide network of clinics providing fully comprehensive service can hope to contain infection levels within manageable proportions. Indeed we have to wait till 1972 to hear the view re-stated in America. At the second International Venereal Diseases Symposium held in the U.S.A., Knox (*Lancet*, 1972) queried whether resources currently spent on contact tracing and epidemiological treatment would not be better deployed in establishing a widespread clinical service of high quality. He saw such a service as the basic essential of control. It called for good doctors, good medical education, well-organised research and public education to make it an effective reality.

The first post-war, newly constructed clinic in Britain was described by Catterall and Seale (1965). The use of the mass survey as a continuous method of detection of syphilis in the U.S.S.R. was described by Rossitanskii (1965); and, in Brazil, by Mellone and Pagenotto (1965). This last study revealed about 2 per cent reactive specimens in 62 572 blood donations. The need for laboratories to notify all positive results to the local venereologist was emphasised by Burgess (1966). He saw very clearly that there was a real danger of cases being found by the laboratories but not being treated for want of close co-operation between specialists. He also brought irrefutable evidence to show that follow-up of family and of sex contacts of detected cases was a very worthwhile activity. A similar view was taken by Pickett (1967) who found that over a 9-month period about a third of all detected syphilitics were found by routine laboratory screening methods.

Proposals to improve and establish out-patients services were discussed by Caletti and Serena (1965). Schepers (1966) emphasised the need for back-up laboratory services if clinics were to be fully effective. He saw early and accurate diagnosis as playing a key role in V.D. control. An ambulatory clinic in Germany was described by Dewald (1966) and co-operation between civilian and U.S.A. military services by Brown (1967).

Freedman (1966a) saw the mechanism of control as multifactorial and based on case findings, adequate clinical facilities, health education, the public health approach and legal aids as supporting contact tracing. Freedman (1966b) followed this up by pointing out that in the U.S.A., where much more than half of all the infected are treated privately, these endeavours have little chance of fulfilling their potential. He calls for greater identification of the private physician with the whole concept of epidemiological control. This point has been taken up by several others in the U.S.A., who have made suggestions for better orientation in the public sector, for example, Vora (1966), Gorlick (1966), Cowan (1966), Johnson (1966) and Porter (1966). The problem continued to exercise writers through 1967. Cleere et al (1967), for example, in a survey of the attitudes of 6 000 private physicians found that the many who did not report, or only selectively reported cases, were concerned about divulging confidential information and were frequently under pressure from their patients not to do so. Thus only 24·8 per cent of gonorrhoea cases and 6·2 per cent of cases of syphilis were reported. An editorial in the *Journal of the American Medical Association* (1967) developed the theme of co-operation between public and private sector in V.D. control.

Such efforts appear to have some effect. Brown (1968) reported improvement in reporting in the U.S.A. from 45 per cent in 1962 to 55 per cent in 1967. In terms of investment in syphilis detection and treatment, Callin (1968) reckoned that for every dollar spent 7·5 were saved. Currently many millions of serological tests for syphilis are carried out annually in the U.S.A.

The prevention of treatment by quacks, illegal in many developed countries, was considered by Lomholt (1968). That treatment of any kind is not without hazard was dealt with by Luger (1967). The treatment regime used by the British Navy was described by Wilmott (1968). Starck (1968) in Sweden considered possible improvements and Rockl et al (1968) the errors that precipitate iatrogenic illness.

Willcox (1968) again discussed the role of epidemiological treatment, when initial testing of named contacts proved negative. King (1968) gave his reasons for a contrary view declaring that there were few reasons for departing from the principle that diagnosis should precede treatment. These opposing views were again aired by these two writers at an international meeting in Venice (Willcox, 1973; King, 1973). Willcox (1972) dealt with epidemiological treatment with reference to gonorrhoea control.

The division of care between private and public sectors is a constant and recurring theme in the literature. The nationwide network of some 6 000 clinics for the care of the venereally infected in the U.S.S.R. was described by Rakhmanov and Turanov (1967). They noted that Russia has 88 professorial chairs in dermato-venereology. Christmas (1968) reported from New Zealand that twice as many patients sought private care as attended public clinics. Teague (1969), a public health worker in Kentucky, U.S.A., showed that for every case of syphilis reported by private physicians he was able to secure the attendance of 11 others. Brown (1970a) noted that the majority of cases not reported by private U.S. physicians were in the lower socio-economic strata. More than 134 633 private physicians responded to a questionnaire sent out by Fleming et al (1970). No less than 4 370 (3·2 per cent) had treated cases of syphilis according to McKenzie-Pollock (1970). These studies reveal that 80 per cent of syphilitics are treated in the private sector and only one in every nine is reported. Kennedy (1969) reports how a public health nurse called on private practitioners who did not report treating venereal disease.

The massive problem and virtual absence of epidemiological control due to self-treatment, quack treatment and pharmacist and private practitioner treatment current in the Western Pacific and South-east Asia regions of W.H.O. was reviewed by Willcox (1970). The literature in this year was replete with articles reflecting concern about the continuing rise in gonorrhoea and syphilis. Papers from some countries admit failure; others talk of epidemic levels of incidence; new developments are generally old control ideas with a new look on their first application in a new area (Lancet, 1970).

Skogh (1968) points to the need for venereology to be regarded as a separate speciality. This he sees as the starting point of effective control. Brown (1970b, c) discusses why control of gonorrhoea and more lately control of syphilis has been lost in the U.S.A.

Quality of public services as well as the quantity is seen as under seige in the U.K. by Catterall and Morton (1970). They review the facts and figures regarding the unrelenting growth of clinic caseloads. They see a crisis situation as inevitable if renewal, replacement and enlargement of clinics, and their staffs, is not undertaken as a matter of urgency. Failure to keep pace with demand they see as leading not just to breakdown of public service, when it is most needed, but to a dissipation of such control as exists. As a product of these and other efforts, improvements have been effected both in London and in the provinces. Wigfield (1972) has shown that nearly 30 years of sustained application of high quality clinical care and contact tracing in the north-east of England has been effective in maintaining a morbidity rate some 20 per cent below the national average. An editorial in the *British Medical Journal* (1971) describes the treatment of venereal disease in general practice. The plans and working of a new purpose-built department for the care of those with sexually transmitted diseases in London's St. Mary's Hospital is described by James et al (1973). The department is designed and staffed to deal with 20 000 new patients per annum.

So common has gonorrhoea become in the U.S.A. that mass screening, using culture methods, is seen as essential in family planning, antenatal and gynaecological clinics, both public and private. Positive cultures for gonorrhoea have varied between 2·6 and 7·3 per cent; see, for example, Zackler et al (1970), Charles et al (1970) and Hart (1971). Such mass screening methods are of course bound to be most productive in countries where control measures are least well developed and morbidity rates are consequently high. Rees and Hamlett (1972) have shown that there is as yet no urgent need for such measures in the U.K where the gonorrhoea morbidity level is about a fifth of that in the U.S.A.

How to set about developing and effectively utilising clinical services is dealt with in reports of two W.H.O. Regional Symposia, one for the Western Pacific (1969) and one for South-east Asia (1972). These offer governments and venereologists guidelines on how best to deploy resources, finance, staff, training, drugs, experience, time, *etc*. In particular the Weston Pacific Report is wide-ranging and raises and answers questions of individual patient management as well as how to deal with the seemingly insurmountable epidemiological problems. An example of application of the principles, in terms of a single country, is contained in a follow-up report by W.H.O. (Morton, 1971).

Much the same objective approach was recently used in the U.S.A. The findings and recommendations are included in the 'Report of the National Commission on Venereal Disease' (1972) issued by the U.S. Department of Health, Education and Welfare. Apart from such findings as the failure of public and professional education and a review of current laws concerning venereal diseases, the most trenchant condemnation is reserved for the scarcity and inadequacy of clinical services. Although the report lacks the motivation and drive of the liberal traditions of Northern Europe, that see some social problems as too big and important to be left to the private sector, there are hints in this report that an age of enlightenment about venereal disease is possible in the U.S.A. Certainly no government can have had a more forthright, frank and wide-ranging assessment of its shortcomings and needs. It will be of interest to see if American politicians can match their commission in social sense and awareness.

Catterall (1973) gives a review of recent developments and changing patterns in organisation and management of clinical services in the U.K. Hopes and suggestions on how to deal with the ever-expanding caseload are set down. Similar reports are available from Uganda (Arya, 1973); East Germany (Elste, 1973); Greenland (Olsen, 1973); the U.S.A. (Webster, 1973) and Portugal (Norton-Brandão, 1973).

For developed countries there is need for sophistication of progress by a more objective approach to planning preventive as well as curative services. Morton (1973) calls for collation and correlation of all forms of social pathology by statisticians and the development of informative, evaluative and predictive social indicators. He appears to believe that faced with facts, politicians, lay and medical administrators and public alike will demand, and make available, the means to cope with the socially inept, whether anti-social, asocial, or venereally infected.

REFERENCES

ALLISON, J. R. (1965). *J. S. Carolina med. Ass.*, **61**, 239.
ARYA, O. P. (1973). *Brit. J. vener. Dis.*, **49**, 134.
BERNFELD, W. K. (1967). *Brit. J. vener. Dis.*, **43**, 53.
Brit. med. J. (1971). Editorial, **2**, 670.
BROWN, W. J. (1966). *Brit. J. vener. Dis.*, **42**, 110.
BROWN, W. J. (1967). *Milit. Med.*, **132**, 316.
BROWN, W. J. (1968). *J. Amer. med. Ass.*, **205**, 800.
BROWN, W. J. (1970a). *Brit. J. vener. Dis.*, **46**, 118.
BROWN, W. J. (1970b). *Ann. intern. Med.*, **72**, 278.
BROWN, W. J. (1970c). *Ann. intern. Med.*, **72**, 280.

BURGESS, J. A. (1966). *Brit. J. vener. Dis.*, **42**, 116.
CALETTI, G. and SERENA, A. (1965). *Ann. Sanità. Publ.*, **26**, 1051.
CALLIN, A. E. (1968). *Salud. Publ. Méx.*, **10**, 611.
CATTERALL, R. D. and SEALE, J. R. (1965). *Brit. med. J.*, **1**, 1305.
CATTERALL, R. D. and MORTON, R. S. (1970). *Brit. med. J.*, **3**, 699.
CATTERALL, R. D. (1973). *Brit. J. vener. Dis.*, **49**, 126.
CHARLES, A. G., COHEN, S. et al (1970). *Amer. J. Obstet. Gynec.*, **108**, 595.
CHRISTMAS, B. W. (1968). *N.Z. med. J.*, **67**, 188.
CLEERE, R. L., DOUGHERTY, W. J. et al (1967). *J. Amer. med. Ass.*, **202**, 941.
COWAN, J. A. (1966). *Mich. Med.*, **65**, 552.
DANDOY, S. and MCKENNA, E. M. (1964). *Publ. Hlth Rep.*, **79**, 1015.
DEWALD, W. (1966). *Dtsch. Gesundh.*, **21**, 1178.
ELSTE, G. (1973). *Brit. J. vener. Dis.*, **49**, 146.
FLEMING, W. L., BROWN, W. J. et al (1970). *J. Amer. med. Ass.*, **211**, 1827.
FREEDMAN, C. W. (1966a). *Med. Anm. Distr. Columbia*, **35**, 355.
FREEDMAN, C. W. (1966b). *Med. Anm. Distr. Columbia*, **35**, 382.
GILLESPIE, E. J. (1965). *Bol. Asoc. Méd. P. Rico*, **57**, 72.
GORLICK, H. S. (1966). *R.N. Oradell. N.J.*, **29**, 39.
GOURLAY, E. (1966). *Nurs. Times*, **62**, 242 and 298.
HAGEN, W. (1965). *Dtsch. med. Wschr.*, **90**, 2217.
HALL, G. E. (1966a). *J. Amer. med. Ass.*, **195**, 309.
HALL, G. E. (1966b). *Arch. Envir. Hlth*, **13**, 388.
HART, M. (1971). *J. Amer. med. Ass.*, **216**, 1609.
JAMES, D. T., JEFFERISS, F. J. G. and WILLCOX, R. R. (1973). W.H.O./VDT/73, 385.
JOHNSON, A. N. (1966). *Arch. Envir. Hlth*, **13**, 393.
J. Amer. med. Ass. (1967). **202**, 981.
KAIL, E. and STEPPERT, A. (1964). *Wein. klin. Wschr.*, **76**, 609.
KENNEDY, H. K. (1969). *Canad. J. Publ. Hlth*, **60**, 482.
KING, A. J. (1968). *Brit. med. J.*, **4**, 581.
KING, A. J. (1973). *Brit. J. vener. Dis.*, **49**, 122.
Lancet (1970). Editorial, **2**, 250.
Lancet (1972). Editorial, **1**, 1109.
LIETCHI, R. (1964). *Praxis, Berne*, **53**, 1714.
LOMHOLT, G. (1968). *Lakartidningen*, **65**, 2156.
LUGER, A. (1967). *Wien. klin. Wschr.*, **79**, 529.
MELLONE, O. and PAGENOTTO, J. (1965). *Revta Hosp. Clin. Fac. Med. Univ. S. Paulo*, **20**, 165.
MENDL, E. and LUND, P. V. (1964). *Z. Haut. Geschlechtskr.*, **37**, 278.
MCKENZIE-POLLOCK, J. S. (1970). *Brit. J. vener. Dis.*, **46**, 114.
MORTON, R. S. (1971). Assignment Report, W.H.O./WPRO/328/70.
MORTON, R. S. (1973). *Brit. J. vener. Dis.*, **49**, 155.
NORTON-BRANDÃO, F. (1973). *Brit. J. vener., Dis.*, **49**, 148.
OLSEN, G. A. (1973). *Brit. J. vener. Dis.*, **49**, 130.
PICKETT, G. (1967). *Mich. Med.*, **66**, 1416.
PORTER, W. L. (1964). *Delaware med. J.*, **36**, 199.
PORTER, W. L. (1966). *Med. Times, Manhasset.*, **94**, 1218.
PRATHER, E. C. (1967). *J. Florida med. Ass.*, **54**, 1038.
RAKHMANOV, V. A. and TURANOV, N. M. (1967). *Vestm. Akad. Med. Mauk S.S.R.*, **22**, 64.
RANGIAH, P. N. (1964). *Antiseptic*, **61**, 535.
REES, E. and HAMLETT, J. D. (1972). *J. Obstet. Gynaec. Brit. Commonw.*, **56**, 1127.
REPORT OF THE NATIONAL COMMISSION ON VENEREAL DISEASE (1972). U.S. Dept. Hlth Educ. and Welf. Publication No. 72–8125.
ROCKL, H., SCHPÖPL, F. and MULLER, E. (1968). *Munich med. Wschr.*, **110**, 2010.
ROSSITANSKII, N. L. (1965). *Vestn. Derm. Vener.*, **39**, 61.

SCHEPERS, G. W. H. (1966). *Med. Am. Distr. Columbia.*, **35**, 357.
SKOGH, M. (1968). *Lakartidningen*, **65**, 1296.
SMITH, W. H. Y. (1965). *J. med. Ass. Alabama*, **35**, 392.
STARCK, V. (1968). *Lakatidningen*, **65**, 2356.
TEAGUE, R. F. (1969). *J. Kentucky med. Ass.*, **67**, 22.
VORA, M. P. (1966). *J. Indian med. Ass.*, **46**, 370.
WEBSTER, B. (1973). *Brit. J. vener. Dis.*, **49**, 141.
W.H.O. (1969). Regional V.D. Seminar. W.H.O./WPRO/0144.
W.H.O. (1972). Regional V.D. Seminar, W.H.O./SEARO/72/267.
WIGFIELD, A. S. (1972). *Brit. J. vener. Dis.*, **48**, 37.
WILLCOX, R. R. (1968). *Brit. med. J.*, **4**, 388.
WILLCOX, R. R. (1970). *Brit. J. Clin. Pract.*, **24**, 97.
WILLCOX, R. R. (1972). W.H.O. Document, W.H.O./VDT/72, 381.
WILLCOX, R. R. (1973). *Brit. J. vener. Dis.*, **49**, 107 and 116.
WILLMOTT, F. E. (1968). *J. R. Nav. med. Serv.*, **54**, 254.
ZACKLER, J., BROLNITSKY, O. and ORBACH, H. (1970). *Publ. Hlth Rep.*, **85**, 681.

46 Health Education

F. St. D. Rowntree

Introduction

Of the methods of control which can be applied to the venereal diseases, health education has the greatest potential for expansion. Continuous reference is made to this fact in the literature and authors constantly emphasise the need for developing the health education aspect of preventive work. This emphasis is not new and since the beginning of the century both clinical and social workers have stressed the need for public education. Unfortunately, their interpretation of 'education' was, and sometimes still is, a purely informational activity concerned with the indiscriminate and didactic dissemination of facts about the consequences of venereal disease and medical services available for its treatment. Many early writers expressed the view that venereal disease is a moral rather than social problem. They demanded provision of some form of reinforcement for declining moral codes. For example, in the Final Report of the Royal Commission on Venereal Disease (1916), a call was made for instruction in 'moral conduct in relation to sexual relations'. These views were reflected in early educational and publicity programmes which were frequently directed at creating behaviour changes through the development of moral guilt, anxiety or shock. This type of approach was undoubtedly responsible for many of the failures to produce the hoped for behavioural changes necessary to bring about reductions in the incidence of sexually transmitted disease, for the lack of acceptance and continuance of treatment, and for the unhealthy degrees of anxiety produced in venereal and non-venereal patients of the type reported by Kite and Grimble (1963).

Despite the growing demands for education there was little agreement on the form that it should take, or on the time, place and circumstances of its provision. The approaches used in educational campaigns were based on intuitive guess work and lacked the support of empirical evidence. The purpose of the education was not clearly defined and, because specific objectives were not precisely delineated, there was confusion on the part of both the educators and the educated. Evaluation of success or failure was made difficult or impossible because of the multiplicity of objectives.

PUBLIC EDUCATION

The early 1960s brought changes that were to have far-reaching effects. In 1959 the International Union against Venereal Diseases and Treponematoses (I.U.V.D.T.) recommended study into epidemiological factors, especially the effect of behaviour, on the spread of venereal disease. In 1962 the World Forum on Syphilis and other Treponematoses included a section on Behavioural Science in its programme for the-first time. There was consequently a call for an increase in use of the concepts and techniques of behavioural science in the field of venereal disease control. In the United States this culminated in the formation in 1963 of a Behavioural Sciences Section as an integral part of the United States Public Health Service (Forer, 1965). Attention was repeatedly drawn to the importance of health education in Behavioural Medicine courses and to the need for behavioural diagnosis and educational treatment (Burton, 1969).

There was no immediate and universal acceptance of these new approaches which aimed at studying human behaviour and interactions with a view to applying the information gained to control measures including health education. However, studies concerned with assessing associations between knowledge, attitudes and behaviour in sex matters, and the type of knowledge and its source, were undertaken in various parts of the world. These studies established the value of the behavioural sciences approach and led to critical appraisal of the earlier, naive acceptance of the demands for indiscriminate distribution of information. Amongst the earlier reports were those concerned with the knowledge of male venereal disease patients (British Federation against Venereal Disease, 1958); the contents of sex education books (Dalzell-Ward, 1960); the attitudes to sex of venereal disease patients (Dalzell-Ward et al, 1960); non-attending patients (Prebble, 1962); sources of venereal disease information (Deisher and Mills, 1963); immaturity as a risk factor (Keighley, 1963); poor educational record as a risk factor (Laird, 1963); use of prostitutes (Willcox, 1962); teenage knowledge (Ponting, 1963; Toribio and Glass, 1965); presence and absence of fear of venereal disease (Wheldon, 1964; Seale, 1966); young people and V.D. (British Medical Association, 1964). Not all of the workers in these enquiries supported one another. For example, Wheldon found fear of venereal disease as a factor affecting sex behaviour, whereas Seale found this not to be the case. None the less the findings established a corpus of knowledge acquired in a scientific manner and which provided information on patterns of sex knowledge, attitudes and behaviour in differing human groups.

The identification of the case of need in the late 1960s

The continuing demand for information led to further enquiries, some of which used sophisticated and costly techniques in the collection and analysis of data. For example, the study of the sexual behaviour of young people carried out in Britain sought information on every aspect of the sex behaviour and knowledge of adolescents, by means of in-depth interviews of hundreds of young people drawn from nation-wide samples (Schofield, 1965). The enquiry found that sexual inter-course had been experienced by a large minority of adolescents, *ie* 30 per cent of boys aged 17 to 19 years and 11 per cent of 15 to 17 year old boys, with lower figures for girls in the same age groups. Whilst the numbers at risk of contracting a sex disease were not considered great, the report revealed considerable ignorance of the risks of pro-miscuous sex and of the symptoms of sex disease; 75 per cent of the boys and 80 per cent of the girls said they would not have known if they had been infected, even if symptoms had existed in the case of the girls. Fear of venereal disease was found to be low, and the contribution of parents to the sex education of their children was virtually negligible.

The role of the parents was examined by Bird (1965) who found that sex was little discussed with young people; even in homes where the expectation would have been that parents would have provided some sort of sex education. Morton (1967) in a study of 330 venereal disease patients found that less than one-third had had any sex education and few had seen pamphlets on venereal disease. Holmes and her co-workers (Holmes et al, 1968) found that only 23 per cent of a control group, matched with young patients attending a venereal disease clinic, had any knowledge about sexually transmitted disease. They found the most outstanding characteristic of the patients was the early age at which they left school. They concluded, 'any education about venereal disease which is to prove useful to the group most at risk should be given before the age of 15 years'. Statham (1968) noted a lack of knowledge amongst late presenting males with gonorrhoea. These patients had had urethral discharge with or without dysuria for several weeks. Arya and Bennett (1968) in an African study noted that both venereal disease patients and controls had insufficient knowledge but that the controls had acquired their information earlier. Juhlin (1968) found half the teenagers visiting his clinic at Uppsala had had intercourse by the age of 15 or 16 years. Elias and Gebhart (1969) demonstrated differences in sex know-ledge according to social class. For example, in the lower socio-economic groups 96 per cent of adolescent boys knew about intercourse, but only 4 per cent knew about fertilisation. There was a similar pattern in the girls from the same social group. The opposite was true of higher socio-economic groups where larger percentages were acquainted with the facts of fertilisation but not the details of intercourse. Psychiatric factors were studied by Peddar and Goldberg (1970) who regarded 30 per cent of all new admissions to a special clinic as 'probable' psychiatric cases on the basis of Goldberg's general health questionnaire. Hossain (1969) investigated the knowledge of immigrant Pakistani males residing in Britain and found an ignorance of the risk of venereal disease. Unfavourable family and social backgrounds were noted by Ekstrøm (1970) in a sociological study of girls and young women with gonorrhoea. Verhargen and Gemert (1972) showed that migration, caused by changes in economic conditions, was a more common factor in patients than controls. Promiscuous sex activity was found to be more likely following the consumption of alcohol (Rowntree, 1972). Sigger (1972) in a study of patients at a venereal disease clinic found that misinformation and ignorance outweighed correct knowledge.

Such findings emphasise the pluralistic nature of human society, the variability and vital importance of the identification of vulnerable groups and the consequent need for a variety of approaches if health education is to play an important part in venereal disease control.

Ways and means of meeting the needs

The communication of health information and the development of attitudes and behaviour patterns starts early and continues throughout life. There are many participants in the process, providing both positive and negative health influences. Communication takes place through *personal* interactions in face to face situations such as conversations and discussion between individuals and groups and through *impersonal* means such as the printed word, radio and television, all of which make a contribution to the matrix of knowledge and beliefs of the individual. Behavioural science theory stresses that the prime source of influence is the family followed by the other sub-groups to which the individual belongs. These together with the cultural complex in which they are set are the *informal* sources of influence. *Formal* influences are provided through deliberately planned health education activities which, from the point of view of the Health Care Delivery System, has a number of aims including:

  (a) initiation of health-promoting behaviour,
  (b) reinforcement of existing health-promoting behaviour,
  (c) avoidance of behaviours hazardous to health,
  (d) counteracting anti-health influences, including correcting mis-
      information.

Health behaviour is influenced by social norms and value-orientation patterns laid down in childhood and not, on a large scale, subject to drastic alteration during life by social pressures, sanctions or by knowledge of an intellectual type (Parsons, 1951).

Health education has tended to concentrate on the provision of knowledge using a variety of methods and media. Didactic and formal teaching often associated with exhortative evangelism is now largely discredited in favour of more effective methods based on the theories and practices of pedagogy, advertising, publicity and mass communications. Utilisation of these techniques in venereal disease control is dependent on the development of a climate of public opinion which not only accepts but demands education about venereal disease, as part of a preventive programme rather than as a measure of last resort following epidemic incidence. The development of favourable opinion takes considerable time, involving repeated personal interactions between health educators, policy makers and leaders of public opinion. These efforts are well justified and can lead to the development of comprehensive programmes of education and publicity which utilise the services of health workers, educationalists, other professional personnel and lay people able to make contributions at varying levels.

In Sheffield in 1960 the development of a long-range comprehensive programme began following meetings both at policy making and grass roots level (Rowntree, 1966). This programme involved all types of personnel and utilised many different forms of teaching and publicity aids, including provision of background and information notes, teaching kits, talks, lectures, quiz sessions, the printed word, leaflets, posters, booklets and books; slides, film strips, tape recordings, a permanent travelling exhibition, press articles, radio broadcasts, television films and telerecordings; a recorded telephone answering service with facilities for the provision of personal advice and information through live telephone talks and personal interviews. These various techniques were progressively introduced into a programme which has been expanded over a 14-year period and frequently re-designed to meet the needs of specific groups, for example, school children, adult leisure organisations and sections of the public not members of formal groups or who were unresponsive to one type of approach or another. This continuous project is integrated within the total health education programme provided for the city.

An alternative type of programme offered in the United States is that of the short duration Public Awareness Campaign, which actively involves a variety of community agencies, to draw attention to the dangers of venereal disease (American Social Health Association, 1968). Considerable research on the use and effectiveness of different communication and teaching methods in health education of the adult general public, young people and patients has been undertaken. A series of comprehensive reviews of this research has been published in the United States by the Society of Public Health Educators in its series of Health Education Monographs (Young, 1967; Young and Simmons, 1967; Young 1967a, 1968, 1968a, 1969). The International Union Against Cancer also reviewed Research Findings and Theoretical Concepts in Public Education (U.I.C.C. 1967). All these publications are worthy of detailed study for their relevance to venereal disease education programmes.

A number of reports on the use of particular methods and media in venereal disease education have been published (Morton, 1966). Impersonal methods such as books, posters and pamphlets are widely used and in some instances these have been found as successful as personal discussions. As a means of increasing information, they should therefore be useful in reaching those inaccessible through personal contact (Rosenblatt and Kabasakalian, 1966). Combined programmed and conventional instruction produces the best results according to Glass and Campbell (1965) though the opportunities for such methods would be limited to formal learning situations. Where wide-ranging courses of sex education have been developed, discussion methods involving small groups of school children and mixed teams of teachers have been found of value (Hollins and Dicks, 1968). The individual interview within the clinical situation is another important method of communicating and imprinting information and an important aspect of the medical profession's role in health education (Baric, 1969). One wonders how many venereologists fail to take the opportunity presented to educate during contact with patients. Kelus (1973) found that gonorrhoea patients had only slightly better knowledge of syphilis than the general public.

The integration of sex education, including venereal diseases education, into the general curricula of schools is an important step forward in many countries though the approach may have a bearing on the outcome (Rowntree, 1971). In Sweden sex education has been compulsory since 1956 but the gonorrhoea rate continued to rise steadily. There was, for example, little use of condoms as protectives. Their use increased following the wide display of a humorous poster illustrating a giant condom. It was felt that the less authoritarian approach increased the effectiveness of communication (Starck-Romanus, 1973). A fall in the gonorrhoea rate during and after the campaign was attributed to its effect.

The mass media have considerable value in reaching wide sections of the community who cannot be contacted through formally organised groups. Newspapers, journals, radio, films and television all have a part to play in education, though the *active* partnership of the medical profession is required to ensure accuracy, balance and credibility. In the U.S.A. and U.K. particularly, films are widely used in support of venereal disease education, though the lack of 'suitable' films has been constantly remarked upon. The use of unsuitable films does, perhaps, more damage than no educational effort at all. An example of the partnership between practising health educators and expert communicators was the production by the British Broadcasting Corporation of a television film on venereal diseases in their '20th Century Focus' series for schools (British Broadcasting Corporation, 1973).

This film goes some way to matching the American venereal disease education film '$\frac{1}{4}$ Million Teenagers', now '$\frac{1}{2}$ Million Teenagers', produced by Los Angeles Public Health Department, and which has been successfully used for so long in venereal disease education programmes (Churchill, 1969). The B.B.C. film, which provides a more up-to-date presentation of the subject, was transmitted following pre-tests with small groups. It was found to be acceptable to parents, teachers and pupils alike and was considered suitable for youth and adult audiences following nationwide transmission (Croton, 1973). The film has been made available for sale and hire and is being increasingly used in educational programmes in the United Kingdom (B.B.C., 1973). The production of both these films exemplifies the advantage of co-operative ventures between the medical profession, health educators and the communications media.

Exposure to the message alone, irrespective of the medium used, is no index of success, and a measurement of total message transmission bears no direct relationship to its acceptance or any resulting behavioural change. People select and retain from the messages transmitted to them only those factual and abstract things which fit in with their prior beliefs, judgements, constructs of reality and perceptions of seriousness and relevance. Many programmes of education appear to fail because they appeal to values which differ from those of the target population and 'because we would like them to strive for things which are simply not important or perhaps not understandable to them' (Hochbaum, 1960). For this reason consumer participation is being recognised as an increasingly important factor in all aspects of the organisation of health care programmes, for 'without consumer involvement there is the danger of a professional decision-making apparatus which may not reflect the goals of society' (Levin, 1969).

Evaluation of health education on sexually transmitted diseases

Education of the public about venereal disease is not easy to evaluate because of the multiplicity and complexity of the problems and the factors involved and because individual programme goals have rarely, been defined at the programme planning stage. It is necessary in considering evaluation of health education programmes to distinguish between objective measurement of specific parameters, and general, subjective judgements or opinions. Some specific parameters such as levels of health knowledge can be measured comparatively easily, others such as attitude changes and alteration of covert behaviour patterns are more complex and less amenable to quantitive and qualitative assessment. Both general and specific evaluation is necessary, both in the immediate and long term, and should be embodied in the objectives of any health education programme. Evaluation is important both to study the immediate effects of the methods used and as a means to improve future activity. It is a diagnostic tool which can assess not only reasons for success or failure, but disadvantages as well as advantages deriving from any form of intervention. Without such objectivity the phenomenon of iatrogenic disease is as possible in preventive as in curative medicine. Unintended consequences may arise as a result of a misunderstanding of a communication or because of selective perception of messages.

The changing public attitude to sex and sexually transmitted disease as a subject of acceptable public discussion, and particularly as a school education subject, is an indication of the increased awareness of the problems created by sex behaviour. The fact that this awareness exists is an index of success in communicating one group of messages, namely those concerned with the seriousness of the present epidemic situation.

The index of success most often demanded is that of a reduction in disease rates (though not all of the factors reponsible for venereal disease are amenable to health education action, for example, individual inadequacy or psychopathy). There is little evidence that the indiscriminate dissemination of information has any effect on behaviour though programmes of information with discussion can lay the foundations on which enlightened public opinion can grow (Burton, 1969).

A number of other studies have indicated the potential that health education may have for venereal disease control. Smith and Kane (1970) found that the ability to perceive the seriousness of a symptom was related to the health knowledge possessed, symptomatic perception being defined as the ability to discriminate the perceived severity of a symptom in terms of its requiring health action. Syphilis was included in the list of diseases they considered. Green (1970) investigated the effects on adolescents of single short talks about sexually transmitted disease, and found that months afterwards knowledge was higher amongst those who had received education than those who had not. The more specific the questions the more evident became the difference between the groups.

Subjective evaluation has been carried out by venereologists who report that the public, and particularly young people, are better informed about venereal disease than ever before and that their attitudes about sexual matters in general reflect the enlightened climate of opinion. Morton (1973) in a report to the Third International Symposium on V.D. Control, tries to measure the effect of public education in the control of venereal and other sexually transmitted diseases. After employing four approaches he admits their limitations in terms of objective assessment.

In Britain the Health Education Council has undertaken a programme of 'Forward Planning for Venereal Diseases Education'. This includes the evaluation of films and other aids together with the examination of multi-disciplinary approaches to the overall promotion and improvement of education for personal relationships, emphasising personal responsibility (Dalzell-Ward, 1970). A more specific evaluation of a venereal disease education programme has more recently been designed by the Health Education Council. A primary objective is defined, namely that of improving the contact tracing rate in the case of gonorrhoea. Baseline studies of the demographic characteristics of the area of the campaign were undertaken for the purposes of later comparison. This includes identifying V.D.-prone groups. A second aspect of this research concerns the impact of the communication methods on the target groups. This project was initiated in June 1972. Fuller results are awaited with interest. An interim report (H.E.C. Newsletter, July 1973) gives baseline data. (Dalzell-Ward, 1973). The findings of this study, and other well-designed evaluation projects involving inbuilt evaluation from the initial stages of planning, should provide valuable data for the development of more effective educational programmes.

PROFESSIONAL EDUCATION

The post-war decline in the incidence of venereal disease led to a fall in interest in the teaching of the subject in professional courses, and a generation of doctors and other medical and social workers grew up with little training or awareness of the seriousness of venereal diseases and of the importance of prevention. Worldwide attention was drawn to medical ignorance and the inadequacy of training by Webster (1966), Ravenholt (1966) and Adams (1967). The comparative indifference shown by some medical schools was demonstrated by Webster (1966a) who in a world survey found the average hours spent learning the subject were fewer in Britain (17 hours) and the United States (19 hours) than other areas (47 hours); despite the fact that Great Britain is probably the only country in the world where venereology is practised as a speciality (Alergant, 1970). In the United States the recognition that *all* health workers could come in contact with venereal disease patients at some time or other, and therefore needed education and objectivity, led to the design of special professional teaching kits (Lenz, 1966). By the mid-sixties there was a call for the integration of social and behavioural sciences into medical curricula to provide medical workers with an understanding and awareness of the variety of causes of individual and social pathology (James, 1967; Royal Commission, 1968). Burton

(1969a) emphasised that the effectiveness of clinical and public health workers depends to as great an extent on their understanding and participation in the life of the community in which they work, as on their technical ability. By 1970 as a result of joint W.H.O. and I.U.V.D.T. activity there was more interest in teaching undergraduates about venereal disease, including the public health and social aspects (Webster, 1970). The teaching of Behavioural Science in Health Education by faculties of medicine has been extensively developed in progressive universities such as Manchester (Baric, 1972). This example is being followed but slowly elsewhere.

The preparation of school teachers is nowhere adequate. Neser and Weichman (1967) in the United States found only 54 per cent of education majors had had sex education. Surprising gaps in the knowledge of those teaching about venereal disease have also been demonstrated (Glass et al, 1968). Personal experience has shown that in most instances it is rare for intending school teachers to be provided with adequate health education, particularly in sexual matters, to meet their own individual needs let alone the needs of their future students. This is true also in the case of those undertaking short post-graduate courses in education following degree training in other subjects. A similar lack of knowledge about venereal disease, and awareness of training in the importance of prevention, can be demonstrated amongst many other professional groups with a potential to contribute to public education, ie health visitors and nursing personnel generally (Fluker, 1966).

Doctors practising venereology as a speciality have not been as active or enthusiastic as might have been expected in their co-operation or support for both public and professional education programmes. All too few mirror the support for health education provided by their professional organisations or government and official agencies. Morton (1966) in a survey of the attitudes of British venereologists discovered that of those who completed his questionnaire (69 per cent returned) 17 per cent were not certain that venereal disease education of the public 'did any good' or felt it did 'more harm than good'. In another survey (Rowntree, 1968), venereologists were invited to co-operate in the assessment of the suitability of a television broadcast for use as a film for public education. Two of the respondents indicated 'they had better things to do with their time'. Such responses indicate only one end of the spectrum. At the other are those venereologists who actively involve themselves with professional and public education about sexually transmitted disease, through practical teaching or as writers of articles, booklets and books designed to interest and educate the general public and through their appearance and broadcasts on television and radio. Where such support has been manifested and co-operation extended in the implementation of local and national health education programmes, rapid steps forward have been made in the development of public awareness and the acceptance of venereal disease education. This has been adequately demonstrated in specific instances, for example, by Rowntree (1966).

General conclusions

Unfortunately, the medical profession, with venereologists in particular, remains divided and uncertain on the purpose, scope and methodology of health education, and the contribution its effective application can make to the prevention and control of disease. Many take the simplistic view that the transmission of knowledge will of itself alter the behaviour of 'the public' who they regard as a homogeneous whole rather than a pluralistic dynamic system of groups and individuals in a constant state of interaction. There has been some progress however, and there are signs of increasing interest and awareness of the contributions that exploitation of the behavioural sciences can make, for example, to the detection of 'at risk' groups and the development and implementation of health education programmes most likely to reach them.

The lesson of recent advances is clear: only by full utilisation of the behavioural sciences, long-range planning of comprehensive programmes, with clearly delineated and measurable objectives, and systematic evaluation at all stages is it likely that increasingly effective contributions to venereal disease control will be made by health education. The opportunities and rewards for health education have been demonstrated in many other aspects of health care and provide a challenge to venereology.

Coda

The challenge to venereology of the last decades of the twentieth century will not be met unless present day complacency is eradicated and clinical expertise matched by sociological insight, prophylactic zeal by proselytising fervour and rhetoric by research. Doctors, nurses, teachers, social workers and health educators will only effectively begin to exercise their complementary skills in the prevention of venereal disease when they understand the dynamics of the society in which it occurs, together with the importance of health education as the operational aspect of preventive medicine. Extension to the pathetically inadequate present-day training of each of these professions is needed to equip them with an insight and understanding of the behavioural aspects of disease, an awareness of the role of the social environment in disease causation and the consequences of social dysfunction.

Early research findings must be followed up to provide more accurate indices and indicators of vulnerability. The role of the medical profession as legitimisers of the 'at risk' as well as sick roles must be given closer study, and the existence of precursor pathology should be more precisely determined to provide earlier identification of 'at risk' groups. There must also be recognition and acceptance of the fact that the roles of the medico-social pathologist, the behavioural scientist and the health educator may be more important in the control of sexually transmitted disease in the latter part of the twentieth century than that of the clinical bacteriologist today.

REFERENCES

ADAMS, A. (1967). *Med. J. Aust.*, **1**, 145.

ALERGANT, C. D. (1970). *Brit. J. vener. Dis.*, **46**, 162.

AMERICAN SOCIAL HEALTH ASSOCIATION (1968). *Today's V.D. Control Problem.* American Social Health Association, New York.

ARYA, O. P. and BENNETT, F. J. (1968). *Brit. J. vener. Dis.*, **44**, 160.

BARIC, L. (1969). *Int. J. Hlth Educ.*, **12**, 24.

BARIC, L. (1972). *Int. J. Hlth Educ.* **15**, 1.

BIRD, M. S. (1965). *Brit. J. vener. Dis.*, **41**, 217.

BRITISH BROADCASTING CORPORATION (1973). 20*th century Focus—V.D.* B.B.C. Television, Non-Theatric Sales, Villiers House, London W5 2PA.

BRITISH FEDERATION AGAINST VENEREAL DISEASE (1958). *Med. Offr.*, **99**, 163.

BRITISH MEDICAL ASSOCIATION (1964). *Young People and V.D.* British Medical Association, London.

BURTON, J. (1969). *Hlth. Educ. J.*, **18**, 81.

BURTON, J. (1969a). Health education in behavioural medicine. In *Theory and Practice of Public Health*, 3rd ed. (ed. W. Hobson). Oxford University Press.

CHURCHILL FILMS (1969). 662 North Robertson Boulevard, Los Angeles, California, 90069 (available for sale only in the United Kingdom from Boulton-Hawker, Hadleigh, Ipswich, Suffolk, England).

CROTON, G. (1973). Private communication.

DALZELL-WARD, A. J. (1960). *Proc. Ann. Hlth Cong.* Royal Society of Health, London.

DALZELL-WARD, A. J., NICOL, C. S. and HOWARD, M. C. (1960). *Brit. J. vener. Dis.*, **36**, 106.

DALZELL-WARD, A. J. (1970). *Brit. J. vener. Dis.*, **46**, 159.

DALZELL-WARD, A. J. (1973). *Brit. J. vener. Dis.*, **49**, 171.

DEISHER, R. M. and MILLS, C. A. (1963). *Amer. J. Pub. Hlth*, **53**, 1928.

ELIAS, J. and GEBHARDT, P. (1969). *Phi Dalta Kappan*, **7**, 401.

EKSTRØM, K. (1970). *Brit. J. vener. Dis.*, **46**, 93.

FLUKER, J. L. (1966). *Brit. J. vener. Dis.*, **42**, 244.

FORER, R. (1965). *Pub. Hlth Rep.* **80**, 1015.

GLASS, L. and CAMPBELL, C. E. (1965). *J. Sch. Hlth*, **35**, 322.

GLASS, L., ATKINSON, L. and RICKETT, M. (1968). *Educ. Res.*, **11**, 135.

GREEN, W. J. (1970). *Health Education on the Sexually Transmitted Diseases.* Unpublished dissertation. Faculty of Medicine University of Manchester, England.

HOCHBAUM, G. (1960). *Health Education Monographs*, No. 8. Society of Public Health Educators, New York.

HOLLINS, F. R. and DICKS, S. (1968). *Med. Offr.*, **120**, 261.

HOLMES, M., NICOL, C. and STUBBS, R. (1968). *Educ. Res.*, **11**, 38.

HOSSAIN, A. S. M. T. (1969). *Pakistan Med. Rev.*, **4**, 18.

JAMES, G. (1967). *J. Amer. Med. Ass.*, **202**, 415.

JUHLIN, L. (1968). *Acta derm.-venereol., Stockh.*, **48**, 82.

KEIGHLEY, E. (1963). *Brit. J. vener. Dis.*, **39**, 278.

KELUS, J. (1973). *Brit. J. vener. Dis.*, **49**, 167.

KITE, E. DE C. and GRIMBLE, A. (1963). *Brit. J. vener. Dis.*, **39**, 173.

LAIRD, S. M. (1963). *Brit. J. vener. Dis.*, **39**, 280.

LENZ, E. P. (1966). *Pub. Hlth Rep.*, **81**, 996.

LEVIN, L. (1969). *Pub. Hlth Rep.*, **84**, 252.

MORTON, R. S. (1966). *Brit. J. vener. Dis.*, **42**, 238.

MORTON, R. S. (1967). *Nurs. Times.*, **63**, 657.

MORTON, R. S. (1973). *Report to the International Symposium on V.D. Control* held at New Orleans, U.S.A., (in the press).

NESER, W. B. and WEICHMANN, G. H. (1967). *Pub. Hlth Rep.*, **82**, 917.

PARSONS, T. (1951). *The Social System*, p. 208. Routledge and Kegan Paul, London.

PEDDER, J. R. and GOLDBERG, P. D. (1970). *Brit. J. vener. Dis.*, **46**, 58.

PONTING, L. I. (1963). *Brit. J. vener. Dis.*, **39**, 273.

PREBBLE, E. E. (1962). *Brit. J. vener. Dis.*, **38**, 86.

RAVENHOLT, O. (1966). *Arch. Envir. Hlth*, **13**, 367.

ROSENBLATT, D. and KABASAKALIAN, L. (1966). *Amer. J. Pub. Hlth*, **56**, 1104.

ROWNTREE, F. ST. D. (1966). *Brit. J. vener. Dis.*, **42**, 246.

ROWNTREE, F. ST. D. (1968). Unpublished Report.

ROWNTREE, F. ST. D. (1971). The new role of Sex Education. In *Communication and Behavioural Change*. Proc. 7th Int. Conf. International Union for Health Education, Geneva, Switzerland.

ROWNTREE, F. ST. D. (1972). *Drinking Behaviour of Industrial Adolescents.* Unpublished Thesis, Faculty of Medicine, University of Manchester, England.

ROYAL COMMISSION ON MEDICAL EDUCATION (1968). *Final Report of the Commission.* H.M.S.O., London.

ROYAL COMMISSION ON VENEREAL DISEASE (1916). *Final Report of the Commission.* H.M.S.O., London.

SCHOFIELD, M. (1965). *The Sexual Behaviour of Young People.* Longmans, London.

SEALE, J. R. (1966). *Brit. J. vener. Dis.*, **42**, 31.

SIGGER, V. (1972). Unpublished Report. Whitelands College, London.

SMITH, L. and KANE, R. (1970). *Social Sci. Med.*, **4**, 557.

STARCK-ROMANUS, V. (1973). *Brit. J. vener. Dis.*, **49**, 163.

STATHAM, R. (1968). *J. Inst. Hlth Educ.*, **6**, 29.

TORRIBIO, J. A. and GLASS, L. H. (1965). *Pub. Hlth Rep.*, **80**, 1.

U.I.C.C. (1967). *Public Education about Cancer: Research, findings and theoretical concepts.* Springer-Verlag, Berlin, Heidelberg and New York.

VERHAGEN, A. R. and GEMERT, W. (1972). *Brit. J. vener. Dis.*, **48**, 277.

WEBSTER, B. (1966). *Arch. Envir. Hlth*, **13**, 367.

WEBSTER, B. (1966a). *Brit. J. vener, Dis.*, **42**, 132.

WEBSTER, B. (1970). *Brit. J. vener. Dis.*, **46**, 156.

WHELDON, G. R. (1964). *J. R. Nav. Med. Serv.*, **50**, 109.

WILLCOX, R. R. (1962). *Brit. J. vener. Dis.*, **38**, 37.

YOUNG, M. A. C. (1967). *Review of Research and Studies Related to Health Education Practice* (1961–1966). *What People know, Believe and Do About Health.* Health Education Monograph No. 23. Society of Public Health Educators, New York.

YOUNG, M. A. C. and SIMMONS, J. J. (1967). *Review of Research and Studies Related to Health Education Practice* (1961–1966). *Psychosocial and Cultural Factors Related to Health Education Practice.* Health Education Monograph No. 24. Society of Public Health Educators, New York.

YOUNG, M. A. C. (1967a). *Review of Research and Studies Related to Health Education. Communication. Methods and Materials* (1961–1966). Health Education Monograph No. 25. Society of Public Health Educators, New York.

YOUNG, M. A. C. (1968). *Review of Research and Studies Related to Health Education Practice* (1961–1966). *Patient Education.* Health Education Monograph No. 26. Society of Public Health Educators, New York.

YOUNG, M. A. C. (1968a). *Review of Research and Studies Related to Health Education Practice* (1961–1966). *Program Planning and Evaluation.* Health Education Monograph No. 27. Society of Public Health Educators, New York.

YOUNG, M. A. C. (1969). *Review of Research and Studies Related to Health Education Practice* (1961–1966). *School Health Education.* Health Education Monograph No. 28. Society of Public Health Educators, New York.

47 Contact Tracing

R. S. Morton

Contact tracing is a two-part exercise—interview and action.

Interviewing endeavours to obtain the fullest personal details of the patient's primary or source sex partner as well as the same concerning any secondary contact or contacts, that is, those the patient may have infected following his contaminating exposure. The principle applies equally to male and female patients and their contacts. The work calls for many personal qualities, not least, tact, patience, persistence and a persuasive manner. The second part, action on the contact data, may be undertaken by any or all of the following:

(a) The patient using a contact slip.
(b) The interviewer using the telephone or writing.
(c) A health worker visiting the contact or contacts at home, work, or elsewhere.

To be maximally effective, the whole operation needs to be executed with speed, regularity, assertiveness and confidentiality. The guiding principle is a basic epidemiological one. For every infection found at least one other should be sought.

Other endeavours may be seen as extensions of contact tracing; for example, the mass surveys already described, special surveys of 'at risk' groups and 'cluster testing'. This last means inviting the social contacts, as well as the sexual contacts, of infected persons to have tests.

Contact tracing, assertively and thoroughly pursued, is generally agreed to be the most effective method of venereal disease control presently available.

In planning control by contact tracing Willcox (1965) points to the importance of paying attention to the 'feed back' mechanism, by which he means the continual renewal of the pool of occult gonorrhoea in females; and thus the maintenance of high infection rates. Willcox et al (1966) presented the results of their contact tracing efforts, starting with the contact data of 330 male West Indians attending St. Mary's Hospital, London, with gonorrhoea. About a quarter of the primary source contacts attended. Of secondary contacts nearly 90 per cent of those named as wives or regular girl friends were seen, but only 14 per cent of promiscuous and little-known primary contacts. Burgess (1966) noted that 449 syphilitics produced 517 sex and family contacts and that 77 (14·9 per cent), including three children, were found to be infected. The role of the social worker in this type of work was considered by Stubbs (1965). Gupta et al (1965) and Robertson (1965).

In the U.S.A. a *Medical News Report* (1965) stated that the public health authorities re-affirmed their intention to eradicate syphilis by 1970 by Special Task Force endeavours. The rise in the incidence of syphilis since the Task Force began its operation some 5 years earlier was considered a sign of successful case finding. The services offered to the private practitioner in this scheme were outlined and evaluated by Ball (1964). Brown (1966) stated that 20 per cent of the total number of persons attending with early syphilis did so through contact tracing, based on 700 000 reactive test results out of the country's annual number of serological tests for syphilis, judged to be 32 million. Friddell and Flye (1966), reporting from Tennessee, showed how one case of syphilis reported by a private practitioner resulted in a further 30 cases being traced and treated. This was underlined by Johnson (1966) who considered that the contact tracing services of public clinics should be made available and used by private practitioners. He demonstrated that much improved co-operation and effective working was possible if the practitioner knew the social worker personally. Successful efforts along these lines were also reported by Porter (1966).

A social worker operating in the U.K. calculated that in a single year, 1965, one in eight of all males with syphilis attended as a result of contact tracing. The figure was one in five in the case of gonorrhoea (Lamb, 1966). Muspratt and Ponting (1967) also working in the U.K. showed that as a result of issuing 799 contact slips to patients, and instructing them on their use, 453 (56·7 per cent) contacts attended for examination. A working party set up by the Department of Health examined current contact tracing methods in the U.K. and made recommendations. It also prompted changes in the law (The National Health Service (Venereal Disease) Regulations, 1968) which protects health workers from charges of libel or slander, provided of course that they act confidentially and in good faith on the contact data available to them.

Olsen (1966) working in Greenland described an outbreak of syphilis and showed how contact tracing in conjunction with other measures, such as routine serological testing and quarantine, were used in effective control. Co-operation with other specialists in case finding in Czechoslovakia was discussed by Potuznik (1967). According to Martin-Bouyer (1967) 14 per cent of gonorrhoea in males occurred through contact with asymptomatic prostitutes. The special problems these women pose to the contact tracer are discussed. Brown (1968) in the U.S.A. noted that whereas in 1962 only 45 per cent of privately treated gonorrhoea was reported, the figure in 1967 was 55 per cent. This improvement he saw as offering a springboard for control. Prather (1967) lamented the rising incidence of syphilis and gonorrhoea in the U.S.A. He sees contact tracing as the only hope of containing the increasingly depressing situation.

In 1970 there are some heartening reports. Hare et al (1970) working with social workers in London, and from a starting point of 119 men with gonorrhoea secured the attendance, by a variety of contact tracing techniques, of 40 per cent of 117 primary or source contacts and 82 per cent of 28 secondary contacts. The value of re-interviewing patients about their contacts was noted by Capiński and Urbańczyk (1970) in Poland. They were able to increase their 'yield' of attending contacts significantly. In the judgement of Brown (1970a) if one-third of all new cases of syphilis could be traced and treated before they exposed a secondary contact to infection, control to the point of eradication would be a real possibility. He lists the reasons preventing this. The same author, Brown (1970b), considered gonorrhoea in the U.S.A. out of control and likely to remain so until mass screening methods and a serological test for the disease became available. The role of the contact tracer in the U.S.A. was described by Mathias and Shook (1971).

Successful contact tracing in the control of gonorrhoea in parts of the U.K. was claimed by Morton (1970) and Dunlop et al (1971). Morton showed that a fall in the male : female ratio in gonorrhoea was restricted in its value as an indicator of successful contact tracing. The same trends existed in all other sections of his clinic population. He shows how the successful pursuit of contact tracing results in a growing number of infected females attending. The really significant break-through point comes when this rising female total results in a fall in the annual number of infected males. The paper by Dunlop et al states that whereas in 1960 only 6 per cent of source contacts attended; the figure in 1969 was 36 per cent. This tied up with the observation that whereas in the earlier year 31 per cent of the men claimed to have been infected by a paid prostitute, usually difficult to trace and identify, the figure in 1969 was 14 per cent. Morton (1972) takes up this point. He suggests that at least in the U.K. a higher percentage of infected people nowadays know their source contact. Furthermore in this age of sexual freedom people are much more frank and honest in the interview situation so that contact data for effective action has never been so plentiful. Thus, although contact tracing is called for more than ever before, it has never been easier or so full of potential as today.

In Denmark, Pedersen and Harrah (1970) looked at the productivity of contact tracing in another way. They noted that 88·5 per cent of 748 named male contacts were found infected. All but 19 (2·5 per cent) had been treated when traced. By contrast, of 583 named females contacts 77·7 per cent were found infected and of these 222 (38 per cent) had not previously sought examination or treatment.

Bernfeld (1971) found 22 cases of gonorrhoea following the attendance of an infected lorry driver. Lesiński et al (1971) in Poland, starting with a case-load of 171 syphilitics, 75 with early infectious disease, traced a further 34 infected persons. Pemberton et al (1972) in reviewing the socio-medical characteristics of patients attending a venereal diseases clinic in Northern Ireland point out that there is a group of women, highly promiscuous and frequently named as source contacts, who are only infrequently traced. The importance of identifying, tracing and treating these women is seen as a vital part of the whole operation of contact tracing, the establishment of control and its subsequent maintenance.

Thin (1972) reported on the contact tracing methods used by the British Army in the Republic of Singapore. The close liaison with civilian services helped to give a remarkably high yield of source contacts.

Elste (1968) described the exchange of contact data between European countries. A growing number of countries are establishing international contact tracing bureaux. At a meeting in Copenhagen under the auspices of W.H.O. (*Brit. J. vener. Dis.* (1973) **49**, 89) the problem of dissemination of infection throughout the European continent was discussed. Arrangements were agreed to improve international contact tracing.

In the U.S.A. Bloont (1972) reported on the costs of interviewing and contact-visiting. Nearly 10 000 patients were concerned. Males attending of their own accord each produced a contact at a cost of $6.16. Females attending a family planning clinic and being found infectious had their contact data successfully acted on at a cost of $7.04. These two groups give the extremes of costs of what appears to have been very successful contact tracing. Marino et al (1972) questions just how worthwhile contact tracing is. Interviewing 799 women for 5 to 8 minutes produced data on 945 men of whom 833 attended for examination. The group could be divided into three more or less equal parts: those already treated; those in need of treatment; and those found uninfected. Male contacts were frequently asymptomatic. Those with symptoms, sometimes for as long as 30 days, often continued to indulge in sexual intercourse. The same study also concerned itself with a study from the interviewing of 1 550 infected men. They gave contact data on 2 322 women of whom 1 865 attended. Gonorrhoea was diagnosed in 56 per cent. Thus of the total gonorrhoea treated in Marino's department 41·4 per cent attended by invitation. Karolyi (1972), from Hungary, suggests that there is need to direct control efforts to the countryside where the incidence of infection is rising much faster than in the capital city, Budapest.

Perdrup (1973) outlines the 200 years of venereal disease legislation in Denmark. Contact tracing in that country may well involve police action. The view of Danish venereologists is that this is an outmoded approach and should be replaced by public education to engender a greater awareness of social obligation, one person to another.

Some of the details of contact tracing procedures as pursued in the U.K. are outlined by Morton (1972).

Final coda

W.H.O.'s Director-General Dr. Marcolino Candau in his annual report for 1972 notes that venereal disease is spreading so rapidly that it is threatening to become completely out of control. Quick action, he says, is essential to avert this.

Many of the control measures reported have not been pursued everywhere with a force and vigour likely to fulfil their potential. The responsibility falls heaviest on the clinicians. Matters can be improved only if they publicise the facts and press their epidemiologists, demographers and medical administrators to act on an appreciation of what is needed by way of facilities and services.

Dr. Candau says, 'In almost all countries the annual increase in prevalence [of gonorrhoea] is as high as 10 per cent'. The situation is 'perhaps a little less alarming' in regard to syphilis.

Few medical administrators and no politicians have shown such awareness. International bodies have done little. The International Union against the Venereal Diseases and Treponematosis (I.U.V.D.T.) has called from time to time for action by governments. The World Medical Association does not appear to be aware of the problem. There is a need for these bodies to act with more vigour and effectiveness.

Through Dr. Candau the W.H.O. has identified the problem but it has shown no new initiatives. Such bodies as the I.U.V.D.T. should be calling for these. Leadership is needed in every field of V.D. control. Action is required for speedier dissemination of epidemiological data, for the establishment of more reference laboratories, provision of many more training scholarships and provision too of an early warning system, reporting regular monitoring of the antibiotic sensitivity of the gonococcus. Also needed is greater and more direct pressure on medical schools to provide professional education about venereal diseases and to stimulate research. Not least, W.H.O. could do even more by way of ensuring that accepted methods and recent advances are used.

Better prospects for implementing such measures would be available if W.H.O. reverted to its original policy of providing each of its regional offices with an adviser specifically trained and experienced in V.D. and its control. The problem is again too big to be left to general epidemiologists. If W.H.O. fails to involve itself deeply in active leadership now, the outlook will indeed be bleak. Early action could make the next edition of 'Recent Advances in Sexually Transmitted Diseases' less depressing than this one.

REFERENCES

BALL, R. W. (1964). *J. Amer. med. Ass.*, **193**, 13.
BERNFELD, W. K. (1971). *Brit. J. vener. Dis.*, **47**, 54.
BLOONT, J. H. (1972). *Amer. J. Publ. Hlth*, **62**, 710.
BROWN, W. J. (1966). *Bol. Sanit. Pan-am.*, **60**, 93.
BROWN, W. J. (1968). *J. Amer. med. Ass.*, **205**, 800.
BROWN, W. J. (1970a). *Ann. intern. Med.*, **72**, 278.
BROWN, W. J. (1970b). *Ann. intern. Med.*, **72**, 280.
BURGESS, J. A. (1966). *Brit. J. vener. Dis.*, **42**, 116.
CAPIŃSKI, T. Z. and URBAŃCZYK, J. (1970). *Brit. J. vener. Dis.*, **46**, 138.
DUNLOP, E. M. C., LAMB, A. M. and KING, D. M. (1971). *Brit. J. vener. Dis.*, **47**, 192.
ELSTE, G. (1968). *Dtsch. Gesundh.*, **23**, 2489.
FRIDDELL, T. J. and FLYE, R. E. (1966). *J. Penn. med. Ass.*, **59**, 141.
GUPTA, B. L., MATHUR, A. S. and SAYENA, K. N. (1965). *Med. Digest*, **33**, 178.
HARE, M. J., LAMB, A. M. and KING, D. M. (1970). *Brit. J. vener. Dis.*, **46**, 485.
JOHNSON, A. N. (1966). *Arch. Envir. Hlth*, **13**, 393.
KAROLYI, I. (1972). *Derm. Vener. Halad.*, **16**, 3.
LAMB, A. M. (1966). *Brit. J. vener. Dis.*, **42**, 276.
LESIŃSKI, J., SERWATKO, M. et al (1971). *Przegl. Derm.*, **58**, 163.
MARINO, A. F., PARISER, H. and WISE, H. (1972). *Amer. J. Publ. Hlth.*, **62**, 714.
MARTIN-BOUYER, G. (1967). *Bull Inst. Nata. Sanit.*, **72**, 1021.
MATHIAS, T. W. and SHOOK, J. B. (1971). *H.S.M.H.A. Hlth Rep.*, **86**, 107.
Medical News (1965). December, p. 5.
MORTON, R. S. (1970). *Brit. J. vener. Dis.*, **46**, 103.
MORTON, R. S. (1972). *Venereal Diseases*, 2nd ed. Penguin Books Ltd., Harmondsworth, London.
MUSPRATT, B. and PONTING, L. I. (1967). *Brit. J. vener. Dis.*, **43**, 204.
OLSEN, L. A. (1966). *Ugeskr. Laeg.*, **128**, 1071.
PEDERSEN, A. H. B. and HARRAH, W. D. (1970). *Publ. Hlth Rep.*, **85**, 997.
PEMBERTON, J., MCCANN, J. S. and MAHONEY, J. D. H. et al. (1972). *Brit. J. vener. Dis.*, **48**, 391.
PERDRUP, A. (1973). *Brit. J. vener. Dis.*, **49**, 174.
PORTER, W. L. (1966). *Med. Times, Manhasset*, **94**, 1218.
POTUZNIK, V. (1967). *Cesk. Derm.*, **42**, 217.
PRATHER, E. C. (1967). *J. Florida med. Ass.*, **54**, 1038.
ROBERTSON, E. A. (1965). *Canad. J. Publ. Hlth*, **56**, 142.
STUBBS, R. K. T. (1965). *Brit. J. vener. Dis.*, **41**, 214.
THIN, R. N. T. (1972). *Brit. J. vener. Dis.*, **45**, 542.
WILLCOX, R. R. (1965). *Acta derm.-venerol., Stockh.*, **45**, 302.
WILLCOX, R. R., JEFFERISS, F. J. G. and NAUGHTEN, E. M. (1966). *Brit. J. vener. Dis.*, **42**, 167.
W.H.O. Meeting in Copenhagen (1973). *Brit. J. vener. Dis.*, **49**, 89.

Appendix

Reference sources

Excepta Medica
Abstracts of Hygiene including the annual review *Perspectives in Venereology* by R. R. Willcox.
Abstracts of Current Literature on Venereal Diseases published by the U.S. Department of Health, Education and Welfare.
British Journal of Venereal Diseases.
Reference lists provided by W.H.O.
Reference lists provided by the Royal College of Physicians, Edinburgh.
Cumulative Index Medicus
Penicillin in the Treatment of Syphilis (1972). O. Idsøe, T. Guthe and R. R. Willcox. W.H.O.
Treponematosis Research (1970). W.H.O. Technical Report Series, No. 455.

Other works consulted

Clinical Rheumatology (1971). J. A. Boyle and W. W. Buchanan. Blackwell.
Medical Mycology (1970). 2nd ed., C. W. Emmondes, C. H. Binford and J. P. Utz. Lee and Febiger, Philadelphia.
Benign Diseases of the Vulva and Vagina (1969). H .L. Gardner and R. H. Kaufman. Mosely, St. Louis.
Recent Advances in Venereology (1964). A. J. King. Churchill Livingstone, London.
Venereal Diseases (1969) 2nd ed., A. J. King and C. S. Nicol. Ballière-Tindall and Cassell, London.
Current problems in Dermatology (1968). A. Lugar, Vol. 2, Karger, Basle and New York.
Venereal Diseases (1972). 2nd ed., R. S. Morton. Penguin Books, London.
Sexual Freedom and Venereal Diseases (1971). R. S. Morton. Peter Owen, London.
Microbes and Morals (1972). T. Roseberry. Secker and Warburg, London.
Sexually Transmitted Diseases (1972). C. B. S. Schofield. Churchill Livingstone, London and Edinburgh.
Progress in Venereology (1953). R. R. Willcox. Heinemann, London.
A Text Book of Venereal Diseases and Treponematoses (1964). 2nd ed., R. R. Willcox. Heinemann, London.

Index

Abortions, septic, and *Corynebacterium vaginale* infection 357
Actinospectacin, in gonorrhoea 79
'Adenexitis' in trichomoniasis 211
Adolescents, gonorrhoea in 18
  sexual behaviour 390
  venereal infections in 372
American Social Health Association 392
Amies' carrier medium 48
Aminobenzylpenicillin *see* Ampicillin
Amnionitis, gonococcal 35
Ampicillin, in gonorrhoea 72
  in syphilis 168
Antibiotic resistance and gonorrhoea 12
  sensitivity testing for gonococci 48
Antibiotics, relationship to candidiasis 236
  therapeutic use in non-specific urethritis 296–299
Antibodies, immunoglobulin, in syphilitic sera 141
  thermostability 143
Antibody types in treponemal infection (Table) 127
Antifungal agents, use in candidiasis 246
Antigens, gonococcal 63
Anti-lipoidal antibody, tests for 128
Aortic incompetence in syphilis 105
ART *see* Automated Reagin Test
Arthritis, Chlamydia and 290, 291
Arthritis, gonococcal 35, 36, 37
Artificial insemination, and gonorrhoea 39
Aspirin, therapeutic use in Reiter's disease 314, 315
Automated Reagin Test (ART) 129
Automation of screening tests 128
Australia antigen 350–352

Bactrim, in gonorrhoea 82

Balanitis, candidal 241
Balano-posthitis 231
  in candidiasis 240
  therapy 246
Bartholin ducts, gonococcal infection 38
Bashke–Lowenstein tumour 340
Bedsonia *see* Chlamydia
Behavioural aspects of venereal disease 375
Benign gonococcaemia 37
Benzyl benzoate, in treatment of scabies 348
Bertholinitis 258
BIC globulin, in secondary syphilis 99
'Bioanalyst' 129
Biochemical test media for gonococci 47
Biogen fermenter 54
Biopsy in granuloma inguinale 196
Bismuth, in syphilis therapy 165
Blood–brain barrier in secondary syphilis 104
British Federation against Venereal Disease 389

Candida albicans 232
Candida krusei 232
Candida parapsilosis 232
Candida stellatoidea 232
Candida tropicalis 232
Candidal balano-posthitis 231
  therapy 246
Candidiasis, clinical aspects 240–242
  epidemiology 231–233
  following drug therapy 235–238
  laboratory aspects 243, 244
  lichen simplex in 242
  oral contraceptives and 236, 237
  perianal 240, 241
    therapy 246
  vaginal plaques in 242
  predisposing factors 235–238

411

Candidiasis (*contd.*)
  pregnancy and 233, 235
  social aspects 231–233
  therapy 246–248
  trichomoniasis and 212
  vulval erythema in 241
  vulval pruritis in 241
Carcinoma, cervical and genital herpes 333
Carcinomatous change in granuloma inguinale 196
Cardiolipin *F* antibody 130
Cardiovascular aspects of Reiter's Disease 310, 311
Cardiovascular syphilis 105
Case reporting of gonorrhoea 8
Cell culture, of Chlamydia 280
Cell mediated immunity in syphilis 156, 174
Cephaloridine, in syphilis 169
Cephalosporins, in gonorrhoea 82
Cerebro-spinal fluid examination in secondary syphilis 104
Cerebro-spinal fluid, FTA tests on 136
Cervical cancer and genital herpes 333
Cervical cancer and trichomoniasis 205
Cervical cytology examination in trichomoniasis 206
Cervical erosion and trichomoniasis 206
Cervicitis 258
Cervicitis, in herpes genitalis 329
Chancroid 185–187
Children, gonorrhoea in 39
  leucorrhoea in 39
  Reiter's disease in 309
Chlamydia 188, 190
  arthritis and 290, 291
  culture in yolk sac 275, 284
  cell culture of 280
  experimental infection of animals 290
  and eye diseases 262–264, 275–278, 283–286
  genital reservoir of infection 290
  gonorrhoea and 286
  group and non-specific genital infection 262–265, 283–286
  infections, chemotherapy 299
  infection, tests for 275–283
  laboratory aspects 275–286
  lympho granuloma venereum (?) and 291
  micro-immunofluorescence test 281–283

non-specific genital infection and 291
  non-gonococcal urethritis and 285
  pathogenicity 283–286
  radio-isotope precipitation test 283
  Reiter's disease and 287–289
  terminology 278–280
  urethritis and 285
Chloramphenicol, in gonorrhoea 81
  in syphilis 168
Chronic biological false positive reaction in syphilis tests 174–181
  mechanism of 177
  significance of 175
Clinical aspects of syphilis 97–119
Clinical services in venereal disease 380–385
  legal aspects 381
'Cluster testing' in contact tracing 402
Condylomata accuminata, genital 338–341
Condylomata lata in secondary syphilis 310
'Condylomatosis', genital 338
Congenital syphilis 112
  deafness in 117
  eighth nerve involvement 117
  nephrotic syndrome in 115
  radiological diagnosis 116
  therapy 166
  thrombocytopenia in 116
Conjunctivitis, acute follicular, complicating non-specific genital infection 258
  Parinaud's 291
Contraceptive pill and gonorrhoea 12, 23
Contact tracing 402–407
  costs 405
Contact treatment in venereal disease 381–384
Corticosteroids, association with candidiasis 236, 241
  contra-indication in secondary syphilis 102
  in syphilis 165
  therapeutic use in Reiter's disease 316, 317
Corynebacterium vaginale infection 354–359
  treatment 358
Co-trimoxazole, in gonorrhoea 82
'Crab' lice, genital 342, 343
Crede's method 38
Cryoglobulins in syphilitic sera 143
Cultivation, gonococcal 57

Culture media for gonococci 46
Columbia blood agar base 47
Cystine trypticase agar 47
Cystitis, acute abacterial 258
    haemorrhagic 258
Cytochalasin 61
Cytology, cervical, in trichomoniasis 206
Cytomegalovirus infection 361–363
    mononucleosis 362

D.D.T., use in phthiris pubis infestation 342, 343
Deafness, in congenital syphilis 117
    in secondary syphilis 103
'Delayed' test for gonorrhoea 46
Denmark, gonorrhoea in 19–21
Di-iodohydroxyquinolone pessaries in candidiasis 247
Disseminated gonococcal infection 35, 37
Doctors, training in venereal disease 396–398
Donovania granulomatis 194
Donovaniosis 194–197
Dysplasia, and trichomoniasis 206
Dysuria, trichomoniasis and 210

Ecological forces in venereal disease (diagram) 17
Eighth nerve involvement in congenital syphilis 117
Electron microscopy, Treponema pallidum 148
Elephantiasis, vulval, in lymphogranuloma venereum 189
Emotional instability, and venereal disease 28
Endocervical hyperplasia and trichomoniasis 206
Endotoxin, gonococcal 63
Epidemiological treatment in venereal disease 381–383
Epidemiology, of candidiasis 231–233
    of cytomegalovirus infection 361
    of gonorrhoea 7–14
    of granuloma inguinale 194
    of herpes genitalis 325–329
    of lymphogranuloma venereum 188
    of non-specific genital infections 253–256
    of non-specific urethritis 253–256
    of Reiter's disease 303
    of scabies 345
    of syphilis 91–93
    of trichomoniasis 203–208
Epididymitis 258
    in trichomoniasis 211
Erythema, vulval, in candidiasis 241
Erythromycin, in gonorrhoea 81
    in non-specific urethritis 298
    in syphilis 168
Evans' blue 45
Experimental infections, gonococcal 61
    syphilis 148–153
Eye, diseases, and chlamydia 262–264, 275–278
    in syphilis 111

False positive reactions in granuloma inguinale 196
    in lymphogranuloma venereum tests 191
    in syphilitic tests 175
Females, incidence of gonorrhoea 23
Films in venereal disease education 393, 394
Fimbriae, role in gonococcal virulence 57, 64
Fitzheigh–Curtis syndrome 39
Flazo orange 45
Fluorescein isothiocyanate 45, 137
Fluorescent antibody technique for candidiasis 244
    antibody testing 45
    antibody testing in secondary syphilis 99
    treponemal antibody test 133, 175
    on cerebro-spinal fluid 136
Fortus, cytomegalovirus infection and 363
Frei skin test for lymphogranuloma venereum 190
FTA see Fluorescent treponemal antibody

Gamma benzene hexachloride, in treatment of scabies 348
Gas chromatography, Treponema pallidum 149
General paralysis of insane (G.P.I.) 107
Genital 'condylomatosis' 338
Genital herpes see also Herpes genitalis
Genital herpes virus, in gonorrhoea 38
Genital infection, non-specific 251–300
Genital tract, male, in candidiasis 240
Genital warts 338 341
Gentamicin sulphate, in gonorrhoea 83
Gentian violet, use in candidiasis 247

Glycosuria, candidiasis and   235
Gonococcal antigens   63
  arthritis   35, 36, 37
  complement fixation test (G.C.F.T.)
      44, 49, 50
  conjunctivitis, neo-natal   37
  dermatitis syndrome   35
  endotoxin   63
  meningitis   39
  perihepatitis   39
  pharyngitis   33
  proctitis   32
  research   54–67
  salpingitis   34
  septicaemia   35
Gonococci, antibiotic sensitivity (table)
    71
  antibiotic sensitivity testing   48
  biochemical test media   47
  colony types   55, 56
  cultivation   54
  culture media   46
  destruction and phagocytosis   60
  L forms, culture   47
  sensitivity to penicillin (Table)   70
  serological tests   49, 63
  transport media   48
  type variation and virulence   55
Gonorrhoea, adolescents and   18
  antibiotic resistance and   12
  artificial insemination and   39
  asymptomatic male carrier   32, 40
  case reporting   8
  and children   39
  Chlamydia in   286
  clinical aspects   32–41
  complicated infection   34–39
  contraceptive pill and   12, 23
  control   371–377
  crab louse infestation and   342
  diagnostic problems   40
  dissemination of infection   7
  experimental infections   61
  genital herpes virus in   38
  immigrants and   26
  epidemiological aspects   7–14
  in Denmark   19–21
  in Hungary   21, 22
  incidence in females   23
  increased incidence   371–377
  international variables   10
  joint lesions   37
  laboratory procedures   44–51
  penicillin dosage schedules   69
  penile infection   38

  radiobioassay   65
  recurrence   72
  research developments   54–67
  seafarers and   24
  seasonality   12
  skin lesions   37
  social aspects   15–31
  strain markers   66
  therapy   69–84
  urethritis and   253, 254
  vaccine possibilities   65
Granuloma inguinale   194–197
Group anti-treponemal antibody   130

Haematospermia, in trichomoniasis   211
Haemophilus ducreyi   185
Haemophilus vaginalis   354, 357
Haemophilus vaginalis, in non-specific
    urethritis   254
Halberstaedter–Prowazek inclusion body
    276
HBAg see Australia antigen
Health care delivery system, aims   391
Health education   388–399
  evaluation of   394–396
Health Education Council   396
Health information, communication of
    391
Helminths, sexually transmitted   365–
    366
Herpes genitalis   325–334
  cervical cancer and   333
  clinical aspects   329–331
  laboratory tests   331, 332
  neonatal infection   328, 329
  sexual transmission   328
  treatment   332, 333
Herpes virus, genital, in gonorrhoea   38
Herpes virus hominis   325, 334
Herpes virus, photodynamic inactivation
    333
Homosexuals, helminths in   365
  protozoa in   365
  syphilis in   94
  venereal disease in   26, 373
  viral hepatitis B and   350–352
Humoural   immune   mechanisms   in
    syphilis   155, 174
Hungary, gonorrhoea in   21, 22

5-IDU see 5-Iodo-2-deoxyuridine
IgM FTA tests in diagnosis of neonatal
    syphilis   136
Immigrants, venereal infections and
    374

Immunisation, against syphilis 158
Immunity in syphilis 155–160
Immunochemical staining of spiro-
    chaetes 152
Immunofluorescence *see also* Fluores-
    cent antibody testing
Immunofluorescence methods for detec-
    tion of *T. pallidum* 138
  technical advances in 138
Immunoglobulin class of antibodies in
    syphilitic sera 141
'Indirect' test for gonorrhoea 46
Indomethacin, therapeutic use in Reiter's
    disease 316
Infection, gonococcal, dissemination 7
Inguinal adenitis in chancroid 186
International contact tracing bureaux
    405
International Union Against Venereal
    Diseases and Treponematoses
    389, 397, 406
International variables, in gonorrhoea
    10
Interstitial keratitis in syphilis 117
Interviewing in contact tracing 402
5-Iodo-2-deoxyuridine, use in herpes
    genitalis 332
Iso Vitalex 47

Jarish–Herxheimer reaction 165, 168
JH reaction *see* Jarish–Herxheimer
    Reaction
Joint lesions, in gonorrhoea 37

Kanamycin, in gonorrhoea 78
Kellogg's gonococcal colony types 55
Keratitis, interstitial, in syphilis 117
Koebner phenomenon, and chlamydial
    infection 286

L forms of gonococci, culture 47
Laboratory aspects, of Chlamydia 275–
    286
  non-specific genital infections 267–
    274
  Reiter's disease 304–306
Laboratory tests for candidiasis 243,
    244
  for neurosyphilis 110
Laminectomy in tabetic spinal arthro-
    pathy 108
Latent syphilis 104
Legal aspects of venereal disease control
    381

Leucorrhoea, in children 39
  in *Corynebacterium vaginale* infection
    357
  trichosomiasis and 210
Leukaemia, association with scabies
    347
Lichen simplex in candidiasis 242
Lipid composition of treponemes 149
Lipopolysaccharide haemagglutination
    test 50
Lissamine rhodamine labelled albumin
    45
Lupoid sclerosis 176
Lymph channels, venereal disease of
    188
Lymphocyte transformation reaction in
    syphilis 157
Lymphogranuloma venereum 188–192
  Chlamydia and 291

Malnutrition, candidiasis in 235
McLeod–Reyman medium 48
Mass surveys of venereal disease 381–
    384
Meningitis, gonococcal 39
Metabolism, abnormal, association with
    candidiasis 236
Methotrexate, therapeutic use in Reiter's
    disease 317, 318
Metronidazole, predisposing to candi-
    diasis 236
  in trichomoniasis 202
'M' fluorescence 178
Micro-immunofluorescence test, for
    Chlamydia 281–283
Micro-immunofluorescence typing test
    for *Lymphogranuloma venereum*
    191
Molluscum contagiosum 336, 337
Mononucleosis, cytomegalovirus 362
Morbus gallicus 376
Mycoplasma fermantans 268
Mycoplasma hominis 258–261, 272, 273
Mycoplasmas, in newborn 259
  in non-specific urethritis 258–262
    laboratory aspects 268–272
  nomenclature 268
  non-specific urethritis and 268–274
  post-gonococcal urethritis and 269–
    271
  sexual intercourse and 268
Myelography in neurosyphilis 108

National Health Service (Venereal
    Disease) Regulations, 1968 403
Neisseria gonorrhoeae 34

Neisseria lactamicis 34
Neisseria meningitidis 34
Neonatal syphilis, IgM FTA tests for 136
Nephritis, association with scabies 347
Nephrotic syndrome, in congenital syphilis 115
  in secondary syphilis 99
Neuralgic amyotrophy, in Reiter's disease 311
Neurosyphilis 107–111
  diagnostic criteria 109
  laboratory tests 110
  therapy 165
Newborn, eye diseases, and Chlamydia 262–264, 276, 277
  and Mycoplasma 273
  herpes genitalis and 328–330
  mycoplasmal infections in 259, 273, 274
  trichomoniasis infection in 207
NGU *see* Non-gonococcal urethritis
Non-gonococcal urethritis, Chlamydia and 285
Non-specific genital infection 251–300
  and Chlamydia 262–265, 283–286, 291
  chlamydial, eye diseases and 262–265, 283–286
  clinical aspects 257–265
  epidemiological aspects 253–265
  laboratory aspects 267–274
  sexual intercourse and 253
  social aspects 253–256
Non-specific urethritis, asymptomatic 258
  clinical aspects 257, 258
  detection of Chlamydia in 264
  diagnosis 264
  epidemiology 253–256
  in *Haemophilus vaginalis* 254
  mycoplasmal association 268–274
  mycoplasmas in 258–262
    laboratory aspects 268–272
  therapeutic aspects 296–299
Non-venereal treponematoses 124
Norwegian scabies 346
NSU *see* Non-specific urethritis
Nystatin, therapeutic use in candidiasis 246–248

Obesity, candidiasis in 235
Ophthalmia neonatorum 37
  Chlamydial 263, 264, 276, 277, 283, 290

mycoplasmal 273
Oral contraceptives and candidiasis 236, 237
Out-patient services in venereal disease 382

Parinaud's conjunctivitis 291
Penicillin, adverse reactions to 167
  allergy to 167
  by injection, in gonorrhoea 73
  gonococcal sensitivity (Table) 70
  in syphilis 162
    dosage 164
  oral, in gonorrhoea 72
Penis, gonorrhoeal infection 38
  oedema, in lymphogranuloma venereum 189
Peri-anal candidiasis 240, 241
  therapy 246
  warts 340
Pelvic infection 258
Perihepatitis, gonococcal 39
PSU *see* Post-gonococcal urethritis
Phagocytosis and destruction of gonococci 60
Pharyngeal/tonsillar infection, gonococcal 33
Phimosis, in chancroid 185
Photocolposcopy, in trichomoniasis 212
Photodynamic inactivation of herpes viruses 333
Phthiris pubis infestation 342, 343
Phytohaemagglutinin 157
Pleuropneumonia-like organisms 267
Polymorphs in urethral pus 59
Post-gonococcal urethritis 253, 255
Post-gonococcal urethritis, detection of Chlamydia in 264, 284–286
Post-gonococcal urethritis, mycoplasmal association 269–271
Posture, therapeutic, in Reiter's disease 314
Potassium hydroxide preparation for diagnosis of candidiasis 243
PPLO *see* Pleuropneumonia-like organisms
Precipitin test 49
Prednisone, in congenital syphilis 118
Pregnancy, candidiasis in 233, 235, 242
  T-mycoplasma in 260
Pre-menstrual urethritis 258
Primary syphilis 97
  diagnosis 98
Probenecid, in syphilis 163

Proctitis, gonococcal 32
in lymphogranuloma venereum 189
Prostatitis 257, 258
in trichomoniasis 210
Prostitutes, venereal disease in 25, 375
Protozoa, sexually transmitted 365–366
Pruritis, in trichomoniasis 210
vulval, in candidiasis 241
Pseudo-bubo in granuloma inguinale 195
Psychiatric factors in venereal disease 391
Pyuria, abacterial 258

Rabbits, experimental syphilis in 152
Radiobioassay, in gonorrhoea 65
Radio-isotope precipitation test, for Chlamydia 283
lymphogranuloma venereum 191
Rapid plasma reagin (RPR) card test 128
Reagin, tests for 128
antibody, sensistivity of tests for 129
Rectum, stricture, in lymphogranuloma venereum 189
Reiter protein complement-fixation test (RPCF) 130
Reiter's disease 36, 303–318
aetiological factors 305, 306
cardiovascular aspects 310, 311
in children 309
Chlamydia and 287–289
clinical aspects 308–312
complicating non-specific genital infection 258
differential diagnosis 310
epidemiology of 303
genetic aspects 304
laboratory aspects 304–306
neurological complications 311
therapy 314–318
'Repeaters' 27
Report of the National Commission on Venereal Disease (1972) 385
Research developments in gonorrhoea 54–67
Reticulo-endothelial involvement in secondary syphilis 103
Rheumatoid factor in syphilitic sera 143
Rhodamine conjugated anti-staphylococcal serum 45
Rifadin, in gonorrhoea 83
Rifampicin, in gonorrhoea 83
Rimactone, in gonorrhoea 83

RIP test see Radio-isotope precipitation test
Rovamycin, in gonorrhoea 81
Royal Commission on Venereal Disease (1961) 388
RPCF see Reiter protein complement-fixation
RPR see Rapid plasma reagin

Salpingitis, gonococcal 34
mycoplasmas and 272, 273
'Saxophone penis' in lymphogranuloma venereum 189
Scabies 344–348
clinical aspects 346
laboratory aspects 347
treatment 348
Schaudin, Franz Richard 377
School teachers, training in sex education 397
Screening tests, automation of 128
Seafarers, gonorrhoea and 24
venereal infections in 374
Seasonality, and gonorrhoea 12
of trichomoniasis 204
Secondary syphilis 99–104
BIC globulin in 99
blood-brain barrier in 104
cerebro spinal fluid examination 104
condylomata lata in 103
corticosteroid contra-indications 102
deafness in 103
diagnosis from viral hepatitis 100
fluorescent antibody testing 99
negative serological tests 103
nephrotic syndrome in 99
reticulo-endothelial involvement in 103
Septicaemia, gonococcal 35
Septrin, in gonorrhoea 82
Serological tests for gonorrhoea 49, 63
negative, in secondary syphilis 103
Serology, syphilis 127–143
Serum immunoglobulin levels in syphilis 140
Servicemen, venereal infections in 374
Sex education 390–394
Sexual behaviour of adolescents 390
Sexual intercourse, as cause of non-specific genital infection 253
helminths and 365–366
herpes genitalis and 328
mycoplasmal infection and 268
protozoa and 365–366
viral hepatitis B and 350–352

Sexual transmission of trichomoniasis
    207
Silver impregnation staining methods
    for *Treponema pallidum* 152
Skin lesions, in gonorrhoea 37
Slide flocculation test 50
Social aspects of candidiasis 231–233
    of cytomegalovirus infection 361
    of gonorrhoea 15–31
    of granuloma inguinale 194
    of herpes genitalis 325–329
    of lymphogranuloma venereum 188
    of non-specific genital infections
        253–256
    of scabies 345
    of syphilis 93–95
    of trichomoniasis 203–208
Soft sore 185–187
Spectinomycin, in gonorrhoea 79
Spectinomycin sulphate, in syphilis
    169
Speech discrimination test 119
Spiramycin, in gonorrhoea 81
    in syphilis 169
Sterility, T-mycoplasma and 261
    in trichomoniasis 205
Strain markers, gonococcal 66
Streptomycin, in chancroid 186
    in gonorrhoea 78
    in granuloma inguinale 196
Stricture, urethral 258
Stuart's carrier medium 48
Students, venereal disease in 26
Sulmycin, in gonorrhoea 83
Sulphonamides, for chancroid 187
    in lymphogranuloma venereum 191
Synovial fluid, in Reiter's disease 306
Syphilis, ampicillin therapy 168
    aortic incompetence in 105
    bismuth therapy 165
    cardiovascular 105
    cell mediated immunity 156, 174
    cephaloridine in 169
    chloramphenicol therapy in 168
    chronic biological false positive reac-
        tion 174–181
        mechanism of 177
        significance of 174
    clinical aspects 97–119
    congenital 112
    control 371–377
    corticosteroids in 165
    epidemiology 91–93
    erythromycin in 168
    experimental 148–153

eye and 111
false positive reactions 175
history of 376
homosexual spread 94
humoural immune mechanisms 155,
    174
immunisation against 158
immunity in 155–160
increased incidence 371–377
latent 104
lymphocyte transformation reaction
    157
neonatal, IgM FTA tests for 136
penicillin as therapy 162
    dosage 164
primary 97
probenecid in 163
secondary 99–104
serology 127–143
serum immunoglobulin levels in 140
social aspects 93–95
visceral 105
spectinomycin sulphate in 169
spiramycin in 169
tetracyclines in 169
therapy 162–171
yaws eradication and 95
Syphilitic sera, cryoglobulins in 143
immunoglobulin class of antibodies in
    141
rheumatoid factor in 143
sensitivity of tests on (Table) 135

Tabes dorsalis 107
Tetracyclines, in gonorrhoea 80
    in granuloma inguinale 196
    in lymphogranuloma venereum 191
    in non-specific urethritis 297–299
    in syphilis 169
    Thayer–Martin medium 48
Thermostability of antibodies 143
Thin-layer chromatography, *Treponema
    pallidum* 149
Third International Symposium on V.D.
    control 395
Thrombocytopenia, in congenital syphi-
    lis 116
Thrombophlebitis, in Reiter's disease
    308
T-mycoplasma 255, 256
    biological characteristics 267
    laboratory aspects 267–274
    in non-specific urethritis 258–262,
        270–274
    in pregnancy 260

in sterility 261
T-mycoplasma-uria 260
Torulopris glabrata 232
TPI *see* Treponemal immobilisation test
Trachoma, and Chlamydia 262, 263, 276, 278
Transgrow medium 48, 51
Transport media for gonococci 48
Treponema pallidum 124, 127, 132
immunofluorescence methods for detection 138
methods of identification 148
Treponema pertenue 148
Treponemal agglutination tests 139
Treponemal haemagglutination tests 139
Treponemal immobilisation test (TPI) 127, 131, 174
Treponemal infection, antibody types in (Table) 127
Treponematoses, endemic 124
TRIC agent *see* Chlamydia
Trichomoniasis 201–227
Trichomoniasis, 'Adenexitis' in 211
asymptomatic 206, 210
candidiasis and 212
cervical cancer and 205
cervical cytology in 206
cervical erosion and 206
clinical aspects 210–212
complications 212
diagnosis as cystitis 207, 210
diagnosis as urethritis 207
dysplasia and 206
dysuria in 210
endocervical hyperplasia and 206
epidemiology 203–208
epididymitis in 211
haematospermia in 211
leucorrhoea in 210
neo-natal infection 207
photocolposcopy in 212
prevalence rate 205
preventive measures 208
prostatitis in 210
pruritis in 210
seasonal incidence 204
sexual transmission 207
social aspects 203–208
sterility in 205, 211
urethritis in 211
vaginal discharge in 210
Triphenyltetrazolium chloride medium for diagnosis of candidiasis 244
Trobicin, in gonorrhoea 79

Ulceration in granuloma inguinale 195
Unheated serum reagin (USR) test 128
United Nations Convention on Prostitution, 1959 29
United States Public Health Service, Behavioural Sciences Section 389
Urea, metabolism by T-mycoplasma 267
Urethral stricture 258
post-gonococcal 38
Urethritis, Chlamydia and 285
in trichomoniasis 211
non-specific *see* Non-specific urethritis
post-gonococcal *see* Post-gonococcal urethritis
pre-menstrual 258
USR *see* Unheated serum reagin
Uveitis, anterior 257
complicating non-specific genital infection 258

Vaccine possibilities in gonorrhoea 65
Vagina, plaques, in candidiasis 242
Vaginal discharge in trichomoniasis 210
Vaginitis, in *Corynebacterium vaginale* infection 357
VDRL slide test 128
Venereal disease, adolescents and 372
behavioural aspects 375
clinical services 380–385
legal aspects 381
contact tracing 402–407
control 369–377, 406
health education and 388
ecological forces (diagram) 17
emotional instability in 28
historical aspects 376
in homosexuals 26, 373
immigrants and 374
professional education 396–398
in prostitutes 25, 375
psychiatric factors 391
seafarers and 374
servicemen and 374
in students 26
Venereologists, health education and 398
Vesiculitis 258
Viral hepatitis B 350–352
'Virulence factor', gonococcal 55
Virus hepatitis, diagnosis from secondary syphilis 100
Visceral syphilis 105

Vulva, elephantiasis, in lymphogranu-
loma venereum 189
Vulva, warts 341
'Vulvular dysuria' 241

Warts, genital 338–341
peri-anal 340
vulvar 341
Wassermann, August von 377

West Indian immigrants, gonorrhoea in
26
W.H.O. Report . . . on V.D. Control
in the Western Pacific 13
World Forum on Syphilis and . . .
Treponematoses 389

Yaws 124
eradication and syphilis 95

Printed by Adlard & Son Ltd, Bartholomew Press, Dorking